Pill Hill

Books by Helen Copeland

Meet Miki Takino
Lothrop, Lee and Shepard Co., New York

Duncan's World
T. Y. Crowell, New York

This Snake Is Good
T. Y. Crowell, New York

Festival in the Park
Crown Publishers, Inc.
Young Books from Crown, New York

Endangered Specimen:
and other poems from a lay naturalist
St. Andrews Press, Laurinburg, North Carolina

Pill Hill

⁊ *Growing Up with the Mayo Clinic* ₰

July 9, 2005

Helen Masson Copeland

To Damon Balfour —
I remember your handsome grandfather as one I sometimes rode horseback with. And I often get the generations mixed up! Your great grandparents I remember fondly as Uncle Don and Aunt Carrie. Enjoy this bit of your own background in this book,

Helen Masson Copeland

Heritage Letterpress, LLC
Charlotte, NC

PRIVATE EDITION

Copyright © 2004 by Helen M. Copeland

Cover design by Jack Desley

Library of Congress Control Number: 2004105230
ISBN 0-9754234-0-1

Manufactured in the United States of America
Heritage Letterpress, LLC
Charlotte, North Carolina 28208

First Edition

"Contented industry is the mainspring of human happiness."

Dr. William J. Mayo

In memory of my mother,
Marion Knowles Masson.

Contents

Preface and Acknowledgements ... ix
Prologue ... xiii
1. Early History of the Mayo Clinic ... 1
2. The Courtship of My Parents ... 21
3. The Heroic Age of Surgery ... 41
4. The 1914 Building and Beyond ... 53
5. Pill Hill Children ... 67
6. Kendall's Movies ... 83
7. Halloween and Belva L. Snodgrass ... 91
8. The Dreams of Youth ... 101
9. Exploring the Mayo Clinic ... 109
10. Sunday Picnics ... 117
11. In Hunting Season ... 125
12. Grateful Patients ... 137
13. Cedar Beach ... 151
14. The Women's Clubs ... 167
15. Prohibition and Social Drinking ... 183
16. In Times of War ... 195
17. The Great Depression ... 211

Contents

18. A Century of Progress   219
19. World War II and the Korean War   231
20. On the Social Side   251
21. Tracks in the Snow   267
    Notes   275

Preface and Acknowledgments

Rochester, Minnesota, is my hometown. My story is a personal memoir as well as an anecdotal account of how a small Minnesota town became home to the world-famous Mayo Clinic. It baffled the world's scientific communities that a modern medical center took root in a field of wheat.

My brothers and I lived with our parents, Dr. J. C. Masson, a former horse-and-buggy doctor from Canada, and his Massachusetts wife, Marion Knowles Masson, on the hilly southwestern side of Rochester. Most of the early doctors who joined the practice of Dr. William Worrall Mayo and his two sons, William James and Charles Horace Mayo, built homes and raised families on that high part of Rochester that came to be known as "Pill Hill." The land rose steeply behind Saint Mary's Hospital and rolled with many dips and humps and one dramatic ravine, Kendall's Canyon, down to the surrounding farmland and the serpentine Zumbro River.

Although much has been published about the Mayo Clinic and its history, I know of no account of how it felt to grow up in the shadow of the struggling new Mayo Clinic. Looking back, I find myself at home in my parents' world of Mayo Clinic families in the 1920's to the 1940's.

I was eight years old in 1928 when the carillon bells at the top of the Mayo Clinic Building rang their melodies for the first time over the Zumbro River valley and that tall, stately building was dedicated to the ideals of the Mayo brothers, known fondly to the world as Dr. Will and Dr. Charlie. There is no better assertion of those ideals for the medical profession than that the duty of the physician to the patient is to live by the Golden Rule; medicine's place is to serve mankind.

But for a flick of fate, the Mayo Clinic might never have flourished on that black Minnesota soil. When the Civil War was over and President Lincoln no longer needed a doctor to assess the health of Minnesota's soldiers, a wanderlust gripped "the little doctor," as William Worrall Mayo was known. He had an explorer's yen to see beyond the horizon. He told his wife and children they were moving to St. Paul, away from the pokey little town of Rochester.

Louise Abigail Wright Mayo put her foot down. "No, dear," she told him, "I like it here, and remember, I'm having another baby."

What gratitude is owed that staunch lady who, with her energetic husband, raised two good daughters and two renowned sons who put Rochester, Minnesota, on the map of the world's distinguished communities!

I remember the tone of the times in Rochester when its population totaled 20,000 persons. Wars, epidemics, false rumors and financial depressions put a strain on the rapidly growing Mayo medical practice, the first group practice in the world. I recall meeting world-famous men and women who came to the Clinic for consultation and treatment. And how could I ever forget the charm and warmth of my first heroes, outstanding men of medicine, the friends of my parents, the fathers of my friends.

Assembling the facts and anecdotes for this book was a joy I hadn't fully expected. To put some of my memories into words brought tears to my eyes. Inspiration came from many sources. My mother kept a diary. In her elegant handwriting she noted nature's quirks, her own world and the world at large. I am eternally regretful that she never knew it was her fun with words that led me to write this book with loving memories of her on every page.

I appreciate help from many Pill Hill friends, especially Barbara Benedict Hanlon, who answered my many questions, reminding me of things I had forgotten, such as Halloween on Ninth Avenue. Other Rochester friends who wrote me letters include Margaret Helmholz Burchell, Carol Haines Anderson, Olivia Haines Blackburn, Mary Louise Hargesheimer Gibson, Jean Davis Warman, Betty Willius Kirby, Bob Roesler, Lawrence Derksen, Hugh Kendall, Jack Pemberton and Bob New. Bob was a friend of many family picnics, now a retired Episcopal priest who wrote the paragraph "About the Author" for the cover of this book.

I remember a long, hilarious phone conversation with Carolyn Walters Brown about my mother's late arrival at a meeting of the Magazine Club

Preface and Acknowledgments

at Dr. Will and Mrs. Hattie's home. I am indebted to Mary Elizabeth Giffin, M.D., for her insights into her relationship as a young polio patient with her doctor, Will Mayo. Belatedly, I want to thank Dr. Edmund C. Burke who advised me on how, respectful of Mayo policy, to prudently write of the death of a young Edison school friend.

My brothers Jay and Stan told me of previously secret adolescent pranks accomplished in our Mayo Clinic, now the Plummer Building. Stan gave me his untold story of being a penicillin guinea pig in World War II, and Jay wrote about the Clinic's role as he experienced it in the Korean War. My cousin Allan Masson of Oakville, Ontario, offered a lot of good laughs and one poignant story for this book, and I wish he were still around so I could thank him in person.

I am truly fond of my memory of Dr. Frederick A. Willius, whose book *Aphorisms* was the source for the insightful quotations of the Mayo brothers that I use at the start of each chapter.

Most helpful of the books in my father's library was the extraordinary 822-page volume, *The Doctors Mayo*, by Helen Clapesattle, published in 1941 by the University of Minnesota Press and reprinted for the fourth time in 1990. From that book I learned much about the earliest Mayo Clinic doctors. I have also gleaned important information from The Olmsted County Historical Society and from pamphlets published by the Mayo Foundation. Carolyn Stickney Beck, the Clinic archivist during my research, loaned me old copies of *Mayovox* and *Mayo Alumnus* magazines and clippings from the Rochester *Post Bulletin*. She graciously checked my first draft manuscript for accuracy.

The only person who searched my manuscript for errors in punctuation was Karen Parsons, the copy editor of Heritage Letterpress. She corrected any remaining quirky spelling, and with her fine red ink she made all punctuation consistent. She then gave me the daunting job of finding for the endnotes the sources for all quotations in the text, for which I am now grateful. Karen was a delight to work with.

Here in Charlotte, North Carolina, I have been greatly benefitted by my talented writers' workshop group, who gave me helpful appraisals of each chapter in its first draft: Mignon Ballard, Margaret Caldwell, Jane Grau, Miriam Herin, Mary Kratt, Rebecca Schenck and Ruth Moose. Another group of mostly poets who gave me their critical insights was Liz Carroll, Irene Honeycutt, Mary Ann Thomas and Leslie Tompkins. Other local writers and friends in Charlotte who encouraged this project

Preface and Acknowledgements

include: Paul Baker Newman, Katherine Springs, Florence Chapman, Nancy Cox and Fern Culbreth. Joe Elliott and his wife Audrey told me of the perks and happy times they had enduring Minnesota winters and poverty with their peers in a Mayo Clinic three-year fellowship.

It was a happy day for me to discover as a neighbor Rose Naiman, a medical writer and lecturer. She enthusiastically helped me organize the Pill Hill material and I appreciate her suggestions and friendship.

My old friend David Pennington of Rochester, formerly a Mayo Department of Development officer and president of the Olmsted County Historical Society, is just naturally a generous man. Busy as he is with family and community involvement, he has spent much time advising me by e-mail and providing pictures from the Olmsted County Historical Society files for use in this book. It was he who steered me to former Mayo artist Jack Desley of Lewisville, North Carolina, who created the delightful cover art for this book and the map of Pill Hill in the days before the Mayo Clinic of Rochester became a cluster of glistening new buildings dedicated in perpetuity to medical education, research and the service of today's patients and the dispirited ill of future generations.

Among my list of wellwishers I want to applaud the young man most responsible for helping me manage my computer, Randy Marshall of Rock Hill, South Carolina. Patiently, he guided me through the insubordinations of my iMac, till it and I can almost be friends. Randy was a good friend, and it saddens me that he died last year of heart failure.

In 1994 Robert W. Olmsted, the managing editor of *Northwoods Journal*, published a short story of mine, "Tracks in the Snow." It was a fictional account of the true events related in the last chapter of this book. I loved that story and regretted that I gave it up to a little magazine. But now that I have brought the true story to life, my last visit home to see Dad, as the ending for this book, I want Robert Olmsted to know how much I appreciate his gracious words to me and the opportunity he gave me to publish in the *Northwoods Journal*.

As Louise Abigail Wright Mayo might have remarked, one has to be of a forward-looking disposition to take on a long-range job. I have been buttressed in the writing of this historical account of life as it was back in the '20's and '30's on Pill Hill by the expectations of my four children—Howard, Marion, Bill and Jamie—who, with the cooperation of their varied and interesting spouses—Patti, Jeff, Christine and Carolyn—

Preface and Acknowledgements

raised my grandchildren, eight Copelands—Douglas, Wendy, Margaret, Beatrice, Eugenia, Marion, Lucian and Willie—and three Mitchells—Alison, Helen and Charlotte. I thank them all for their loving encouragement.

Lastly and especially I want to express a bouquet of thank-yous to my friend and printer, William E. Loftin, Sr., who heads Heritage Printers. Recently, he gladly adopted into the firm a young, enthusiastic new owner of the newly renamed Heritage Letterpress, Will Hardison. As Bill Loftin represents three generations of printers in his family, in this book we honor the three generations of Doctors Mayo who carried forward the medical ideals of the patriarch, Dr. William Worrall Mayo.

> Whosoever finds whimsy in this book,
> may you sleep with a smile
> and forgive the author's
> digressions.

Prologue

> In America our idealism is not unusual, nor does it differ much
> from that of the medical faculty of other countries; if we excel in anything,
> it is in our capacity for translating idealism into action.
>
> Dr. C. H. Mayo, 1931[1]

My last visit home to see Dad was in 1974. He was ninety-three years old, still living in the house on Fourth Street where I grew up, across from the Foundation House. He was weakened by prostate cancer but his mind was acute, except when thoughts were painful or mixed with dream fantasy. The doorbell was answered by a thin little maid I hadn't met before. The great oak door groaned back over its threshold. I walked in on the polished tile, stamped snow off my boots and took them off. The maid stood in my way. I took her hand and introduced myself, the doctor's daughter, and slid past her. She backed away, a startled look on her face.

"Mrs. Masson isn't in," she said. "She was planning to meet you at the airport."

"Oh—my flight from Chicago was canceled. I was put on an earlier one. It's all right, I got a taxi."

The girl, looking through straight brown bangs, seemed even more alarmed when I picked up my suitcase and headed for the stairs. Then Mabel, our exuberant cook, burst through the kitchen door and threw her arms around me. The maid disappeared.

"My God, Helen, it's good to see you!" That was always Mabel's hearty greeting on my annual visits home. Mabel Macken was the best cook in town. She worked as much as she wanted to, which was all the time. She had two professions: cooking for parties and dressmaking. Also, she stretched her schedule to include two very old doctors whose meals she prepared, my father and Dr. W. F. Braasch, formerly head of the Mayo Clinic's section of urology and a brilliant bridge player.

"Go on up," Mabel said. "He's been waiting all morning. Mrs. Masson has gone to get her hair done at the Kahler. I'll see you later." She hung my coat in the closet on her way to the kitchen.

I listened to the tick of the grandfather clock, my hand on the oak newel post. The smiling face of the clock's moon was rising into a crescent of blue sky above the gold Roman numerals. The hands pointed to five minutes past eleven. As a child I used to watch my father wind the clock on Sunday evenings. The key, like a roller skate key, was fit into its socket. As he wound it around, the heavy brass weights rose, first one, then the other. He would give me the key then, and I would put it back behind the glass door where the weights hung and the disk-like brass pendulum swung sedately back and forth.

I felt the solidity of this house, my love for it, as my hand slid up the banister. A few of the stairs creaked, as they always had. I left my suitcase at the top of the stairs, my heart beating in anticipation, and went to the open door of the Big Room. Dad was in his hospital bed, the head of it slightly elevated. He was looking out the picture window as snow fell steadily.

"Dad?" I said, not knowing if he could hear me.

His head turned on the pillow, and his hands rose off the sheet like fluttering doves. "Ah, here she is, my good little pony!" I went to his bedside and put my cold cheek next to his warm one. His face was pink and smooth, his eyes as blue and clear as they always were.

"Dad, you look wonderful. How're you feeling?" I pulled up a chair and sat by his bed.

"Pretty good for an old feller." He looked at me intently, trying to see clearly through a mist of cataracts. He gave my hand a squeeze and held it. "I wish I could have met you at the station, Dear." He was remembering a girl with long blond hair who used to come home from college on the old Minnesota 400.

A pretty red-haired nurse came into the room with juice and crackers on a tray. My father smiled and pointed a finger at her. "This girl Betty takes pretty good care of me," he said. "Look what she's brought me now.

Prologue

It's just water, I think. I used to get a little Scotch before dinner, but I'm thankful for small blessings."

Betty laughed and raised the head of the bed, then gave him the glass. He took a sip. "I sure do like your dad," she said to me. "I wish I'd known him when he was a young horse and buggy doctor up in Canada."

Dad gave me a nudge with the back of his hand. "Well, well, did you hear that? If I heard this girl right, I'd say that if she'd been around then, she might have asked me to marry her, and I just might have done so."

"Oh, Doctor!" Betty said, blushing. "I forgot you had on your new hearing aid." She fluffed up the pillow behind his head and said, "It must have been tough practicing medicine in those days."

"It wasn't for sissies, that's for sure. My little daughter here always asked about my mare Trixie. She was a marvel. After I'd seen the last patient on my route and we headed home, she'd step along lively, and I'd fall asleep. I'd wake up when I heard her nosing the latch on the barn door.

"Many of my patients were farmers," he said. "Dunnville was a pretty small town. Somebody on horseback would race into the yard, yelling for me to come. I'd get out there fast. Sometimes it would be childbirth. Too often somebody would be tangled with a piece of farm machinery. Those early inventions weren't safe."

Dad stopped talking and looked out the window. "Little Lucy Love," he said softly.

"Who was Lucy Love?" I asked.

"She was a child. Her arm got caught in a wringer." He turned to the window again, as if that memory could be lulled by the slow dance of snowflakes that gently clung and slid down the big pane of thermal glass.

I remember the harmony of being in the Big Room with Dad on that November day of a heavy snowfall. But I would never have remembered these conversations with the three of us, and later with others, had I not gone to my room and written them in a notebook as a family memoir, as Mother kept her diary. When I came back, Dad seemed asleep, lying on his side, facing the falling snow.

"Your dad is very much on the ball for ninety-three," Betty said, "but now and then he seems to step into a dream world. It worries Mrs. Masson, but I think he enjoys his memories. They're like bridges to the past." Betty sat in a Victorian rocker from Mother's old home in Massachusetts. Her knitting needles clicked. It seemed strange for a modern young

xvii

woman like Betty to be knitting a sweater. "I enjoy it," she said. "I do a lot of waiting around while my patient sleeps." She asked how my father happened to come to the Mayo Clinic from Canada.

"I came in 1913," Dad said. "It wasn't the Mayo Clinic then." He opened his eyes. "I'm not asleep, just resting. The Clinic was a small family practice then, so busy they invited other doctors to join the family. Then the newspapers got interested. For a while, some jealous types said the Mayos were quacks and worse. But word got around, and those whiners eventually slunk away with their tails between their legs."

He smiled and turned to me. I knew that metaphor reminded him of something. "Helen, did you ever hear about my last patient?"

Betty came from the bathroom with a small cup. "Time for your medicine, Doctor."

"Whatever it is, I'll take it from your little hand."

He drank from the cup Betty held. She patted the rim of white on his upper lip with a tissue. "What about your last patient, Doctor?"

"It's a good story, if I do say so myself." He gave me a grin. He knew I'd heard it before, but he would tell it to Betty. "It was a few years after my retirement in 1946. Marion, my first wife, and I were visiting the Bell Ranch in Texas. Bell was a former patient. He brought in this lovely golden retriever he wanted me to see. She trotted up to me looking first-rate, I thought, but, by golly, when I reached around and felt her belly, there was this big fatty tumor, a benign lipoma, hanging down from her abdomen. It was as big as an apple."

Betty's eyes widened. "Doctor Masson! Don't tell me you were also a vet!"

"Whenever I was asked, I was. Operated on the kitchen table with chloroform. A skinny little cowboy was my anesthetist. I told him what to do, and he did it. I shaved the dog with a straight razor and then cut in a curve."

I knew this story from previous tellings. I could visualize that kitchen and the bloody scene, the poor dog limp on her back, her head in the hands of the cowboy who put her to sleep with a few good whiffs of chloroform soaked in a pad of bandage. Dad was wearing the ranch cook's apron, holding a knife he had brought along in his emergency kit. Mr. Bell stood by with a soup bowl. Mother and Mrs. Bell were nowhere in sight; they had watched the preparations, but left quickly for the fresh

Prologue

Texas air on the patio. Dad drew a neat elliptical incision on the retriever's soft belly. After a little probing he lifted the bloody tumor into the soup bowl held by the nervous Mr. Bell. It slid around and nearly fell on the kitchen floor. "... Then I clipped off the excess skin," Dad said, "and sewed her up."

Dad wished he had *always* traveled with a kit of emergency supplies. Once he returned from a medical meeting in Kansas City severely shaken. He had been in a train wreck. He was asleep in one of the last Pullman cars when the tragedy happened, a head-on collision with an engine left by mistake on the wrong track. Many people were killed and injured. Dad was devastated by the fact that he was unprepared to help relieve the suffering of so many people. It wasn't like him to tell us children tragic things that happened. He would tell a few facts and let it go at that; nothing more. But that time he couldn't ignore our pleading for answers. Mother tried to calm us and comfort him; he had done his best. But it wasn't enough to hold hands and talk, he said; what he needed was morphine. After that, he never went anywhere unprepared for an emergency.

So, on that trip with Mother to the Bell's ranch, he had in his luggage the equipment to remove a tumor from a "good old mother dog," as he referred to the golden retriever.

"Holy cow!" Betty blurted out. "Doctor, you amaze me. Did the dog live?"

"Sure she did. A lipoma is easy to fix." He smiled up at Betty and his dentures slipped.

"That's some story," Betty said. "If you're going to keep on talking, we have to fix those teeth."

He nodded. "I'll give it some thought. I used to fix a lot of things myself." He stroked my hand. His nails were ridged and neatly manicured. "I fixed your bicycle when the chain came loose. Your brother Jay and I made kites out of balsa wood and drafting paper, long tails from dressmaking scraps. And, do you remember Stanley's pushmobile? He and Sylvester made it out of junkyard parts. I helped fix it after he smashed it up. It was fast, the wheels well greased." He looked out the window again, snow mounding up on the sill and on the limbs of the big oak tree.

My brother Stan remembers that accident in the pushmobile. Sixty years later he pulled up his pants leg and showed me the purple bruise that never went away. He was racing down Fourth Street when the steering mechanism broke and the wheels turned sharply into the curb. He and the cart flew up in the air in front of the Gooding's house.

"Somebody helped him home," Dad said. "I think it was Norman Kendall. Stan had a deep cut all the way to the tibia. Your mother and I took him to Saint Mary's for an x-ray."

His gaze drifted back to the big, lazy snowflakes that twirled and danced against the glass. "Little Billy had his share of disappointments," he sighed, his eyes closed. Betty pushed the button to lower the head of the bed.

Perhaps he was shutting out memories that hurt, memories of his youngest boy after he graduated from the University of Minnesota and moved to Los Angeles. All should have gone well with Bill, a brilliant young engineer. He had a job at Avionics Research, a delightful girlfriend named Gloria, a motorcycle, a green Porsche sportscar and a compact little house on a hill overlooking Los Angeles. Also, in a garage at the bottom of the hill, he kept an old Lincoln Continental that somebody had totaled. Bill restored its motor so it could be driven again. He told me when he came to visit in North Carolina—all the way on the motorcycle—that he bought the Lincoln because he felt sorry for it, such a wonderful old car, wrecked. He paid a hundred dollars for it before they could tow it to a junk yard.

Dad was asleep when the doorbell rang. I put my suitcase in the guest room and went down to greet Ruthie, my stepmother.

In the six days after this early snowfall in November, 1974, I learned more about my younger brother Bill and how three wars and a depression had dealt with the Mayo Clinic and its people. I see in my memory the tall, stately building of my childhood rising above the sidewalks of Rochester into the blue sky, our only skyscraper. We called it the Mayo Clinic, now named the Plummer Building after the genius who designed it, Dr. Henry Stanley Plummer. Gradually over the years the Plummer Building, with its carillon tower of many tons of resonant bells, has attracted sparkling new construction to the blocks encircling it.

The Mayo Clinic has become a midtown campus of medical specialty buildings designed to further the dreams of the Mayo brothers, Dr. William James and Dr. Charles Worrall Mayo. In these buildings and at the

Prologue

two satellite Mayo Clinics in Jacksonville, Florida, and Scottsdale, Arizona, men and women are at work to further the health and happiness of this and future generations. These lofty ideals are the backbone of the stories I have had the pleasure of writing down.

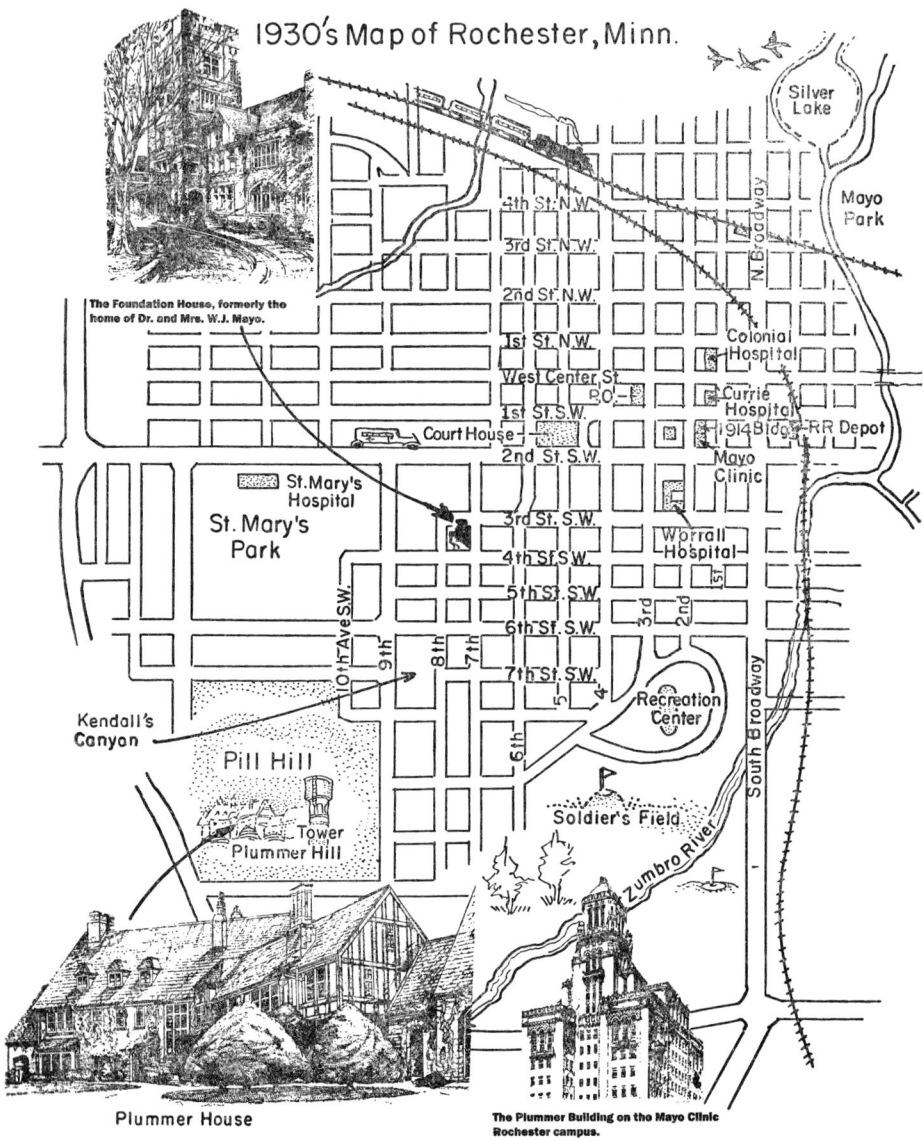

Pill Hill

1

The Early History of the Mayo Clinic

> It is the hope of the founders of this building that in its use
> the high ideals of the medical profession will always be maintained.
>
> Dr. William J. Mayo
> Laying the cornerstone, 1912[1]

IN 1854 stage coaches began traveling the Dubuque Trail, rattling over a log bridge spanning the Zumbro River and stopping in Rochester. Weary travelers disembarked with their luggage and trudged into Head's Tavern or one of the newer log houses with rooms for hire that had sprung up beside the long, straight, dirt road that had been cleared by George Head, Rochester's first settler, and his team of oxen. George Head and his wife Henrietta named the road Broadway and the place Rochester, out of nostalgia for their former home in New York. Some of those travelers caught the next stage for St. Paul or farther west. Others, wanting land to farm, liked the looks of Minnesota's rich black soil and staked a claim with the local "regulators."

Rochester grew with the vigor of its wheat, wheat so tall it was said a man on horseback could hide in it. A few years later Broadway was still muddy after rains, but it was a thoroughfare, lined with wooden walkways and shops. A photograph in *The Rochester Story* by Mearl W. Raygor[2] shows the street in front of the "Boot and Shoe Store" crowded nose-to-axle with covered wagons drawn by long-horned oxen. A flock of sheep, rounded into a tight circle on Broadway, was tended by a good sheep dog. The arrival of railroad tracks in the fall of 1864 made Rochester the center for distribution of hundreds of thousands of bushels of wheat from the surrounding fields to the seemingly endless demand of markets in the east.

Pill Hill

Ninety miles northwest of Rochester in Le Sueur on the Minnesota River, a restless young doctor, William Worrall Mayo, an immigrant from Salford, Lancashire County, England, had settled with his wife Louise Abigail Wright Mayo, two daughters, Gertrude and Phoebe, and an infant son, William James. This baby, born in 1861, along with his brother Charles, would become founders of the world-famous Mayo Clinic.

Dr. William Worrall Mayo onboard ship to America had recorded his profession as "taylor." However, the mentor of his early years in England who inspired his interest in all fields of education was the internationally renowned schoolmaster and scientist John Dalton, a founder of the Pine Street Medical School of Manchester, England. Young Mayo became his apprentice. He studied briefly in hospitals in Glasgow and London, then went on to open a tailoring shop in the 1840's. At that time England was in political turmoil. America held out a beacon of opportunity to young people, and William Worrall Mayo signed on for a crossing to New York City. He arrived on June 16, 1846, and with another man started a tailoring establishment. It blossomed into "The Hall of Fashion" with a department in ladies' clothes designed to give "grace and elegance to the female form." When he had money to live on, he sold his share of the business, married Louise Abigail Wright, a maker of hats for fashionable ladies, and moved into the orbit of Lafayette, Indiana's distinguished citizen and physician, Dr. Elizur H. Deming. He received his degree in medicine from Indiana Medical College in 1850 after one year of training. Credit was given him for previous work he had done in European hospitals and for the knowledge he displayed in written and oral examinations.

Young Dr. W. W. Mayo's energy and feistiness more than made up for his small stature. He was barely five feet four inches tall. He had a black beard, piercing dark eyes, and a strong, agile body. He brought his family out of Indiana to escape an epidemic of an unknown fatal disease, possibly malaria.

In those days, before the life-saving discoveries of Joseph Lister and Louis Pasteur, the practice of medicine was poorly paid, if at all, and fraught with heartbreak. Surgery, such as amputation after injury, was always followed by infection; the patient usually died. To support his family Dr. Mayo farmed his land in Le Sueur, did veterinary work and operated a ferry boat across the Minnesota River.

In the area a settlement of Sioux Indians also lived. Relations between the Indians and the settlers were generally cordial, but, as news traveled fast on horseback it was apparent to the young Dr. Mayo in Le Sueur that interaction between the settlers and their Native American neighbors had a tragic effect on the Sioux population. They had no immunity against the white man's disease of small pox; many of them, especially their children, died, causing the group to move to new grounds. Mearl Raygor in *The Rochester Story* writes that Rochester's first lawyer, James Bucklin, who was also a maker of coffins, was given a young Indian girl, Winona, to bury. But she was alive, and James Bucklin nursed her back to health. He sent word to the Indians that Winona was well and able to travel, and her family came for her with gifts for Mr. Bucklin—"a pair of moccasins and a fine knife case."[3]

But relations were often strained between the settlers and their Sioux neighbors. Anger flared when a Sioux child came down with smallpox or when buffalo hunting was unsuccessful. On one occasion the promised allotment from the United States government was late in coming and the Indians attacked the town of New Ulm. Dr. Mayo was a ready volunteer and left with his satchel of medical tools to aid his neighbors, leaving the care of home, farm and the ferry boat to Louise Abigail Mayo. When he was gone, she would anxiously watch for his return. If she saw a lame or wounded man passing by her house, she would run to him and ask who had dressed his wounds. She would be filled with relief when she was told, "It was a little doctor." Then she knew her William was alive.

Those were turbulent times, when covered wagons with families were not the only people traveling the dirt roads. There were also unscrupulous young men on the lookout for a prize, a horse. One day Dr. Mayo was riding his horse on his way to the farm of a patient when two young Sioux braves, thinking Dr. Mayo was a mere boy they could frighten, attacked him. But the little doctor was not about to be bullied out of his horse or his case of precious medical tools and supplies. His defense was so fierce his attackers turned and fled.

The saddest of times in our country's history was surely the Civil War years when the evil of slavery, the economic foundation of the agricultural South, was challenged by the industrial North. Rochester was only seven years old when the Civil War began. Olmsted County, with a population of 10,000, sent 1,250 men to preserve the Union in answer to the call from President Lincoln. Dr. William Worrall Mayo was summoned by the president to report to Rochester to examine enlistees from southern Minnesota. To keep his young family together while he served his new country, Dr. Mayo went immediately to Rochester, bought property and built a cottage in time for their second son, Charles Horace, to be born there on July 19, 1865. Helen Clapesattle, writing in *The Doctors Mayo* in 1940, notes that the bedroom where Baby Charlie was born was located where "the fountain bubbles in the lobby of the present Clinic building."[4] (Now, that would be between the Plummer Building and the Siebens Building.)

When the war was over and his duties as examining surgeon were finished, Dr. Mayo put a small notice in the newspaper:

Dr. Mayo
Office on Third Street
Rochester, Minnesota

Dr. Mayo's first Rochester patient was a poor farmer with a sick horse. Soon paying patients began coming to his office. However, when the price of wheat fell at the end of the 1860's, the area doctors suffered like everyone else. Hard times socked in like a blizzard. People still got sick and Dr. Mayo's patients still came to him and he went to them, but often he was paid in potatoes or a load of wood. Money wasn't the issue with him; he cared about his patients, whoever they were, and they knew it. But he brooked no argument from family members who persisted in old-fashioned ways such as covering an injury with goose grease. His instructions on cleanliness were strictly to be obeyed. He owned and used a microscope twenty years before they were available to students in prestigious medical schools.

Dr. Mayo soon became involved in Rochester politics. He was passionate about education and served on the school board. He insisted Rochester should have a library, and donated many of his own books. To improve the minds of the farmers, he helped plan a series of talks by visiting lecturers, including Horace Greely, the founder and editor of the *New York Tribune*. Dr. Mayo spoke out in behalf of a water works, a gas works, an electric light plant and a system of sewers. Dr. William Worrall Mayo's influence as a member of the Rochester Board of Health included oversight of "pest houses" for use during an epidemic, removal of animal carcasses and piles of offal at slaughterhouses and butcher shops, the impounding of runaway cattle, pigs and sheep. He urged citizens to clean up their privies and stables.

By 1869 he was well known to Minnesota politicians. He had stepped on the toes of several St. Paul physicians when he let it be known he thought the state medical society was wishy-washy. He was no doubt a prickly man to have around. Such men make troublesome enemies and solid friends.

The two young Mayo boys, Will and Charlie, grew up noting the compassion, energy and civic-mindedness of both parents. Their father tended everyone who needed him. He never sent a bill to a poor patient. At public meetings he said what he meant and people paid attention. Their mother spent hours listening to the woes of family members of patients as they sat in her parlor. Louise Abigail was an avid reader. Her hobby was studying the stars with her prized possession, a telescope.

Will Mayo and his brother Charlie were inseparable, though very different. Will was tall, thin, light-haired, blue-eyed and self-confident. He had a quick temper which he gradually learned to control. He loved his pony and was an excellent horseman. Charlie was mechanically inclined; he liked motors and farm machinery. He was short like his father, dark-haired and affable, sometimes a mischief-maker. As an adult he was often compared with the wise and witty Will Rogers. Both boys were fascinated by their father's profession. Dr. Mayo was unusually successful with what was euphemistically called "female problems."

One of Dr. Mayo's patients had a huge ovarian cyst, which was generally thought impossible to remove safely. The little doctor had the self-confidence to experiment. He tried draining the fluid through a small abdominal incision. When the patient lived, the case was written up in the Rochester newspaper. Immediately his office was deluged with female patients, mostly farmers' wives who had had many children. They came with benign ovarian cysts, some as large as a basketball. The operations were performed in the patient's home, or in Mrs. Carpenter's boarding house where an operating table could be moved from room to room. Chloroform was administered by Dr. David Berkman, a veterinarian who eventually became the husband of Dr. Mayo's daughter Gertrude. Always listening outside the operating room were the two young Mayo boys.

Will and Charlie attended Central High School in Rochester and then were sent east to medical school. Will attended the University of Michigan, graduating with a degree in medicine in 1883. Four years later Charlie graduated from Chicago Medical School at Northwestern University.

At that time, and as early as 1866, although the elder Dr. Mayo didn't know of Pasteur's bacteria and Lister's ideas on antisepsis, a great debate was raging. Was Sir Joseph Lister right or was he mistaken that carbolic acid must be applied unsparingly to open wounds and sprayed in the very air around the patient as a defense against Pasteur's invisible bacteria?

Dr. William Worrall Mayo, like his sons in medical school, followed the debate with interest. He was not content to simply muse over the rumors. His record was good, but he realized there were too many fatalities among his patients. He needed to know more. So he packed his bags and went to New York City for a three-month trip to study the surgeries of the noted doctors of the day. In Lancaster, Pennsylvania, he visited two brothers famous for their experience with ovarian tumors, Drs. John and Washington Atlee. One of the Atlee brothers had done 300 such operations at the time of Dr. Mayo's visit, with an average mortality rate of thirty percent. Not good enough, Dr. Mayo thought. When he returned home he tried new methods and improved on the techniques he had observed.

For several years Dr. Mayo had regularly seen a patient from New York, a Mrs. Waggonner whom doctors agreed could not be helped. She was diagnosed with "falling of the womb." Dr. Mayo, upon examination, found she had a rectocele (a hernial protrusion of the rectum into the vagina). The usual practice of tucking it back where it belonged didn't hold for long. In two years she was again in Dr. Mayo's office. The condition had recurred. Finally, after consultation with a Chicago gynecologist, Dr. William H. Byford, who was also stumped by the unusual case, Dr. Mayo determined he would go ahead with a radical operation.

Helen Clapesattle, in *The Doctors Mayo*, described the procedure:

> With the patient under ether and the hernial bag emptied of its contents, Dr. W. W. Mayo fastened a clamp behind it to shut off the circulation, carefully put in the necessary sutures, and cut off the rectocele close to

the clamp. Quickly he seared the cut surfaces with an iron he had heating in the flame of a spirit lamp nearby. The bleeding was very slight.[5]

This operation was the talk of the town for weeks. "Dr. Mayo cut her wide open," and three days later, the newspaper concluded, "the lady is doing well."

Reporting on this case to the Minnesota State Medical Society, an unexpected aspect of Dr. W. W. Mayo's character was revealed. Without regard to that day's standards of political correctness, he gave credit where it was due regardless of what it might do to his own professional reputation. Most people at that time agreed that the field of medicine belonged to men. Dr. Mayo didn't see it that way. From the podium where he was reading his prepared statement to a large audience he paused, looked up and said, "At this point I wish to make public my gratitude to Miss Harriet Preston, M.D., a graduate of the Women's Medical College of Philadelphia, for her very able assistance to me while performing this and other operations on women."

His remarks were a rebuke to most of his listeners. For the past three years Dr. Harriet Preston's application for membership in the Minnesota Medical Society had been denied. Dr. Mayo championed her cause from the start, as he knew her to be a qualified practitioner. In 1880, after she had moved to St. Paul, the state society reversed its opinion against admitting women to its ranks.

In those days doctors didn't understand the crucial need for cleanliness around a wound. It is not known if the elder Dr. Mayo didn't either, but his record of success after surgery suggests that, being fastidious in dress and person, he may have kept his instruments cleaner than did many doctors of that time, free at least of dried blood, though not sterile. Before removing a mole or lancing a boil or clipping the ragged edges of a wound, he would bathe the area with alcohol.

His patients spread the word that he answered his calls in a hurry. Livery men gave him their fastest horses, their best cutter in snowy weather, the stoutest buggy when roads were clear. On one occasion, he came up fast behind another rig, shouted politely with a wave of apology and ran a young lawyer, Burt W. Eaton, off the road and into a snowbank. Another time, he was zealously speeding along, holding the reins of a pair of skittish horses when the horses took the bits in their teeth. Dr. Mayo tried to slow them down by pulling toward a stand of trees. Going full tilt, the horses straddled a tree. Dr. Mayo was thrown into the dashboard. After calming the horses he borrowed another buggy from a farmer and raced on to attend his patient. It was undoubtedly a shock to the sick farmer to see his doctor in the doorway with a bloody face and coat, concerned for his patient's well-being and unaware that his own nose was broken.

As other doctors began calling him for help and dropping in to watch him operate, it became apparent that Dr. W. W. Mayo had earned the respect of his peers. He gave a running monologue as he worked. His sons, too, when they were home from school, watched, listened and learned everything their father knew, including his adherence to the new ideas on sterilization that settled the debates about Pasteur and Lister.

On a scorching hot afternoon in August 1883, the year William James Mayo graduated from medical school, Will and his brother Charlie were driving a spirited little mare through the woods north of Rochester. They were headed for the slaughterhouse to pick up a sheep's head for practicing eye surgery. The slaughterhouse employees were locking the gates. Black clouds churned on the western horizon. Suddenly, the black mass swirled into a clearly defined funnel shape heading straight toward the boys in their one-horse rig.

They turned the mare toward home and at a gallop crossed the North Broadway bridge just before howling winds lifted the bridge like a toy and dropped it in a field. On each side of the road, buildings were sucked up and spewed out like silage from a shredder. The roof of the Cole Mill was swept away. The grain elevator crashed to the ground. When the cornice from the Cook Hotel whirled down on the dashboard of the buggy, the terrified horse, dragging the broken shafts, ran into an alley. The boys took refuge in a blacksmith shop.

The tornado left almost as quickly as it had come. An ominous stillness settled over the whole northern part of Rochester. Houses were strewn like jackstraws beside gaping basements; streets were a carnage of trees, broken furniture and dead animals. Throughout the night people searched the devastation for bodies. The injured were taken to hotels, offices and the Convent of Saint Francis. Doctors from nearby towns rode in to volunteer their services. Will and Charlie Mayo cared for some of the injured in their father's office while their father tended others at the Buck Hotel. Temporary hospitals were set up wherever possible. At Rommel's Dance Hall wires were strung and sheets hung to separate the patients on the beds. Mattresses were brought in by the people of Rochester.

After the emergencies had been met, a town meeting was held. Deep differences emerged when doctors couldn't agree on the treatment of patients. At one point, Dr. W. W. Mayo challenged a doctor who had assumed authority. "Either he gets out, or I do!" he growled. The city council voted Dr. Mayo in charge.

After tempers were soothed, healing began with a seemingly miraculous conjunction of two usually disparate disciplines: Science and Religion. The mother superior of the Sisters of Saint Francis approached Dr. Mayo with an idea. Rochester should have a hospital. He told her they didn't have the money. But *we* do, said Mother Alfred, and she pledged $40,000 for a building if Dr. Mayo would see that it was built.

Dr. Mayo admired spirit; he saw that this lady meant business. He allowed his concern over money to be overruled and set out to inform himself about the proper building of a hospital. He visited hospitals all over the state and came to the appalling conclusion that not one was worth table salt. With the true grit of a pioneer, he drew his own plans and put them before an architect.

Five years later, in 1889, Saint Mary's Hospital was ready. It was a red brick building with twenty-seven beds, woefully undersupplied with linens and medical necessities, but equipped with gaslight fixtures and running water outlets in the halls in case of fire. The Sisters set October 1 as the date for a formal opening of the building. Dr. Mayo scheduled an operation when the operating room was ready, the day before the official inauguration. Dr. Charlie Mayo removed a cancer from a patient's eye, Dr. Will assisted, and their father administered the anesthetic. Helen Clapesattle, the incomparable Mayo historian, wrote, "With fine disregard for pomp and palaver, they simply began."

The first trained nurse at Saint Mary's was Edith Graham, a sprightly and attractive Rochester girl who graduated from the School of Nursing at Women's Hospital in Chicago. She trained the Catholic Sisters on the proper running of a hospital and became a friend and associate of the three Mayos; she was their anesthetist, nurse, letter-writer and bookkeeper. Her charms were irresistible to Dr. Charlie Mayo. She joined him in his new sport, riding a bicycle. They married in April 1893. On their honeymoon they visited the famed medical centers of New York, Boston and Philadelphia.

Before Edith left her job to start raising a family (she had eight children; two died and she adopted two more), she struggled with the modest Sisters of Saint Francis, who found it disconcerting to lay hands on men as well as women. A paragraph from *The Doctors Mayo* clarifies the personal trauma of Sister Joseph when introduced to the nursing profession:

> Sister Joseph, on her first contact with the necessities of nursing . . . was asked to assist at the examination of a male patient whose ailment required that his entire body be uncovered for observation. While one of the doctors and Miss Graham worked with him, the young sister stood off in the corner, her back turned, quivering with outrage and shame. As she left the room when the task was done she protested vehemently to Miss Graham that she could never do such work, that she would ask Mother Matilda to send her back to teaching at once. But she stayed on, and quickly learned the lesson that the needs of human suffering transcend the dictates of modesty.[7]

Sister Joseph became one of the best scrub nurses my father, Dr. James C. Masson, ever worked with. "She could have been a wonderful doctor," he said. She knew his procedures in the operating room so well he would put out his hand and she would put into it the instrument he needed.

One day Dr. William Worrall Mayo set an operation for the following Sunday on a woman with an ovarian tumor. He sent word of it to some of the doctors interested in watching the procedure, then left for a consultation with a doctor in St. Paul. He meant to be back Saturday night but missed his train. By the hour set for the surgery, about fifteen doctors had arrived to watch. The patient was waiting with several relatives. What, Will Mayo thought, was a good son to do?

With composure and a lot of courage, Will told the woman and the assembled doctors he would do the operation. He assured them he had assisted his father with this operation many times. With the help of his brother Charlie and a doctor from Eyota, he removed the enormous tumor. Helen Clapesattle reported, "It was big enough to fill a washtub."[8] The watching doctors were greatly impressed. Will was pleased too, but very nervous when he met the next train from St. Paul. His father brought with him a former president of the Minnesota State Medical Society, Dr. Alexander J. Stone, who wanted to watch the operation. When Will told his father what he had done, Dr. Stone laughed until tears came at the young man stealing his father's big case.

By 1892 the pace of the Mayo's primarily surgical practice had increased to the extent that partners in other specialties had to be found. First, Dr. Augustus W. Stinchfield was added to the staff as a medical consultant. Two years later Dr. Christopher Graham became the first intern at Saint Mary's Hospital. He soon joined the medical staff as the second consultant. In 1903 Miss Alice Magaw became the Mayo surgical staff's expert anesthesiologist, using ether. She had abandoned the use of chloroform as far too dangerous, even though almost every surgeon in the country was still using it. From all over the world anesthesiologists came to Rochester to observe the work of this nurse-anesthetist. By then, the elder Dr. Mayo had taken on so many consulting and political responsibilities, the practice was mainly in the hands of "the boys."

Expansion of the practice proceeded at such a pace that space had to be found all over downtown Rochester to accommodate more offices, file cabinets, laboratories, the library and sick patients. They moved into the upper floors of the Masonic Temple and Weber & Heintz Drug Store. They rented parts of old schoolhouses and hotels.

Along with all the good feelings and rewards that attend a successful venture, the Mayos soon discovered there were cynics and grumblers out there, eager to discredit the Minnesota Mayos. The Mayos were not squabblers; they had their own ideas on how to deal with trouble-makers. Dr. Charlie said to ignore them: "If you fight with a polecat, you'll smell like a polecat." Dr. Will's advice to a young associate was, "If you hear a certain man is a liar, go see him. Sometimes a good man is cursed more vigorously than he would be if he were bad."[9]

It was that sentiment that sent Dr. Will in 1890 at the age of twenty-seven to Philadelphia to visit Dr. Joseph Price. Dr. Price had been the butt of severe slander by some doctors at a medical meeting. They claimed he was too radical, a braggart who lied about his low fatality rates. For four days Dr. Will was told the doctor didn't accept visitors. When finally he was allowed in to watch Dr. Price operate, Dr. Will was much impressed. He noted how thoroughly he washed his hands, face and beard. He saw the simplicity of his methods, the few instruments he used. He watched Dr. Price operate for three weeks, and on his return home he greatly reduced his own fatality rate from seventeen percent to five percent.

At the start of the twentieth century when newspapers began printing success stories about the Old Doctor and his two sons, malicious rumors circulated among skeptical doctors. The following is an example of how these many rumors got started.

Either Dr. Will or Dr. Charlie Mayo attended a meeting of some august group such as the American College of Surgeons. The young Dr. Mayo in the audience listened to a paper on the removal of the gall bladder read by a well known surgeon, a study based upon nine or ten such operations. The procedure sounded all wrong to the young Mayo. In the discussion period he stood up and said in his straightforward way that he and his brother had found a safer way to accomplish the purpose. All eyes turned in surprise to the tall, unknown young man standing in the midst of the room full of eminent doctors. Dr. Mayo described the procedure he and his brother had successfully used. It was quicker, he said, and the patient's recovery time was shorter.

Such boldness! Who was this brash young man challenging the renowned speaker?

The man at the podium said gently, "Ummm, sir, would you explain please, upon what you base your conclusions?"

Dr. Mayo replied, "My brother and I have done 123 gallbladder removals in the last nine months with no fatalities."

There was shuffling and murmuring: "What nonsense!" "The fellow is a liar!" Similar situations occurred at medical meetings in Boston, New York, Philadelphia and Chicago. But a few of the listeners took seriously the young doctor's invitation to come to Rochester as their guest and see their work.

The press reports and stories in ladies' magazines of the "miracles" that were happening in Rochester, Minnesota, were an embarrassment to the Mayo family doctors. They didn't relish being thought quacks who thrived on publicity, making tons of money. But the Old Doctor, before he died in 1911 at the age of ninety-one, noticed that little by little the image of the fledgling clinic in Rochester was changing.

Misinformation had to be answered, though, without a scrap that would have them smelling like Dr. Charlie's polecat. The brothers answered every cranky letter. They attended medical meetings and wrote papers. They encouraged their Eastern colleagues to come visit. More and more of those doctors who had thought the brothers were "a couple of rubes in a corn patch" did come. They were given royal treatment, and word got around.

It was more than skepticism that caught the attention of Dr. Carl Beck of Chicago. Something new seemed to be happening in Rochester, a group of specialists all sharing space and expenses. Dr. Beck met with Dr. Charlie in a private conversation after a lecture Dr. Beck gave to students of the Illinois College of Medicine. Dr. Beck was dumbfounded by some of the cases Dr. Charlie described to him.

When he shared his disbelief with his mentor, Dr. Nicholas Senn, Dr. Senn told him "that man's brother" had reported cases and results at a meeting of the American Medical Association "such as only very progressive surgeons with large practices could have." He advised his young associate to take off a few days, accept the invitation Charlie Mayo had given him and investigate.

Dr. Beck took the train for Rochester. He saw a town full of buggies, carts, rooming houses and small hotels. He looked up the offices of Drs. Mayo, Stinchfield and Graham at the Cook House.

"A very antiquated hotel," he wrote. "I was greeted by an old gentleman who sat at a desk covered with large books. I introduced myself and, with a smile, the old gentleman turned to a lady who was present and said, 'This is the man Charlie saw in Chicago.'" [10]

After a few days inspecting every aspect of the Mayo practice, Dr. Beck went back to Chicago with nothing but praise for what he had seen.

A story has been told and retold till the names of the original doctors have been lost: An esteemed Southern doctor in personal distress went to see an expert in New Orleans, then to Memphis, then to Cincinnati, only to find that the specialists he sought to cure his abdominal difficulty were either ill, out of the country or on vacation. In desperation, the Southern doctor took the train to Rochester. When he confessed to the hospital superintendent the roundabout route that brought him to the Mayos, he was assured that he could indeed see at least two of those doctors; they were here recovering from surgery.

"How about Dr. L——— of Cincinnati?" the doctor asked. "They told me he was in Europe."

"He may be there now," said the smiling superintendent. "We dismissed him last week after gastrointestinal surgery."[11]

The newspapers in those days often printed stories of who went where for surgery, which added to the number of new patients arriving in Rochester.

But it took more than mere publicity to account for the honor that came to Dr. William James Mayo in 1906. At only forty-five years of age he was inducted into the American Medical Association as president, in the city of Boston where previously skeptics had berated him as a charlatan. Dr. William L. Rodman of Philadelphia, at their annual meeting, referred to him as "one of the ablest, one of the cleanest, one of the best loved of the western profession." In his response, Dr. Will said he accepted the honor as having been earned equally by his brother Charlie and himself.

By the year 1908, the Mayo's business records had become too complicated to handle. A business manager was needed. The perfect man for the job was a young Rochester banker Will and Charlie knew and trusted, Harry Harwick. Together, the three of them agreed on a system of fee charging: those who could afford to pay, did; those who couldn't, didn't.

Dr. Herbert A. Bruce of Toronto, an early mentor of my father, remembers many discussions of what fees should be charged for surgery in which the opinions of the Mayo brothers were cited. The doctors Mayo, he wrote in his autobiography, decided that the basis for making a charge, when the patient was able to pay, should be determined by the amount of income he earned.[13]

Money accumulated. They agreed that extra money should be saved and spent on a park for the city of Rochester.

According to Dr. Will the best day's work he ever did was in 1906 when they hired Dr. Henry S. Plummer. With Dr. Plummer, their medical-surgical practice struck pure gold. His genius went far beyond his interest in thyroid disease. The meeting between the two young doctors in 1901 proved serendipitous. Henry's father, a doctor in Racine, Minnesota, asked the elder Dr. Mayo to come see a patient of his, a woman with leukemia. As Dr. William Worrall Mayo had to be out of town, he sent his son Will in his place. At the station in Racine Will was met by the son of his father's colleague who was sick in bed. It was Dr. Henry Stanley Plummer, age twenty-seven, who gave Will Mayo a buggy ride he would never forget. Henry took his microscope along on the seven-mile drive on country roads.

He talked to Will about the blood and its diseases. At the farm he made smears of the patient's blood and also the blood of a family member and the hired man. Using the microscope he showed Will Mayo the striking differences between normal blood and the blood of the patient.

Back home Will told his father and brother he was flabbergasted that "this gangling boy" knew so much more than he did about the blood. Immediately they decided to invite Henry Plummer to join their practice. It was a lucky day for the future Mayo Clinic when he agreed to come.

Their new recruit immediately pushed for more and better laboratory space. Once, when Will and Charlie hemmed and hawed about the cost, Henry accused them of thinking laboratory men were just a lot of "pee boilers," referring to the usual urological test. In the long run, his arguments were convincing. To plan an expanded laboratory, they consulted with and soon hired the assistant director of the bacteriological laboratory of the Minnesota State Board of Health who was also a professor at the University of Minnesota, Dr. Louis B. Wilson. One of Dr. Wilson's early contributions to the work was a forerunner to the freeze-dry technique for preparing tissue samples for examination. During an operation, Dr. Wilson set a sample of tissue outside the window in the raw winter air where it quickly froze. With a razor blade he then sliced off thin sections of the frozen sample and applied a fast stain to it. He examined the cells under a microscope, and with the patient still on the table he told the doctor if cancer was present.

A prominent Philadelphia physician, Dr. W. W. Keen, came to the Mayo's to be operated on by Dr. Will. Visiting at his bedside at Saint Mary's Hospital, Dr. Will asked for suggestions on improving their service to patients.

"You ought to write more!" Dr. Keen said. "The doctors should write up unusual cases, publish more in the journals to benefit the profession."

Dr. Will discussed this with his brother Charlie. Each member of the staff had a half or full day off for study and reading medical literature, but there was little time for writing. A suggestion came from Dr. Herbert Z. Giffin: each doctor, reading an important article in a periodical, should summarize it in writing for discussion at a weekly meeting to be held in the homes of the staff on a rotating basis. These meetings, enthusiastically attended, also revealed "the ineptness" of the writing skills of many of the doctors.

Dr. Will discussed the problem with his friend Dr. Albert J. Ochsner of Chicago, who had just finished writing a book with the editing help of a doctor's widow, Mrs. Maud J. Mellish. Dr. Ochsner was quick to recommend her to Dr. Will. Mrs. Mellish, a tall, stately woman of forty-three, had met her husband in the course of her nurse's training and the classes she attended at Rush Medical College in Chicago. Dr. Will's proposal that she join the Mayo staff was too tempting to turn down; she would be given full authority as a reference librarian and teacher of English composition to doctors whose research articles lacked clarity and style. She came to Rochester in 1907 and became indispensable to the Mayos.

Thirteen years later Mrs. Mellish would travel to South America with Dr. Will and a group from the Clinic to welcome Latin American surgeons for the first time into the American College of Surgeons of which Dr. Will was then president. Dr. Will's plan for using leisure time on shipboard was to dictate to Mrs. Mellish an outline of the story he had long neglected: how the Clinic and the Mayo Foundation were established. At one point in his dictation he paid brief tribute to Dr. Louis B. Wilson, director of the foundation. In her revisions of Dr. Mayo's statements, Mrs. Mellish added, "L. Wilson is tremendously brilliant. I have met few men his intellectual equal. In addition to his scientific abilities he has a most pleasing personality."[14] Apparently, there was mutual admiration between them. Mrs. Maud Mellish, the widow, became Mrs. Wilson shortly thereafter.

In 1912, the group was desperately in need of more space. A committee of three—Harry Harwick, Louis Wilson and Henry Plummer—was named to plan a building that would put a roof over the whole group on a site in the middle of town that had been the old Mayo homestead. This building represents the official beginning of the Mayo Clinic as we know it today. As Dr. Fredrick A. Willius writes in a biography of his friend and mentor, Dr. Plummer, no committee was needed. Dr. Plummer single-mindedly planned the red brick building that came to be called the 1914 Building. He designed it inside and out, though he had never had formal training in the field of architecture. Through his own efforts, he became a master builder. In what must have been an exciting expectation for the future of this building, a time capsule was prepared for burial inside the cornerstone.

That carved stone is now a historical marker displayed in the Siebens Building, part of the School of Health-Related Sciences, that replaced the 1914 Building. The *Rochester Post Bulletin* of July 7, 1986, reports on the retrieval of the time capsule, a heavy copper box encased in lead.[15] Its contents were said to be "a treasure trove" of memorabilia on early Mayo Clinic days. There were photographs of "serious-faced young doctors" and pages of statistics. New patient registrations for the first ten months of 1912 came to 12,032. The names of all 111 physicians and employees associated with the Clinic since 1889 were listed. Papers on experimental studies then being conducted were included, as well as sketches of the building Dr. Plummer planned. Coins, stamps and that day's newspapers with headlines of U.S. troops in Nicaragua were included.

On the occasion of the laying of the cornerstone for the 1914 Building, Dr. Charlie put the spade in the ground and Dr. Will spoke these words:

> The object of this building is to furnish a permanent house wherein scientific investigation can be made into the causes of the diseases which afflict mankind and wherein every effort shall be made to cure the sick and suffering. It is the hope of the founders of this building that in its use the high ideals of the medical profession will always be maintained. Within its walls all classes of people, the poor as well as the rich, without regard to color or creed, shall be cared for without discrimination.[16]

As the number of new patients needing ear, nose and throat surgery increased, the Mayo brothers invited Dr. Justus Matthews from Minneapolis to join them, as well as a young man trained in dentistry to be his assistant, Dr. Gordon B. New from Hamilton, Ontario. Dr. New later became the head of the plastic surgery section of the Mayo Clinic. To ease the workload of Dr. Will and Dr. Charlie, who did all the general surgery, they invited their young intern, Dr. Edward Starr Judd, to join the staff.

Dr. Judd told his mother, after graduating from the University of Minnesota Medical School, "I'd rather be a Dr. Will than President of the United States."

At this time Saint Mary's Hospital, after two additions, could accommodate 175 patients.

Soon another surgeon was needed, someone the Mayos could train in their methods. They found him in Minneapolis: Dr. Emil H. Beckman. The officials of Minneapolis must have been startled when their able city physician and chief internist of the city hospital resigned both positions to become an assistant to the Mayo brothers in Rochester.

Dr. Beckman began a short apprenticeship doing nothing but dressing the wounds of convalescent patients who were crowding the smaller hotels and boarding houses in Rochester. Then he became a full-fledged associate who rapidly gained nationwide respect for his judgment and skill.

The arduous task of tending the many post-operative dressings was then taken over by a series of young interns who ultimately assumed prominent positions in various specialties in the Mayo Clinic. Young Dr. Melvin Henderson made his rounds of nearly a hundred patients on a bicycle. When the street lights were turned off, he lit his way with an electric torch. The next young doctor to inherit that Herculean task was Dr. Donald Church Balfour, also a University of Toronto graduate in the class of 1906.

When Dr. Will's daughter Carrie Mayo returned from her sophomore year at Wellesley College, she went on a hayride with some of her old friends and met her father's then assistant, Don Balfour. Dr. Balfour was the fourth general surgeon to be trained by the two Doctors Mayo, but, more significant for this personal history, he was the one who caught the eye of the boss's daughter. In very little time, Carrie Mayo and Donald Balfour were married.

In 1912, a year after the Old Doctor, William Worrall Mayo, died, Dr. James C. Masson, a horse-and-buggy doctor from Dunnville, Ontario, came to inspect the Mayo's unusual medical practice and to visit three of his Toronto classmates, Drs. New, Henderson and Balfour. The Mayo's staff then consisted of six surgeons and thirteen medical doctors, all working together and sharing the load of business services. It was soon discovered that Jim Masson's experience in "kitchen table surgery" had prepared him well for the operating room and he was asked to be Dr. Charlie Mayo's first assistant. He was the last of the Mayo Clinic surgeons to be trained by Dr. Will and Dr. Charlie Mayo.

Dr. Jim Masson, wrapped up in his work as Dr. Charlie Mayo's assistant, delayed his return to Canada. Because of that delay, Mayo Clinic history has become part of my personal story.

Sometime during the winter of 1914, Carrie Mayo Balfour invited her Wellesley classmate, Alice Marion Knowles of Worcester, Massachusetts, to come for a visit. Carrie and Don were in cahoots to play cupid.

Years ago when I asked my mother how she met Dad, she painted a picture that stayed with me. A fire crackled on the hearth in the Balfour's home. The doorbell rang. Don greeted Jim and led him straight to Marion. I can see her there, poised and graceful, and feel her response as Jim Masson came forward and took her hand. How handsome he was, his brown hair curled over his forehead. How blue his eyes!

Later that night in her bed at Don and Carrie's home on Sixth Avenue, S.W. Mother must have been afloat with happiness. But then thoughts of her father would have interrupted her sleep: Frank Poole Knowles would scowl if he knew how giddy his favorite daughter felt about this handsome Canadian.

… { 2 } …

The Courtship of My Parents

> If there is a sixth sense, it is intuition, that instinctive summing up of memories and other evidences collected by the special senses and correlated in man's consciousness.
> Dr. W. J. Mayo, 1927[1]

THE courtship of my parents could read like a Victorian romance: *Poor but honest country doctor from Canada falls in love with jealous textile machinery tycoon's daughter.* But, with no expectations beyond the present, what joyful anticipation must have arisen in the hearts of the young couple when that giddy feeling took hold on a cold gray February day in 1914.

My father, Dr. James C. Masson, was thirty-two years old. There had been a few girls in his thoughts before he came to Rochester, but the career he was aiming for always claimed his highest priority. He lacked money to spend on roses. In those years, a prudent man was expected to be earning a living and to save money sufficient to buy a house before he asked a girl's father for the privilege of marrying his daughter.

When my parents met, Jim Masson, a graduate of the University of Toronto Medical School, was an assistant to Dr. E. Starr Judd, a partner in the clinic of the Mayo brothers in Rochester, Minnesota. On that winter day Dr. Judd and he had finished twelve surgical cases and made rounds in Saint Mary's Hospital. Jim looked forward to dinner and relaxation with friends, a former classmate at med school, Dr. Donald C. Balfour, his wife Carrie and a friend visiting "from the East," Don said. Jim rang the doorbell, opened the door, shook the hand of his old friend and was led to the living room where a fire sparkled on the hearth. Don then presented him to their guest, a girl with a mound of light brown hair and hazel eyes, her hand on the Balfour's grand piano. She met Jim's eyes and smiled. He felt breathless. This was a surprise; he thought the guest would be a doctor visiting the Mayos' clinic. He had expected only Carrie's home cooking, some shop talk with Don and his guest and then back to his narrow bed at the hospital to sleep and be ready for dawn, when he would join Dr. Judd to get on with the plan for the day.

With the arrival of "the house guest from the East" at Don's and Carrie's house, Jim was caught up in a whirl of social events such as he had never experienced before. Her name was Alice Marion Knowles, known as Marion. Everyone wanted to entertain Carrie's college friend, and Jim was included in their plans. They kept him well fed and energized, especially the Canadians, Don and Carrie, Mel and Mabel Henderson and Gordon and Ethyl New. On Sundays they went to Henry and Daisy Plummer's weekly "Salon and Bean Feed," a get-together for all the young interns, staff assistants and their wives, plus a number of single young women. Many friendships blossomed into romance at those Sunday suppers. Daisy Plummer remarked that their home had become a matrimonial bureau.

Formal dinners were hosted by the seniors on the staff. It is easy for me, a daughter, to imagine the young Dr. Jim Masson at a dinner given by Carrie's parents, Dr. and Mrs. W. J. Mayo. Jim would be tired after a long day on his feet but gratified at being with his peers where shop talk was the norm. At the top of his mind, however, would be his anticipation of the arrival of the Balfours and the guest of honor, Marion Knowles. He might be listening intently to Dr. Charlie's description of Henry Ford's latest automobile with running boards, or some interesting work on the treatment for exophthalmic goiter, when voices at the Mayo's front door told him *she* had arrived. Feeling a jolt, he might have blushed and missed a part of Dr. Charlie Mayo's story, but never could the dignified Canadian have said to one of his heroes, "Excuse me, Dr. Mayo, I need to speak to a certain lady." Perhaps if cocktails had been served, his inhibitions would have been overcome, but alcohol was never served at Dr. Will Mayo's dinners.

When finally Jim and Marion found some time to themselves and Jim felt, intuitively, that her heartbeat was as rampant as his, he confessed to being quite totally in love.

I don't know what happened next; nobody told me. But being so truly British and bound by the discretion of those times, my guess is that my

The Courtship of My Parents

father was as frustrated as a teenager under the watchful eye of parents. My mother's natural way of putting people at ease and her own affectionate fluster would have lessened the tension.

Near the end of that one-month visit, I know what did happen, probably in the Balfour's front hall or on the veranda as they embraced and said goodnight, Don and Carrie having discreetly gone upstairs. I know there wouldn't have been any laughing then, but emotional tears from Marion at their impending separation. He asked her to marry him and she quickly said yes, but then, with a jolt, she thought, "What will Papa say!"

In those "Life with Father" years it was expected that a young man first request the hand of a young lady from her father before broaching the subject to the daughter. What a breach of manners Jim had committed in his impetuous proposal of marriage! He understood profoundly his gross faux pas. He knew from what Marion had told him of her family that Papa was not only a prominent businessman, but a man of inflexible principles, not to be trifled with.

Jim must have had many a sleepless night fearing that the stern father might rise up like a bad genie and stand between him and his love. He knew he should go east and meet Mr. Knowles, but that was out of the question. Surgical schedules at the Clinic were tight. All six general surgeons were needed: the two Mayos, and Doctors Beckman, Judd, Henderson and Balfour. As Judd's first assistant, Jim couldn't leave. He would write a letter to Mr. Knowles, and Mrs. Knowles too. He would apologize for his rash proposal and humbly request the hand of their daughter Marion.

Jim was a humble sort, but he knew his own worth. He was a good doctor. He had a sure hand with a knife, could work long hours and be calm in the presence of even the most bizarre accidents that came before him. He had delivered hundreds of babies whose mothers were always glad to see him. What worried Jim was not his ability to make a good living and live happily with the woman he loved, but what would happen when Marion got off the train in Worcester and burst out with her news.

Marion Knowles, at twenty-eight, had not been allowed the usual social contacts with her peers. Her domineering father, Frank Poole Knowles, known as F. P., wouldn't permit a Boston debut for his lovely daughter Marion to meet the sons and daughters of Boston society, though her mother and the aunts were all for such a gala affair. He allowed her to go to Wellesley College, though, a women's college and just a short train ride from Worcester. She often came home weekends, bringing school friends with her. When she came alone, she and her childhood friend, Edith Rockwell, would take the trolley to the end of the line and walk up the hill to Highlawn Farm, the Knowles's country home in Auburn, Massachusetts, just beyond the Worcester city limits. The two girls would saddle up Bess and Peggy and ride the trails in the Highlawn woods.

Marion and Edith were alike in what they loved—nature in all seasons, the horses and cows at Highlawn, its white fences, the pasture, its meandering brook and F. P. himself, stubborn though he was. He loved those girls quite selfishly as part of the life at Highlawn.

It comes across in Marion's diaries how much she also loved the life at Wellesley, skating on the frozen pond, play-acting, singing, field hockey, roughhousing in the dorm, writing papers late at night. She took the train to Boston for dates with Harvard men to plays and concerts, all well chaperoned, of course.

Marion assumed graduation day with the class of 1910 would be the highlight of her college years. She would dance the role of the West Wind in the outdoor pageant planned for mid-afternoon. It was a glorious, breezy day, the pungent smell of spring afloat on the green lawn, the culmination of four wonderful years at Wellesley. Barefoot in a swirling chiffon costume, she leaped into the role of the playful wind before a large happy gathering of parents and friends.

But tragedy cut the celebration short for Marion. When she had finished her dance, Edith came out of the crowd alone and threw her arms around her friend. Marion's older brother George, home to recuperate from an undiagnosed illness, had died that morning.

It took a long time for the family to heal, to feel normal again. What helped most was F. P.'s decision to move permanently from the elegant old Victorian home at 838 Main Street, Worcester, to the sprawling farmhouse and the barns of Highlawn in Auburn. The move kept everybody busy, cleaning and packing, keeping F. P. content.

F. P. was a senior officer at a company founded by his father, Frank Bangs Knowles, who invented a shuttle that put a pattern in cloth and,

The Courtship of My Parents

with a Mr. Crompton, established the Crompton Knowles Loom Works in Worcester, Massachusetts. F. P. became less and less interested in his father's company, though, as his success in the field of agriculture became central to his happiness. When he was semi-retired from the Loom Works he gave his enthusiasm to the hobby he loved, the life at Highlawn Farm as breeder of Holstein Fresian cattle and trotting horses. By the start of the twentieth century he had developed a championship herd of cattle which he showed in dairy states all over New England and the midwest. One of his many silver trophies earned by the high milk-producing capacity of his cows is inscribed: "Best Exhibit, Valley Fair 1905, Awarded by Holstein Fresian Register." F. P. was frequently interviewed for articles in *Holstein Fresian World* and other breeders' magazines. He was awarded a gold medal by the Massachusetts Department of Agriculture for distinctive service over a period of forty years.

F. P. had always been possessive about his daughters. He gave a cold reception to visiting males, be they Worcester South High School classmates of Marion, or Harvard men who came to call. The one young man who had Mr. Knowles's approval was the son of a friend and business associate. He was of no interest to Marion. She wrote in her diary that he "bored [her] dreadfully." The really impassioned disputes between Marion and F. P. were caused by her fondness for Will Wier, a high school friend who graduated from Holy Cross College in 1910 when Marion graduated from Wellesley. Marion and Will had much in common. They wrote for their school papers, took part in plays, danced, skated and rode horseback together. The problem for a good Protestant man like F. P. Knowles came when his daughter's friendship continued past the college years and he realized she was in love with a Catholic man.

In those days in New England there was bitter enmity between Catholics and Protestants. It was especially heated in Massachusetts when Governor Curley, a Catholic, dominated state politics. F. P. liked to joke that politics in Massachusetts was worse than crooked; it was Curley. Will Wier was given a thumbs-down by every Knowles but Marion. She wrote in her diary, "... because of Will, everybody is upset with me, especially Papa."

The friendship of Marion Knowles and Carrie Mayo at Wellesley probably became a bond when they discovered how alike their fathers were. Mr. Knowles and Dr. Will Mayo were both imperious about the men who wanted to marry their daughters. Carrie, too, was having a running controversy with her father over a boyfriend named Rob. Carrie's suitor displeased Dr. Will Mayo enough that he brought Carrie home at the end of her sophomore year at Wellesley.

My mother's diary sheds a revealing beam of light on the denouement of Carrie's romantic dream. Carrie, back home in Rochester, soon fell in love with another man:

> . . . a letter today from Carrie Mayo saying she and Rob have broken their engagement. I was shocked, but not terribly surprised, for Carrie's letters lately have been very uncertain, and I expected something to happen. I could have sworn though she loved that man. She has lived for nothing else for over five years. Poor Carrie!

Less than two months later, Carrie came east with her mother Mrs. Hattie Damon Mayo, her Grandmother Damon and her sister Phoebe. Marion's journal described how "diligently" she had finished all papers and assignments before Carrie's visit so she could be free to devote her time to the Mayos. Her entries sum up the meals, cultural events in Boston, walks around the Wellesley lake, a drive to Revere Beach, a train ride to Worcester for "a peek" at Papa Knowles before he left for business in Syracuse, then back to Boston's Hotel Touraine. After a final return to Wellesley for Carrie's goodbyes to old friends and teachers, the Mayo women departed for Atlantic City.

On Monday, May 31, 1909, Mother wrote how much she liked the Mayos and the sound of the man Carrie had agreed to marry, Dr. Donald C. Balfour:

> I do like the Mayos. They are so unassuming. I was right about Carrie. It is a doctor in Rochester, and she is really in love this time—not in a sentimental way but truly. She says Donald is the only man she ever met who could rule her. That is what Carrie needs.

I can easily imagine how quickly Carrie Mayo forgot Rob, her youthful heartthrob, when she went on a hayride one Saturday afternoon and was introduced to Dr. Donald Church Balfour, newly arrived in Rochester from the University of Toronto Medical School. Dr. Balfour, whom I came to know as "Uncle Don," was a very special man—warm, enchanting, attentive, widely read and literate, a master of gentle persuasion. I can imagine Dr. Will Mayo had a secret trap set for his daughter, and Carrie just naturally fell into it.

In the days after Marion Knowles left Rochester on the Chicago and Northwestern train, after her extended visit with Carrie and Don Balfour in March 1914, Jim Masson must have returned often to the Balfours, the only two people who knew how weightless in the clouds he felt. It was Carrie he needed to talk to; she had met Marion's parents at Wellesley and spent weekends with them at both the Worcester home and at Highlawn Farm. Carrie could have entertained the nervous Jim with an account of one of Mr. Knowles's famous Barn Parties, people all eating at a long table with a white cloth between two rows of cows in their stanchions languidly chewing their mash and hay. No matter how clean Carrie told Jim the barns were, he must have thought he had never seen a clean barn. She must have assured him Mrs. Knowles would adore him as a son-in-law, but she would have known Mr. Knowles would not graciously let any man take Marion so far from home.

Jim was at the Balfour's one evening after making rounds at the hospital when he remembered he hadn't written his mother in several weeks. Don sat him down at his desk and persuaded him to get to it, one more thing off his mind. The cost of a letter sent coast to coast in 1914 in the United States was two cents. Unless snow blocked the tracks or an engine broke down, a letter posted in Rochester to Jim's mother in Toronto would be delivered two days later. Jim stamped the envelope and, on Don's stationery, poured out his happy news:

My dear Mother,
You will no doubt be surprised, but I have some real news this week. I am truly in love and now that I am, I know it is the first time in my life. It is almost a case of love at first sight, but I am sure it is the kind that will last. My lady fair is a college friend of Mrs. Balfour, . . . is a graduate of Wellesley College and comes of an old New England family. Her home is in Worcester near Boston and she has been visiting Mrs. B— for the last month. She is twenty-eight years of age and is a fine, well-built,

healthy, beautiful girl, her hair about the color of Lou's. . . . Her father is a textile machinery company executive, and raises Holstein cattle and sends them to all the large fairs throughout the East. Her mother is living but has not been very strong since the death of her only son four years ago. She has one sister a few years younger than herself. . . . She is definitely not a frivolous butterfly girl, the kind you thought I would marry. Her family are Congregationalists.

Of course nothing is definitely decided, but I am sure our affection is mutual and while her family will be surprised, perhaps even provoked, at such a sudden match yet I feel sure we will be married in probably one year's time. By then I will be on a salary able to keep house, and if I decide to, we can return to Toronto in about another year.

I have definitely decided to stay here at least one year from October first as I am going on Dr. C. H. Mayo's service as senior assistant, and it is by all odds the best service out here for experience. Afternoons I am to call on cases in the various boarding houses and hotels throughout the town. I will leave the hospital and (take a) room downtown. I will be on a salary of probably $100 a month, at least enough to pay expenses. Marion, of course knows my circumstances exactly . . . .

I was almost forgetting to tell you her name. She is Alice Marion Knowles, but everyone calls her Marion. I am sure, Mother, you will love her, and I want to arrange for you to meet her soon.

While I cannot give her the luxuries she has been used to, I am sure, provided my health lasts, that I will be able to keep a very comfortable home . . . and I am looking forward with the greatest pleasure to your frequent and long visits to us.

You can tell the family, but please do not tell any others . . . Mum's the word . . . until after Marion's visit again in the summer. . . . Marion is an out-of-door girl and fond of tennis, drives a car and I am sure just the girl and the only girl that will make me happy and I am sure I can do the same for her. She is not extravagant, in fact is very sensible. . . . Carrie (Mrs. Balfour) thinks she is an ideal girl and says they are a very affectionate family.

Now Mother dear, with lots of love and hoping for your blessing, I remain,

    Your affectionate son,
    Jim

The Courtship of My Parents

Marion's trip home that cold March day was the first of many painful goodbyes and joyful returns, shuttling as she did throughout the years between Rochester and Worcester. She couldn't bear separations from those she loved. Her diary is full of these sentiments: "How I dread leaving Jim"; "My heart is in my boots." On leaving Worcester one time, her father having had a recent heart attack, she wrote, "The train moved in little jerks, pulling my heart like a stretched elastic, then giving me a snap of pain as the dear faces on the platform faded in distance."

But, on this first seperation from Jim, Marion was overjoyed to know she would see him again soon. By midsummer she would be on this train again, returning to his arms. She smiled at the view of the Berkshires, not yet glorious with small green leaves, but she saw crocuses pushing through the dry leaves and syrup buckets hung from maple trees. She closed her eyes, remembering Jim's smooth face with its faint, unfamiliar smell of ether, reminding her that he was a surgeon. In the future she would have to share him with other women who needed him too, but she would be his wife! These thoughts made her happy as she lay down in her Pullman berth. But the next day, impatiently browsing around the La Salle Street Station in Chicago, awaiting the connection to Worcester, thoughts of her father loomed like sultry weather. Poor Papa. Her news would sadden and infuriate him.

The next morning when the train pulled into Worcester, Edith Rockwell, her best friend, was with the Knowles family on the platform. Also there to welcome her was the whole Comins family, including eight-year-old Betty Comins who would, if all went well, be a flower girl at her wedding. Mr. Knowles, unaware of the time bomb that would soon go off in his world, was effusive with news of the farm.

Marion listened and hugged everyone. She laughed as they talked all at once. The baggage was collected, her father joked with the porter and tipped him, and Marion whispered to Edith, "Something wonderful happened in Rochester!"

She held it in till all were seated for the midday meal at Highlawn.

Mr. Knowles at the head of the table, dapper and handsome with neat salt-and-pepper hair and white moustache, served the plates with salmon, scalloped potatoes and beets. Mrs. Knowles, my plump grandmother at the other end of the table, served peas and small onions, then passed a tray of celery, carrot sticks and spiced figs. Mildred, the maid, with a big smile for Marion, came through the swinging door from the china pantry with cornmeal muffins fresh from the oven.

Then Marion, with a fast-beating heart, let it all spill out, told it all in one breathless moment: She wanted them all to know what a truly wonderful time she had at Carrie's! She met so many wonderful doctors and their wives ... especially one doctor named Jim Masson, a Presbyterian from Canada, a friend of Carrie's husband, and ... and ... "he's handsome and so kind and good and understanding, and I fell in love with him, and he asked me to marry him, and I said yes! Oh, yes, I'm so happy! I love him deeply."

Silence dropped like rose petals on the linen table cloth.

"Oh, dear," her mother said softly, and looked at her husband.

Stunned, everyone looked toward F. P.—Marion's sister Lillian and her husband Arthur Eldred, a dentist; Mrs. Alice Bigelow Knowles, my grandmother whom I knew as "Monty"; Cousin Edmund and Cousin Lucy Bigelow who were visiting from Kansas City; Edith Rockwell whom I now call Aunt Deedie and Aunt Jean Averill, a widowed friend who lived in the apartment over the garage.

Mr. Knowles lowered his fork to his plate, his eyebrows puckered. "Who," he growled, "is this impertinent young man who so precipitously proposed marriage?"

"No, Papa!" Marion exclaimed, tears glistening in her eyes. "He's not precipitous. He has waited all these years for me. He's thirty-two years old. We love each other. I know you'll love him too, when you meet him."

"I don't care to meet him! I know the type!"

"No, Papa, he's not ..."

Marion, unable to talk, shook her head and cried into her napkin. The women were all sympathy and soft hands. Grandmother Bigelow said, "Mari, dear, please, this is too sudden," and her mother said, "Please don't mention this to the Comins, Dear. They'll be over after dinner. We need to talk. We won't say a word now ...."

"Yes, we will, Mama! I want Auntie Pudge to know. I'm going to marry Jim Masson; Papa can't stop me. Deedie's happy for me, and you should be too!"

When Mr. Knowles stood up, his chair teetered on two legs until he caught it and set it down hard. He strode from the room. He picked up the telephone in the front parlor, lifted the receiver and clicked it several times. In a terse voice, audible to everyone in the dining room, he told the operator to give him Mr. Walter Tyler. Mr. Tyler was a lawyer at the Oxidage Company who handled the books for the Crompton Knowles Loom Works.

According to Edith Rockwell, my grandfather sent a man to Canada to check out the background and character of Jim Masson. What he hoped for, Aunt Deedie told me with a knowing nod, was for some scandal to be found to justify his opposition to the marriage, some black sheep behavior that would cause a doctor to leave his own country and get lost in a small town in the United States. Mr. Knowles, if he could help it, wouldn't allow his daughter to marry "a foreigner."

The Knowles had met Dr. and Mrs. Will Mayo in 1907 when they came to visit Carrie in her freshman year at Wellesley. They hadn't heard of the Mayo Clinic. Their Dr. Sibley was likely to be one of those eastern doctors who couldn't imagine an authentic medical center sprouting up in the midwest.

After Marion's shocking announcement, Mr. Knowles' intolerant disposition made things unpleasant for everyone. He wouldn't let Marion speak of Jim; her mother urged her to be patient. The time would have dragged unbearably without her friend Edith. Evenings with F. P. in the house were long and stressful. The women played card games and Scrabble with friends who came to call. Then Marion went to her room and wrote a letter to Jim. She wrote every day, and on most days she received a letter from him.

One evening after about two weeks, Mr. Walter Tyler came to the front door with a letter in his hand. He had contacted his nephew, Arnot Craick of Toronto, who arranged some undercover sleuthing into what he called "Mr. Knowles's concern about the Canadian doctor." He handed the letter to Mrs. Knowles:

Dear Uncle Walter,

I am now in receipt of a reply from my friend in Dunnville, Ontario, regarding Dr. Masson. He does not tell me anything about his family but says:

Dr. Masson stood very high here socially and professionally. He made more of a specialty of surgery than the other five doctors and built up a large practice. He did such operations as appendicitis himself and did ten of them in three months prior to leaving, not losing one, the other doctors taking such cases to Hamilton.

I knew him very well and he was a most exemplary character in every particular. It was well recognized here that he was too big a man for this town, as a practice here would not lead to anything really big.

I don't know a man in any walk of life whom I could more conscientiously recommend than Dr. Masson.
Yours faithfully,
Arnot Craick

Mrs. Knowles was in tears before she could finish the letter, it was so full of praise for the Canadian doctor. She handed the letter to Edith, who finished the reading. Looking at F. P., Edith repeated the last sentence, "I don't know a man in any walk of life whom I could more conscientiously recommend than Dr. Masson." Aunt Deedie told me she gave the letter to my grandfather, but he gave it back to her with an angry "Damn!" then left the room to the smiling women.

F. P. was a poor loser, but he was forced, finally, to agree to a wedding only a few months off, October 15, 1914.

A telegram and a flurry of letters from Marion put an end to Jim's worries. He relaxed and let two important tasks fill his evenings, writing letters to Marion's parents. At his desk in Saint Mary's Hospital, Jim stamped the two envelopes he had addressed, and on paper displaying the Masson family crest he wrote first to his future mother-in-law, telling her what he thought she would want to hear from a future son-in-law. It is easy to see, by the way he let his feelings loose, how well he understood the feminine mystique. I don't know if these letters were a struggle for him, but his thoughts seemed to flow blissfully into the ink on the paper:

Dear Mrs. Knowles:

It is impossible for me to satisfactorily express myself in this matter and I have no apology to offer for falling in love with dear Marion. It was almost a case of love at first sight with me, and while I honestly tried not to be rash, nevertheless I could not resist any longer. As soon as I realized that I was truly in love, and I had no idea what it meant before, I decided to keep my affections in cold storage until we would meet again, but this I found impossible to do. As soon as Marion gave me the least encouragement and by one little look showed to my heart's content that she at least cared for me and would miss me on her return home, I was quite irresponsible, and I think even before I called her by her first name I revealed my love for her and in the next breath asked her to be my wife.

Words cannot express my pleasure in learning by my dear Marion's letter, which just arrived today, that you so thoroughly understand the situation, and even before you know me personally, or know anything about my family or my past, you are prepared to accept me as a son-in-law simply because you have every confidence in your daughter's judgment. One of my most pleasant objects in life from now on will be to try and keep her happy in the knowledge that she judged me aright.

I had a letter a few days ago from my dear Mother in answer to one I had written with the all important news in it, and I am proud to say that she also is happy in knowing that I am going to have such a perfect wife.

Now, my dear Mrs. Knowles, my every hope and prayer is that you will never have any reason to regret giving your consent to our engagement. I do hope Marion will be able to visit Mrs. Balfour again this summer, and then we will have time to thoroughly consider everything and plan for the future.

Looking forward with great pleasure to meeting you and Mr. Knowles some time in the near future, I remain,

      Yours very sincerely,
      James C. Masson

Two days later Jim wrote a ten-page, handwritten letter to his future father-in-law on paper given him by Sister Joseph at Saint Mary's Hospital. He quickly apologized for falling in love with Marion so suddenly and unreservedly. Then, with more than enough detail for the average non-family member, he summarized his background (included here for the sake of family and genealogy buffs). This is our Canadian connection. Jim named every family member and his or her occupation. He then outlined the route taken in his preparation for a medical career down to his present employment at "the greatest surgical hospital in the world."

Dear Mr. Knowles:

 I am sure you would be surprised and probably somewhat provoked at Marion's and my short love affair. I have no excuse to offer, Mr. Knowles. I simply fell in love with your daughter about the second or third time I met her, and from that day until the evening I proposed I had the greatest difficulty in not showing my intention. My purpose at first was to wait until I would see her again or possibly have the pleasure of meeting you and Mrs. Knowles as well, and in a natural way let you know—what must be very essential to you both—something of my family and my past. However, when the opportunity offered and I thought I had a little encouragement from Marion I could not wait. I knew I loved her and I thought she loved me, and my greatest wish from now until the end of this life will always be to keep her love and respect and to keep her happy.

I am quite sure you are anxious to know something about my family and my past, and while I would much sooner you would find out from someone else, yet I feel that I must give you a little of this information.

Both my grandfathers and both my grandmothers came to Canada from Scotland. My father's parents settled near Belleville, Ontario, and my father was a graduate in arts and law from Queen's University, Kingston. He practiced law in Owen Sound, Ontario, until 1896 when he was appointed senior Judge of Huron County, Ontario, a life appointment. He was Member of Parliament (Ottawa) for North Grey from 1886 until 1896. He died on December 24, 1904.

My mother's father, Duncan Morrison, was a Presbyterian minister, and his first congregation was in Kingston, and later in Owen Sound. He died at the age of eighty-six in Owen Sound. He was a graduate from Glasgow University, Scotland. My mother has two brothers living—one, Duncan Morrison, Picton, Ontario, was a barrister and is now Judge of Prince Edward County. The other, John, is manager of a farm implement or rather a wagon factory in Chatham, Ontario. My father has three brothers living. One is on the old homestead near Belleville, one was a lawyer in Belleville but is now Police Magistrate of that city. The other is a doctor in St. Vincent, New York State.

I am the fifth of eight children, seven of us are still alive and one thing I am sure of and proud of is that we are all above the average in health and strength. My brother that died, Harold, was operated on for appendicitis when that disease was not thoroughly understood and he never regained consciousness. I have two sisters married—one, Emily, known as "Tiny," to A. H. Jeffrey, manager and secretary of the Polson Iron Works, Toronto; the other, Margaret, to D. A. Boyd of Procton, B.C. He is a civil engineer. My other sister, Louise, and she was always my chum while at home, is now a nurse in New York City. My oldest broth-

The Courtship of My Parents

er, Tom, is in charge of a department in a wholesale hardware store in Toronto, and the next one to me, Stanley, has a government position in the Game and Fisheries Department in Toronto. My youngest brother, Duncan Morrison, is a medical student at Toronto University. My mother is living in Toronto at present and is 66 years of age.

Perhaps you are not at all interested in what I am writing, Mr. Knowles, but I want you to know something about me before we meet, which I hope will be in the near future as I am more than anxious that you should all approve of our marriage.

I was born in Owen Sound in 1881, went to Public School there and Collegiate Institute in Goderich, matriculating in 1900. I then entered the Medical Faculty of Toronto University, and, on account of my father's illness, missed one year, graduating in 1906. I was then in the Sick Children's Hospital, Toronto, for one year as intern, then in the Manhattan Maternity and Dispensary, New York City, for three months, then in the Toronto General Hospital for one year. Then I received the appointment as Resident in the Manhattan Maternity on a salary of $100 a month and all expenses. I kept that one year.

Then, after a trip down through the West Indies, I entered partnership with Dr. Moir of Dunnville, Ontario. I was with him two years, then we separated, and I bought out one of the other doctors in the same town. I was in practice for myself just two years, but during my last year I considered I was probably doing about as much work as I could ever do in that district. In fact I was working too hard, and I thought it was better to stop before I got into the rut of a country doctor and probably spent all my days there. I therefore sold out and started in at this hospital—the greatest surgical hospital in the world—and I am well satisfied with my prospects here.

As you can see, Mr. Knowles, I have spent a good many years preparing for my chosen profession and while I will admit that I should have waited until I had completed my course here (which I figure on as three years) before asking for the hand of any lady much less that of your dear daughter Marion, whom I know has had every advantage this world can afford in the way of happiness and comfort, yet I simply could not wait. I know I can return to Canada and in a short time secure a fairly good practice, but since coming here, I am somewhat tempted to remain, at least for a few years. I am assured of a modest living and all the time I will be securing a wonderful experience which would be a great advantage to me in any city. I am satisfied that a surgeon should not practice that branch alone until he is about forty years of age.

You will no doubt be rather shocked at my present financial standing. After my father's death I paid all my college expenses by working during my holidays and borrowing any necessary amounts from my uncle in Picton, Ontario. While Resident in the Manhattan I was able to repay the greater part and while in partnership with Dr. Moir (he left Dunnville one year after we separated) I cleared myself of debt. I have now a little over $6,000 in the bank. (I have never invested it simply because I have not even yet definitely decided how long I am going to remain here) and I have a mortgage on my late property for $2,000 and I have notes amounting to upwards of $1,000 due me. I carry $5,000 insurance, but before I marry intend increasing it to at least $10,000.

Probably I am foolish to write you in this way, Mr. Knowles, but I want you to understand me thoroughly. I know I have nothing but enough to make a start on, but I am certain of my training for my chosen profession and I know I have had a better training than most, and I am absolutely certain I can keep Marion comfortably if by the Grace of God I am spared in health and strength.

      I have the honor to remain
       Yours respectfully,
        James C. Masson

Since my father's autobiographical report to F. P. Knowles included little of the personal side of his growing-up years, I want to add some revealing anecdotes as confessed to me by Jim himself and some of my Canadian cousins.

Owen Sound, where Jim was born, is a lovely small town in Ontario at the foot of the Niagara Escarpment on the shores of Georgian Bay, which opens to the west into Lake Huron. Jim and his brother Tom owned high-front-wheel bicycles, nicknamed the "penny-farthing" after two British coins, the front wheel having three times the diameter of the rear wheel. Uncle Tom's son, my cousin Allan, explained about those bikes: "You'd never have a blow-out on a penny-farthing; their tires were solid rubber. But if you hit a rock going downhill on the dirt roads into Owen Sound, you'd go ass-over-applecart to the bottom."

Jim Masson was a sturdy, good-looking lad of about five feet, ten inches tall with a thatch of soft brown hair that puffed up over his forehead. He

The Courtship of My Parents

had great stamina for sports, many hobbies and firm friends. He and his friends used to ride the penny-farthings to neighboring towns, sometimes a hundred miles from Owen Sound, to participate in athletic competitions during fairs and festivals. A hobby of his was the raising and training of homing pigeons. On some of those bicycle trips he took along cages of pigeons in his bicycle basket and released them at increasing distances to fly home to their loft in the barn. Railroad men helped him continue training the pigeons, taking them to the end of the line before letting them go. (Jim began that hobby again in Rochester in the 1930's when my brother Stanley took an interest in raising homers.)

In winter Jim belonged to the Snowshoe Club and was an enthusiastic hockey player. Marbles was a spring hobby. All summer he practiced marksmanship with homemade slingshots and bows and arrows. When he was twelve years old he owned a .22 rifle and hunted game for the family table. He told us children the worst mischief he ever got into in high school began when he put a firecracker and matches in his pocket. It was too tempting. When the teacher wasn't looking, he lit the firecracker and tossed it toward the open window. It hit the bottom of the window and fell to the windowsill. The explosion filled the classroom with grey-blue smoke and the smell of gunpowder. The girls screamed, the boys yelled and whistled, and the teacher sent Jim to the principal, a big gruff fellow who bent him over a chair and whacked his bottom with a razor strop. As he told us the story he smiled broadly, but advised us never to take a firecracker and matches to school.

An image of my father's father, Judge James Masson, pops readily to mind, though he died years before my brothers and I were born. A portrait of him hung in our dining room. He had, we thought, a fantastic beard. Twin hanks of puffy white whiskers hung from his cheeks. Muttonchops, they were called, but we children called them goat beards.

When Judge Masson had a debilitating stroke, Jim came home from the university to help care for him. In those days there were no disability pensions; the judge's salary was needed to pay whoever took his place. And he had no insurance. He hadn't expected to die young. He was a renter in a house of many rooms that came to be known in Goderich as "the house of the four judges."

Jim's mother and her seven children moved to Toronto where Tom, the oldest son and sole wage earner, had a job with a hardware company. Three years later Judge Masson died, and Jim returned to the university.

Pill Hill

After further study, internships and residencies in Toronto and New York, Jim, thinking it would be a restful change of pace, took a job as ship's surgeon on a cruise to the West Indies. He told us children he did a poor job of helping the seasick passengers because he was so seasick himself. Another short-term job he took was a stint with a survey crew in the far north woods. He grew a beard on that trip.

"How long was it?" I wanted to know.

"It was this long," he said, holding his fist to his chin. "I could grab it like this and wiggle the tip of it with my little finger."

Jim's first thought, when he heard of a Dunnville doctor wanting to sell his practice, was whether he could scrape up the money. He went to look over the situation and found that the practice included a nice little house, barn, horse and buggy, as well as the doctor's patient records. Jim and the doctor shook hands on a deal. He told the doctor he'd go to Toronto to arrange payment. His uncle would advise him on getting a loan. Today's prudent bankers would certainly be amazed to learn how that transfer of a business and real estate was finalized.

"No problem," said the old doctor to the young one, or words to that effect. "I'm going away for a while, so when you get the money just put it in a cigar box and leave it with the clerk at the Dunnville Hotel."

Four days after writing the two necessary letters to the Knowleses, Jim wrote his mother suggesting she join him in Worcester to meet Marion's parents. September was the earliest he could get away for a few days. "I am just afraid Mr. Knowles will be more than disappointed in regard to my financial standing," he wrote, "but I know Marion will be content to put up with little inconveniences to start with. Work here is extra heavy of late. We are running about forty cases every day, and as a rule it is after 2 p.m. when we get dinner. I usually have from eight to ten cases in my room each day. That means a lot of experience."

Soon after Mrs. Knowles received her first letter from Jim and was thrilled by its genteel tone, she received an invitation from Carrie Mayo Balfour to all the Knowleses to come to Rochester to meet Don and Jim and the two little Balfour "kiddies."

One characteristic of Marion Knowles was her ability to take on another job when she already had more than enough to do. Now, as her engagement to "the dearest of men" was about to be announced, she capitulated to a cry of "Help!" from the Wellesley Club of Worcester. In a letter to Mrs. Knowles on March 14, 1914, she explained why she had to delay a promised visit to Toronto. "The main building at Wellesley College has burned to the ground," she wrote. "Alumnae all over the country are trying to raise money for the rebuilding. Our Worcester Wellesley Club has decided to give a Shakespeare play out-of-doors. Since most of our Wellesley girls are teachers, I, as president of the club, have been managing the play."

When at last her visit to Toronto took place, she expressed her appreciation for the invitation of cousin Jessie Jeffrey to stay with her in Toronto. She wanted "not to be entertained but to get to know the people who are already so dear to me and will mean so much to me in years to come." Marion understood perfectly why Mrs. Masson couldn't travel to Worcester with "important events" about to happen in Toronto.

In early June Marion took the train to Toronto. Jim was too busy at the Clinic to even think of asking for time off. The letter Marion wrote on her return to Worcester isn't dated, but since she mentions "the imminent arrival," I know it was written before June 10, the day my cousin Allan, "the little newcomer," was to be born. Cousin Allan would grow up to become one of the principle contributors of Masson information and humor to this book.

3

The Heroic Age of Surgery

The man of science, in searching for the truth, must ever be guided by the cold logic of facts and be animated by scientific imagination.

Dr. William James Mayo, 1928[1]

NEAR the end of the 1870's, although the risk of infection had been lessened by antiseptic procedures described by Joseph Lister, a surgeon had to be courageous to take up the knife and do what he thought necessary to save a life.

Almost every phase of surgical technique was controversial, even the use of rubber gloves and whether or not the appendix should be removed. New techniques for anesthesia were being tried, but the most popular was still the imbibing by the patient of copious drafts of whiskey. Blood transfusion was known, but methods for the actual transfer of blood from one person to another were primitive. There were no drugs to prevent post-operative blood clotting, no swift-acting compounds to do battle against staphylococcus infections. There was no precedent, no written literature on how to treat an ovarian tumor, a common affliction of women. Few surgeons had the nerve to attempt its removal, and when the operation was undertaken, though the tumor was removed, the patient usually died.

In 1880 Dr. William Worrall Mayo was a more courageous man than the usual pioneer surgeon. He had a patient, Mrs. Waggoner, with a painful swelling in her side. Dr. Mayo suspected it was a small ovarian tumor. When she became pregnant and then suffered a miscarriage, a pelvic infection followed and the tumor grew rapidly. Dr. Mayo recommended removal, but Mrs. Waggoner was too frightened to say yes to anything so radical. The next possible solution, Dr. Mayo thought, was to drain off the fluid contents of the tumor. He did that with her permission. It quickly refilled and continued to grow. When the patient became so weak she couldn't eat, she gave consent to the operation. Either way, she thought, she was dying.

"The Little Doctor," as Dr. W. W. Mayo was affectionately known, was a careful planner, a master innovator. He asked his patient's husband, a blacksmith, for help in the forging of instruments he thought he would need for this unique operation. The tools included some clamps fitted with hooks which Mr. Waggoner made from the teeth of an old mowing machine. When the patient was asleep under chloroform, Dr. Mayo made a small incision, and with a trocar, a sharp pointed instrument used with a flexible tube, he penetrated the tumor and drained several gallons of a thick, gluey substance into a tub he had handy for the purpose. Then he applied the homemade clamps which had been sterilized in a charcoal furnace, and pulled the tumor out with forceps, bit by bit. It was a large one, weighing some twenty pounds. All went well until a big pelvic abscess lying behind the growth broke and spilled its contents into the abdominal cavity. That was a setback. Dr. Mayo sponged out the pus, inserted a drainage tube, and stitched up the incision.

One week later news that Mrs. Waggoner was alive spread through the neighborhood: Dr. Mayo had cut her wide open, and she lived! The event made headlines and brought a groundswell of new patients to Rochester seeking Dr. Mayo's healing hands. It was also published, in that painfully modest age, that the doctor's two young sons, Will and Charlie, had "peeked through the door" as their father performed the surgery.

Today it is considered poor taste for a doctor to seek publicity for his or her work, but back then it was customary for doctors to give journalists interesting news like the cure of Mrs. Waggoner. Undoubtedly, these write-ups in the *Rochester City Post* had a lot to do with the rapid expansion of Dr. Mayo's practice. Two other winter rescues by Dr. Mayo were described in the press. A man almost frozen to death in 22-degree-below-zero weather was brought to life when tincture of camphor was dropped between his lips. And it was called "miraculous" when a woman who was hemorrhaging after childbirth lived through the ordeal. The resourceful little doctor went out of the isolated farmhouse where she lived, scooped up snow and packed it into the patient's vagina. The bleeding stopped.

The Heroic Age of Surgery

Up north in Dunnville, Ontario, in 1909, the young country doctor James C. Masson, who became my father, was going it alone in his new practice. With a house and barn of his own for the first time in his life, his whole family—mother, sisters, brothers, aunts, uncles and cousins—came in a steady stream to visit and make sure he was well cared for. They saw to it that he had home-cooked food, his bed was made and the house was clean. His need for a wife or housekeeper was thereby reduced.

Nothing could lessen the weariness my father felt, with no letup in the continuous stream of patients needing his attention. When he hitched his newly acquired mare Trixie to the buggy and headed out on the dirt road to see his first patient, he didn't know it, but he was entering what has been called the Heroic Age of Surgery. Many people needed treatment and there were too few doctors and hospitals. There was no precedent for treating the blunders of farm families using newly invented diggers, planters, threshers and reapers with meshing cogs and whirling, unprotected blades. In the makeshift conditions of kitchen surgery the horse-and-buggy doctor performed many an operation by flickering lamplight, using instruments sterilized in steam from the spout of a tea kettle. Often his only assistance came from a family member or a farm hand pressed into service.

Some years ago, my father's nephew, Allan Masson of Oakville, Ontario, ran across the son of a man named Marshall who remembered the old days in Dunnville, Ontario. Marshall told Allan his father's favorite story was about the young Dr. Jim Masson one summer when an epidemic of influenza was rampant in the area. As my cousin Allan wrote in a letter,

> There was a bad flu bug in the area. Uncle Jim was going night and day. The horse knew the rounds, so he could sleep in the buggy sometimes between calls, but after days of this he was really tuckered out. His friend, Mr. Marshall, said he saw Jim downtown one day and told him that Mrs. Marshall had taken sick. He asked if Jim could call in to see her. Of course he did, and was ushered upstairs to the bedroom. Mrs. Marshall was in a big double bed, her eyes closed. Uncle Jim sat on the edge of the bed and immediately passed out. Mr. Marshall always boasted that the only other man his wife had slept with was Jim Masson, and he really didn't mind.

Because of his three years in the Dunnville practice, when my father began an internship at Saint Mary's Hospital in Rochester, Minnesota, he was soon recognized as an experienced surgeon and was taken on as first assistant to Dr. Charlie Mayo. That was in 1912, before the Mayos adopted the word "Fellow" to classify the residents. Those young men were graduates of respected medical schools taking a three-year hands-on course under Mayo Clinic doctors in all the medical and surgical specialties.

There had always been among the early surgeons a restless urge to improve their techniques. Dr. W. W. Mayo left home for as long as three months at a time observing the surgeries of successful surgeons in the eastern cities and Europe. His sons, Dr. Will and Dr. Charlie Mayo, used to take turns being away on field trips, never both gone at the same time. They checked out reports published in medical journals or delivered from the podiums at meetings of professional associations. The friendships formed among doctors around the world served as a catalyst to the improvement of their profession.

The teaching role of the Mayo's medical practice at Saint Mary's Hospital became organized on June 7, 1906, with the formation of the Surgeons' International Club. It was the brainstorm of Dr. J. L. Wiggins of East St. Louis, Illinois, one of seven doctors from the United States and Japan, all staying at the Cook House in Rochester. In order to get the most out of their trip, after watching the Mayos operate in the morning they would gather after lunch in a rented room to discuss what they had seen that morning. Any visiting doctor could join for 50 cents (later increased to 2 dollars). Each Monday afternoon officers would be elected and two reporters appointed as specified in the club's by-laws. Reporters were to gather information on the next day's clinics and pass it along to members at the club's afternoon session.

The club served as a social mixer as well as a classroom. Within a month the average daily attendance at the club's meetings in its rented room was twenty-five. A third reporter was appointed to make rounds at the hospital with the interns and report on post-operative progress of the patients whose operations the group had witnessed the previous day. Soon another feature was added to those meetings; a code of rules and responsibilities was added to the by-laws and a printed copy given to each new member. This seemed necessary as, it was written, "a breach of the code of rules causes great annoyance to the patients and hospital man-

The Heroic Age of Surgery

agement." The duties of reporters and rules of behavior were spelled out.

The Mayos took no part in the activities of this group, except to suggest a less pretentious name. "International" was removed from the title.

By the end of the summer of 1906 the roster of the Surgeons' Club of Rochester, Minnesota, included more than 300 names. It was a roll call of prominent physicians from every state in the union and many parts of the world. When forty to fifty daily club members became the norm, a larger room was provided with more tables, chairs and a chalk board. A local physician, Dr. J. E. Crew, was hired as permanent secretary. Free copies of medical books and magazines became the start of a library. The afternoon was too short for the amount of material to be covered, so informal talks were scheduled for the evening hours. Often a distinguished visitor or a member of the Mayo staff was invited to speak to the club.

Viewing space in the operating rooms was also too crowded for comfort. An orthopedic surgeon from Edinburgh, Scotland, Dr. Harold J. Stiles, made a suggestion that the group should build a surgical amphitheatre with money they could raise. The Mayos were appreciative, and said so, but they, too, had considered the problem and would rather solve it themselves. Their solution was several metal platforms with wheels and handrails to lean on, plus a number of slanting overhead mirrors that would present various aspects of the operating field.

To prepare the visitors for an operation about to begin, Dr. Will and Dr. Charlie had an assistant read the history of the operation and the patient's history while the anesthesia was being given. An example would be a patient who had suffered years of "stomach trouble." But, as Dr. Will pointed out when he had made the incision and the stomach was visible to all, the stomach looked normal in every way. The surgeon kept up a running commentary as he performed the operation. (I assume the following observations and conversations from operating rooms came to the historian Helen Clapesattle from notes taken by a visiting Surgeons' Club reporter.[2])

"You have heard the history, gentlemen, but you see this stomach," Dr. Will said. "In my opinion there is nothing wrong with it; the trouble is somewhere else. If I am right, in a few minutes you will notice a spasm of the pylorus."[3] (To these doctors he wouldn't need to explain, as he would to laymen, that the pyloris is an entrance from the stomach into the small intestine surrounded by a band of muscle.) Shortly, a spasm of the pyloric muscles was evident to all. "That does not tell us where the trouble is," said Dr. Will, "but it is not in the stomach. I will see if it is in the appendix."[4] He pulled into view a badly diseased appendix.

As he proceeded to remove the appendix, Dr. Will told the assembled doctors that in his own experience with the deceptive pylorospasm, removal of any part of the stomach never gave relief from the pain. The distressed patient usually came back. "If it wasn't the appendix I inspected the gall bladder. A patient who complained of recurrent indigestion very often had a gall bladder full of stones. When the stones were removed the symptoms vanished."

The clarity of Dr. Will's descriptions made his lessons unforgettable. When he said, "Don't monkey with the ovary; either remove it or leave it alone," it was a caution that went home with the listener.[5]

Dr. Charlie Mayo was famous for his homespun analogies. It was said he "kept his audience in a bubble of anticipation."[6] In a morning's work of ten to fifteen cases, he made comparisons to the galls on his oak trees, the eye of the Tuatara lizard, or the hatchet-sharp edge of the liver. Dr. Charlie might give his audience this warning: "Don't remove the parathyroid. It looks like a piece of fat, somewhat harder, the size of a lima bean."[7]

When Dr. Charlie was the speaker at the Surgeons' Club, some member invariably asked to know his secret with exophthalmic goiters, a dreadful condition known as Graves' Disease that causes the eyes to bulge grotesquely. His success with that kind of surgery was hard to explain, he said, except to say a multiple-stage operation was safer. He and Dr. Plummer went on to the next stage when long experience told them the patient "looked ready." Doctors from all over the country, rather than tread on thin ice, sent their exophthalmic goiter patients to Dr. Charlie. By 1908 he had done a thousand such cases with a three percent mortality rate.

Dr. N. P. Mead of Boston recalled a time Dr. Charlie was removing the thyroid gland from a patient with Graves' Disease. The patient was stirring so restlessly that Dr. Mead remarked: "Most surgeons would have stopped operating and sworn, too. Not so, Dr. Charles Mayo. He went right on, where a single false cut might have meant a bad case of bleeding or the severing of a nerve and possible paralysis; he cut true, with a marvelous sureness and dexterity of touch, and the job was soon done."[8]

The Heroic Age of Surgery

When Dr. Henry Plummer was asked to speak to the Surgeons' Club he first explained the Mayo system of diagnosis. His office, he told them, was in the Masonic Temple building at the end of a long hallway flanked by examining rooms. Patients waiting to see the Mayos had wooden benches to sit on and, on the wall to look at, a framed copy of one of Dr. Will's favorite poems, "The House by the Side of the Road" by Sam Walter Foss:

> *I would not sit in the scorner's seat*
> *or hurl the cynic's ban.*
> *Let me live in a house by the side of the road*
> *And be a friend to man.*

Every day through that hallway passed 150 or more patients, their first scheduled stop to see Dr. Plummer. If Dr. Plummer thought a patient seemed a likely candidate for surgery of a kind Dr. Will was most familiar with, he would put a green card over the door of one of the examining rooms. If the patient had an ailment Dr. Charlie was most accustomed to handling, he would put a red card over another door. When the Mayos finished their morning surgery they returned from Saint Mary's Hospital and went from room to room seeing patients. When they weren't convinced a patient needed surgery, they sent him or her back to Dr. Plummer for further evaluation. The Surgeons' Club members considered this arrangement unique and amazing.

The division of labor afforded the most reliable diagnosis possible. Often these were cases of esophageal stricture, long neglected, in which the patient was able only to drink fluids and was slowly starving to death. Dr. Plummer had read all the literature on unsuccessful attempts to remedy the stricture, such as inserting a rubber balloon and inflating it to stretch the distal end of the esophagus which was obstructing the patient's ability to swallow. In his office workshop Dr. Plummer devised instruments, turning them on a lathe to fit a particular patient.

On one occasion members of the Surgeons' Club arriving by train saw a pitiful sight, a wizened, comatose little man being carried from the train on a cot. Two weeks later Dr. Plummer, in speaking to the club about esophageal stricture, brought along this same patient, one of those who had responded instantly to the treatment he had devised in his workshop. Dr. Plummer was describing the case in medical jargon that apparently bored the skinny, thirty-five-year-old patient who had enjoyed two weeks' worth of solid food. He interrupted his doctor with a shout, "I was dying, and he saved my life!" That might have brought applause from the audience, but it is reported that Dr. Plummer was embarrassed.[9]

Sometimes his inventions were grand successes, but to his dismay, he told the Surgeons' Club, he had sent many patients home still unable to eat a meal with the family. Then he discovered that the trouble was caused not by a stricture, but by the presence of diverticula (bulges that form little sacs that trap food). By x-ray and special measuring devices he determined their exact size and location, information he passed along in detail to Dr. Will or Dr. Charlie, who would do the surgery.

Dr. Plummer remembered his failures. When he finally made a breakthrough, he couldn't wait to get those patients back and cure them. He called, and they came. All except one. She was a washerwoman who said she couldn't afford the trip from Ohio, though the treatment would be free. According to Helen Clapesattle, he said to his associates, "Men, we've just got to get that woman back and fix her up." They all chipped in for the patient's roundtrip to Rochester.[10]

I want to include here a bit about the boy who grew up to be Dr. Henry S. Plummer. He was born in 1874, the son of a doctor and a school teacher in rural Racine, Minnesota. Much as the two Mayo boys learned their father's ways and methods, Henry, as young as six, became his father's assistant. When sick calls came at night, Henry was out of bed in a flash. Using a device he put together himself, he pulled a rope at his bedroom window that went through a pulley in the barn and lifted a lever, releasing a measure of oats into the horse's feed box. So the horse, the doctor and his son were ready to go at the same time. Dr. Henry Plummer was more than the genius everyone knew him to be; he was a kind and generous man. When he was in medical school, his roommate was going blind, but Henry wouldn't let him quit school. He read aloud from their textbooks and explained his lecture notes, and in many ways enabled him to graduate and become the psychiatrist he was well qualified to be.

Sometimes the visiting doctors asked to meet and hear from the Old Doctor, W. W. Mayo, the father of Dr. Will and Dr. Charlie. Almost

The Heroic Age of Surgery

ninety in 1908, he would come and entertain them with funny stories of how he raised his sons in the pioneer years of surgery. They followed him around, he said, and he put them to work.

The phenomenally successful Surgeons' Club had risen from nothing more tangible than need, the need of the visiting doctors to learn what the Mayos could teach so they could go home better doctors. A Canadian doctor reported his impressions in the *Canada Lancet*: "The rush of medical visitors [to Mayo's] is unabated; many doctors fresh from continental clinics... say this clinic far surpasses anything they saw on the other side of the Atlantic.... The little western town [is] slowly becoming the greatest post-graduate center of the century, with possibilities practically illimitable."[11]

Many bright young graduates from the University of Minnesota came to Saint Mary's Hospital to observe, hoping to be put to work and learn more about the profession. Dr. Will, Dr. Charlie and Dr. Plummer felt that part of the responsibility of the Mayo Clinic was to train these young graduates so they could begin a principled and effective practice of their own after leaving Rochester. On Dr. Will's visits east to observe the work of other surgeons he noticed the interns were treated as "flunkies." He and his brother named their young assistants "Fellows" and treated them with great respect. Many of them were put to work at Saint Mary's and paid a small remuneration.

My Uncle Morrie, Dr. Duncan Morrison Masson, ten years younger than Dad, came to the Mayo Clinic as a Fellow in 1924. Uncle Morrie, or Moss, as he was known to the Canadians, was a mesmerizing storyteller. He could recite many long narrative poems by Robert W. Service that dramatized the rousing frontier days when gold was discovered in the Yukon Territory. I can see him now, with his dark curly hair and handsome, ruddy face, standing in front of our fireplace on a cold winter night, reciting the rollicking rhymes of "The Cremation of Sam McGee," who hadn't been warm since he left Tennessee.

Once Uncle Morrie told us a bizarre tale he declared was "probably" true. He got it from a medical student whose father was one of a group of students present when the events reported were first witnessed. In those days medical students were required to supply their own cadavers. If the morgue in one's town was fresh out of bodies at room temperature, unclaimed by relatives, it became a serious problem for the student of

Pill Hill

anatomy. "Dead people are hard to find above ground," Uncle Morrie said with a serious grin as he began this story to us eager children.

"A group of med students were on a train returning to school after the mid-winter holiday. They were discussing a common dilemma—none of them had lined up a cadaver. Then another fellow joined the conversation. Yes, he had a corpse, he said. "It's in the baggage car. Thank God it's below zero."

"Where did you get it?" he was asked.

"Shot him," the young man said. He pointed to his rifle on the overhead rack.

The other students laughed and thought he was kidding till they went with him to the baggage car and saw what he had. It was wearing boots. A grain sack was over its head, a rope around its middle.

"The year was 1882," Uncle Morrie said. "The grisly cargo had been acquired in St. Joseph, Missouri, when the student found himself witness to a gun fight. Jesse and Frank James had robbed their last bank. One of their gang shot Jesse for a $5,000 reward. The medical student saw one of the robbers trying to skip out of town on the train."

Uncle Morrie paused. Wide-eyed, we children stared at him. "Then what? What did he do?"

With a grin, Uncle Morrie lifted an invisible rifle, sighted along the barrel, pulled the trigger, and said, "Pow!"

I was a baby and Jay was two when Uncle Morrie and Aunt Laura bought my parents' house across the street from Uncle Don and Aunt Carrie Balfour. We older Massons moved to 724 Fourth Street Southwest. Dr. and Mrs. Will Mayo lived across the street in their stately stone home topped by a tower for viewing the stars through a telescope. That house is now the Mayo Foundation House, given to the Mayo Foundation when Dr. Will and Mrs. Hattie moved into a smaller house they built next door. The Foundation House is used for meetings, hospitality and the display of Mayo memorabilia. Our brick and stucco house with its buckthorn hedge and windbreak of pine trees was built and the trees planted by Dr. Emil H. Beckman.

Dr. Beckman was the second surgeon after Dr. E. Starr Judd invited to join the Mayo brothers' practice. The death of Dr. Beckman in 1916,

The Heroic Age of Surgery

in the midst of a brilliant surgical career, was a severe loss to the young Mayo Clinic. He died of a staphylococcus infection in his nasal passages, a condition he would have survived had antibiotics been available then.

In 1935, Dr. Judd, then Chief of the Mayo surgical staff, died of pneumonia. The next senior surgeon, Dr. J. C. Masson, my father, was then designated Chief of Staff, a position he held until his retirement in 1946 at age sixty-five, when the use of the title was discontinued.

My father had what a good doctor must have, a first-class bedside manner. Sometimes I got to see for myself how he treated his patients. Now and then, when I was the fortunate child in my family, I got to accompany Dad on his rounds at Saint Mary's or the Colonial Hospital. We walked up flights of stairs more quickly than the elevator could lift us. Dad liked the exercise. He was followed down corridors by several younger doctors striding briskly to keep up. I would be trotting by my father's side. He introduced me to his patients, most of them women smiling brightly in bed jackets. They heaped praise on my wonderful father and smiled at me, the little girl holding his hand. Each lady was sure he had saved her life. He responded modestly that any good surgeon could have done as well. Their rooms were often full of flowers, and sometimes I was given a bouquet to take home to my mother.

Once I was startled by a lively male patient who threw back the covers, saying, "Look what your father did to me."

For the life of me, I can't remember . . . was it red or purple, that skin around the bandage? I was embarrassed at seeing so much bare skin on that robust man, I scuttled around behind my father, afraid to look. The patient laughed and Dad pulled the sheet over this uninhibited man.

Surgeons throughout the ages have been asked to perform some strange services for the most humble of patients, but the strangest patient I ever heard of was poor Dickie in the year 1930, told to me by my good friend Marion Rogers of Huntersville, N.C. The Henry Church family of Roseburg, Oregon, was told there was a young male orphan who needed a home. They brought little Dickie to live with them, never suspecting Dickie's secret identity. Their new friend was small and light, with a pleasant, chirpy disposition. When Dickie began to mature, however, they noticed some erratic, fluttery behavior. Dr. Shoemaker was called to determine what was wrong. He came to the house with his bag of tools. Dickie looked tuckered out, prostrate and shivering, the color of jaundice.

When Dr. Shoemaker had Dickie quieted under his warm hand, as the family watched, he took a scalpel sterilized in rubbing alcohol and did what he thought should be done. Then gently he picked up the marble-sized white egg released into his hand and said with satisfaction, "This is the first time I ever did an episiotomy on a bird."

Dickie was not down for long. Soon she was singing like an ordinary canary.

⋇{ 4 }⋇

The 1914 Building and Beyond

One of the chief defects in our plan of education in this country is
that we ... lay too much stress on acquiring knowledge
and too little on the wise application of knowledge.
Dr. William J. Mayo, 1933 [1]

ON a warm day in March 1914, Rochester was experiencing an almost lyrical excitement over the completion of the first Mayo Clinic, the 1914 Building. That grand new red brick building united under one roof all properties, specialties, personnel and patients that previously had camped out all over Rochester. Laboratory and office and equipment, beds, boxes of books, et cetera, were loaded in trucks and transported from the Masonic Temple, two hotels, rooms above a drug store, and cubby holes all over town to the new five-story building planted on the site of the old William Worrall Mayo homestead.

Among the unique schemes devised by Dr. Plummer for this building was an inter-office telephone communication system. When Dr. Plummer asked the telephone company to install such a system to enable the doctors to be instantly in touch with each other as well as with the outside world, the officials looked baffled. That was impossible!

"No, it isn't," Dr. Plummer said. "Call in your engineers and I'll show them how to do it." Dr. Plummer explained his diagrams.

That was the first intercommunicating telephone system in the country, according to my trustworthy source, Helen Clapesattle, the author of *The Doctors Mayo*.[2]

Also, Dr. Plummer devised an inter-office communicating system for contacting a doctor who was not in his office, but somewhere else in the building. He could be notified he was wanted immediately by the ticking of his code number on telegraphic receiver units placed throughout the building.

These were not the first technically amazing innovations installed in a Mayo office. Thirty-five years earlier, on December 12, 1879, a long writeup in the *Rochester Record and Union* announced the arrival of Rochester's first telephone. A line one-mile long between Dr. W. W. Mayo's residence and his office on the upper floor of a drug store was "in position and working splendidly. Parties wishing to summon the doctor between six in the morning and nine in the evening can do so by making their wants known at Messrs. Geisinger & Newton's drug store."[3] After 9 p.m. one would have to get the night watchman to operate the switchboard.

Another technological leap in the 1914 Building was Dr. Plummer's use of vertical vacuum tubes that lifted and lowered patients' histories from one floor to another as if in a small, swift elevator. An even greater stroke of inventiveness was the horizontal delivery of records back and forth between the new Clinic building and St. Mary's Hospital. The histories were placed inside round, heavy-duty transparent plastic capsules about fourteen inches long and six inches in diameter. The capsules were then inserted into a compressed air tube buried in the ground under Second Street Southwest. It was a straight mile from the Clinic to Saint Mary's, and the delivery took fifteen minutes. A parallel tube shot the capsule back on a return trip to the Clinic. Suction was created by powerful fans at the receiving end of the tubes. It baffled patients sometimes that their records arrived in a doctor's office before they did. In later years the equipment was enlarged to accommodate specimen containers.

On the day of the grand opening of the 1914 Building, 1600 persons trooped through the building like tourists with tour guides. They were shown all five floors, from spacious lobby and marble stairs to smoothly running elevators and up-to-the-minute examining rooms and laboratories. The next day, it was back to business, but definitely not business as usual. The patients enjoyed a luxurious environment. Instead of the old hard wooden benches, they had comfortable chairs to sit in, green plants and a bubbling fountain to look at. Instead of the inconvenience of having to trek all over Rochester to find their doctor's office and meet their laboratory appointments, it was all in one modern building.

Long before Dr. Henry Plummer began putting his mind to that building's construction, another question was being mulled over by Dr.

The 1914 Building and Beyond

Will and Dr. Charlie Mayo. What were they going to do with all the money people were paying to this busy private practice? Part of it should go back to the people, they thought. But how? All along the policy being followed was to not spend more money than was needed, to save till a worthy use for it became evident. Two things worried the Mayo brothers—the uncertain future of medical education and the lack of good research. In those years there was no long-term post-graduate course for medical students anywhere in the world. A young man had only to set himself up with his name on the door in any specialty he chose. The patient had no way of knowing his level of competence. The Mayo's practice of allowing graduates of the University of Minnesota Medical School to observe in the operating rooms at Saint Mary's was a good start. Dr. Charlie and Dr. Will, who had learned their basic skills from watching and helping their father, knew how necessary this training was to the young graduates straight out of med school. The students were taught surgery by the Mayo staff at no cost to them, but it wasn't enough. An official post-graduate course of study for which certification was given by the University seemed an excellent idea to the brothers.

Dr. Will, who for four years had been a member of the University of Minnesota's Board of Regents, talked this over with Dr. George E. Vincent, who became president of the University in 1911. They agreed it was a problem. They appointed a committee comprised of the Drs. Mayo, Graham, Plummer, Judd and Balfour. After frequent meetings a plan was agreed upon. A corporation was created—the Mayo Foundation for Medical Education and Research. The Foundation was not to be affiliated with the University or its medical school.

That decided, on the following day, February 9, 1915, three trustees were appointed—Burt W. Eaton and George W. Granger, Rochester lawyers, and Harry J. Harwick, the Clinic's business manager. Dr. Will and Dr. Charlie then turned over to them securities amounting to $1,500,000. The principal of the fund was to be kept invested in perpetuity. The income from it would be used for graduate medical and surgical instruction and research at the Mayo Graduate School of Medicine when established and named under the direction of the University. The teachers would be chosen from the Mayo Clinic staff, which at that time numbered seventeen. Students would receive degrees from the University. That first year sixty students were accepted.

This plan, so happily begun, was well underway when the Doctors

Mayo were given a severe and insulting rebuke. It came not from the usual grumblers who could not believe the Mayo Clinic had prospered honestly in a Midwest prairie town, but from 202 doctors in medical societies of the two largest cities in Minnesota, St. Paul and Minneapolis. They had signed a document requesting that the regents discontinue affiliation with the newly formed Mayo Foundation.

Word spread rapidly that a swindle was in the making. Pamphlets were broadly distributed, one with the headline, "A Phantom Gift to a Trial Marriage." A cartoon portrayed the University Medical School as a girl being dragged into marriage by an evil seducer. Fifteen more county societies went on record against affiliation, only four in favor. A bill was rushed to the state senate forbidding the unheard-of relationship between a university and a private business firm. The struggle became one big hullabaloo. Widespread publicity claimed the "business" of the Mayo Brothers was a sneaky trick, a money-grubbing scheme.

What caused this outcry was the gift of $1,500,000 for the exclusive use of its graduate school in Rochester. The bill that was brought before the state legislature charged the Mayos with a selfish motive and demanded the regents disavow the proposed affiliation.

Dr. Will and Dr. Charlie were profoundly hurt by this burst of enmity from their own colleagues. Dr. Will, as the spokesman for the Clinic, went up to Minneapolis to respond. In the limelight, on the stage in that auditorium, wearing a dark suit and blue tie, he stood tall, still, unsmiling, his hands at his sides with nothing in them. I think now of what Dr. Harvey Cushing of Harvard, one of the world's greatest brain surgeons, said of Dr. Will's hands—"hands which seemed possessed, in an emergency, with an uncanny ability to do, unflustered, just the right thing at the right moment."[4] Inside, Dr. Will felt a holy calm. Not a muscle moved in his intelligent, handsome face as he waited through the sparse applause that followed a quick introduction by one of Minnesota's elected officials.

He spoke from his heart. What he said from that podium in that crowded senate auditorium was not written down in its entirety. It is known as "the lost oration." Many journalists were present to witness and report on the meeting. Among them was Thomas J. Malone of the *Minneapolis Morning Tribune* who reported Dr. Will's speech under the headline "Dr. Mayo's Stirring Address":

Seldom, if ever, in the history of Minnesota has so remarkable an address been delivered by so remarkable a man, under such notable circumstances, as that by Dr. William J. Mayo in the Senate chamber Thursday night.

The occasion itself was impressive. Gathered for discussion of the bill that would compel the University of Minnesota to sever relations with the Mayo Foundation were representatives of the medical profession in the Twin Cities and the State, the president and other members of the Board of Regents, and legislators of both houses.

Placed in a position of peculiar embarrassment by having his motives misconstrued when he sought to serve magnificently the state in which he was born and in which he had earned his world-wide renown, Dr. Mayo took the floor and entered on a straightforward, man-to-man talk, about things which men are wont to talk far less than to think. Simply, candidly, humanely, as one speaking to friends and neighbors, he spoke of his father, his brother and himself, of the growth of 'the business' that had made the little town of Rochester world famous. A silence could be felt in the room as he said why he and his brother wanted to give this gift: "... that these dead shall not have died in vain."

A thrill went through the audience, a thrill that ended in tears for many.

"We have our ideals," Dr. Will said. "Everyone who came into the Clinic and hung up his hat was to get treatment regardless of the cost, and no one was asked if he had the price. We never sue. No mortgage has ever been given on a home to pay a bill ... thirty percent of our patients are charity cases."

Dr. Mayo paid tribute to his father as the inspirer of the ideals that had guided the sons. "All we are and all we have we owe to the people of Minnesota, and we consider that we are holding this fund in trust for the two and a half million people of this state and we want to return it to them...."

The applause that followed the address was even more enthusiastic than that which had preceded it, applause extended plainly by members of opposing factions as regards the dissolution bill and extended to William J. Mayo, physician and man, a son of Minnesota whose life has been witness that he who serves the ills of the body with the ideals of the spirit is performing a benign ministry.[5]

Pill Hill

News of this speech and its reception in Minneapolis put an end to most of the skepticism about the honest character of the Mayos. The Mayos and their Clinic were suddenly more newsworthy than ever. Famous people like Will Rogers and Helen Keller came to Rochester, and the Mayo Clinic was pulled onto the front pages. The Clinic's name was used by fakers with products to sell. Rumors of new Mayo Clinics popped up everywhere, like the story that the Mayos had bought the Ambassador Hotel in Los Angeles with plans to open it as a sanitorium.

This rumor was put to rest by the genius of Dr. Henry Plummer. On the back of the registration card given to every patient was the following unambiguous notice:

> Any person traveling about the country representing himself as in any way connected with this institution or using our name to secure public confidence should be looked on as a swindler. Testimonials or recommendations in which our name is used in advertisements are not genuine. We are not responsible for unsigned statements or articles concerning us appearing in public print.

It wasn't long before the 1914 Building was seriously overcrowded. Planning began again for a new building. Dr. Plummer was given a free hand in its design. This time he went way beyond utility. He fixed his sights on beauty as well. Every square inch of the building, now known as the Plummer Building, was given his scrutiny.

On a trip to England Dr. Will heard the bells of a distant steeple chime. Its pure notes drifted over the countryside for miles around. On his return home he discussed with his brother the idea of giving a carillon with that majestic sound to the city of Rochester. The two brothers took the idea to Henry Plummer who went eagerly to work adjusting his blueprints to include a bell tower with pillars supporting a pyramid-shaped roof and fixtures of a strength to support eighteen tons of bells that would be molded in Croydon, England, by the best maker of bells in the world. In 1928 patients were being treated in the Clinic before the work on the carillon was finished. When it was completed, its spire against the blue sky, it was breathtakingly beautiful, a Romanesque skyscraper. Lucy Wilder, in her book *The Mayo Clinic*, described the new building as

The 1914 Building and Beyond

"... an Aesculapian temple of yellow Indiana limestone. It rears its head so proudly in our unassuming little town."[6]

A great variety of creatures and mythological events, such as St. George slaying the dragon, are carved in limestone relief and set into the exterior walls. There is a marvelous stone cameo of Dr. Henry Plummer himself. His long-limbed frame is squeezed into a square with an owl at his bent knee as he studies a scrolled drawing of the building he has conceived. The bronze front doors, each weighing 4000 pounds, and the doors of the elevators are artfully crafted by the sculptor A. J. Brioschi with floral and plant motifs and figures common to Minnesota. The same artist created colorful octagonal designs for the ceiling above the terrazzo floor in the lobby. All the artistic expression in that building is related to medicine's past, its present and the dawning future. The tower is open to the winds, with arches and Corinthian columns supporting its tile roof. Marble griffons decorate its four corners. Gargoyles and other symbolic statuary, such as a nurse representing her profession, share that lofty space with the bells.

My mother wrote in her diary, September 16, 1928: "This afternoon the carillon in the tower of the new Clinic was dedicated in memory of the heroes of World War I. We took the children and went to a lecture on the carillon in the new Clinic lobby."

The Fellows who came to be trained at the Mayo Graduate School of Medicine were a stalwart breed, willing to work long hours for very little money in exchange for an education unavailable anywhere else in the world. Life for them was a round of fascinating work, congenial associations and shared poverty which seemed to bother none of them.

Once a month on Saturday night the Clinic reserved the Rochester Country Club for a Fellows Dance. Cost, one dollar a couple. Every other dance was free. Dr. Joe Elliott, from Charlotte, North Carolina, was a Fellow in Dermatology from 1947 till 1950. He and his wife Audrey always went to the free dances and saved a dollar. They lived in a one-room apartment at the Reiter Apartments on Second Street on an income of $225 a month. The sum was increased to $325 when Joe was made first assistant. The perks made life exciting, Audrey says.

The Clinic had a strawberry patch at the Experimental Institute with rows of strawberries, labeled by species, which the Fellows and their wives were invited to pick. The Clinic paid the fees for the Mayo Clinic Bowling League which competed with other Rochester leagues. There were free art lessons for the wives and many social events at the Foundation House, such as monthly dinners and teas. For the Fellows there was a Tuesday night seminar where they met with staff leaders to discuss the work of the past week. In winter the Clinic maintained a ski tow at a nearby hill for the skiers among them. It was well known in Rochester that when the pressure was off and it was party time, those Fellows knew how to have a good time. Joe and Audrey Elliott believe they invented the "spritzer" in 1947. Their eighty-year-old landlord gave them his homemade elderberry wine to take to the monthly dance where they mixed it with soda water before that combination had a name.

Dr. O. T. ("Jim") Clagett, in his book *General Surgery at the Mayo Clinic 1900–1970*, gives many interesting details of his work as a Fellow with his various "chiefs," for example, with Dr. Jim Masson:

> I had a particularly extensive experience [with Dr. J. C. Masson], and it was a special pleasure to work with him. He had a large surgical service often doing ten to fifteen or more operations a day, mostly gynecological operations and hernia repairs. Dr. Masson was a very fast, dexterous surgeon. He seemed to perform his operations at a leisurely pace, but there was no indecision or wasted motion, and his procedures were completed in a surprisingly short time.

"Dr. Masson never raised his voice or berated his assistants," Dr. Clagett wrote. The first time they worked together, Dr. Clagett said he was unfamiliar with his routines and didn't know just what he was supposed to do. "After a little," he reports in his book, "Dr. Masson stopped, looked up at me across the operating table and said in a very kindly way, 'Young man, if you aren't going to help me, at least keep out of my way.'"

On another occasion, Dr. Clagett remembered, "Dr. Masson was working deep in the pelvis performing a hysterectomy when a second assistant, peering over his shoulder, asked, 'Dr. Masson, what are you working on down there?' Dr. Masson replied, 'I'm not sure I remember the name of it, but I know where it is.'"[7]

The many surgeons Dr. Clagett assisted during his Fellowship had their different styles and idiosyncrasies. Dr. Masson's gift was for improvisation. Efficiency mattered to him. He liked to fix anything that needed fixing while the patient was on the table for a major operation. He liked

The 1914 Building and Beyond

to oblige his plump ladies and gentlemen by removing many globs of fat that cluttered the operating field. If he learned that the patient also had hemorrhoids he would volunteer to do a hemorrhoidectomy. His procedure was unique. When he had finished the major surgery he would prepare the anal region, make a small slit in a piece of cardboard that was placed over the anal region, and draw the protruding hemorrhoid through the slit. Then he would burn it off with a red-hot cautery flush with the cardboard. This extra service greatly annoyed Dr. Gus Buie and his associates in proctology. They thought they should have a monopoly on the treatment of hemorrhoids. But Dr. Masson's method was remarkably effective and his patients were always grateful. Improvisation for Dr. Jim, as he was called by his young associates, was learned in his kitchen-surgery days when he had to invent ways to make do with whatever was at hand.

The Mayo Clinic has introduced through its instrument shop many devices for improving and simplifying the treatment of patients. A doctor with an idea for an instrument that would facilitate a certain operation would go to the instrument shop and talk it over with a skilled craftsman.

In the 1930's, Dr. Jim had an idea for a better way to obtain strings of fascia for use in internal suturing. He took his idea to Mr. Earl Albert (Al) Quehl at the instrument shop, a master craftsman, and Mr. Quehl created a new tool, the Masson Fascia Stripper.

My father brought home a film of the Fascia Stripper and explained its use to us as he would later at a medical meeting. Through a small incision in the thigh, the instrument, a thin, steel shaft as long as a thigh bone with a small loop and cutting edge at the tip, would be threaded onto a strand of tough lateral fascia covering the muscle and slid down its length to separate and cut out a tough string which would be used for suturing the patient internally. Internal suturing with the patient's own fascia was always more successful since the fascia was eventually absorbed by the body. Removal of fascia in the old way left the patient with a long scar on the thigh rather than a short one.

Dr. Clagett, too, was an innovator. In his autobiography he wrote, "There were no blood vessel clamps available suitable for cross-clamping the aorta during cardiovascular surgery without causing damage to the vessel."[8]

He took the problem to a craftsman in the engineering section. Several new clamps were soon ready for testing, which was done at the experimental institute where he used the new instruments to do vascular surgery on dogs. With minor changes the instruments were ready to be used on human patients.

Dr. Clagett's work as a Fellow is vivid in my mind because of his close association with Dr. Stuart W. Harrington, one of the outstanding thoracic surgeons in the world. I knew Dr. Harrington only as the man who owned a beautiful and friendly collie dog named "Taz," said to be a litter mate of the famous Lassie in the movie made from the Albert Payson Terhune books. Dr. Harrington came to the Clinic in 1914 as one of the first Fellows of the Mayo Foundation. Several years later Dr. Clagett chose Dr. Harrington's service in thoracic surgery in spite of the fact that many of his peers claimed that "Tack" Harrington was difficult to work with, exacting and grumpy. The nickname "Tack" stuck to Dr. Harrington from his days of glory on the Walter Camp All-American football team of 1910.

The friendship of the attractive young Dr. Jim Clagett and the sometimes curmudgeonly Dr. Harrington touches me deeply. Dr. Harrington and his wife Gertrude, a former anesthesiologist at Saint Mary's Hospital, had no children. Hoping to conceive, they put off adoption till they were too old. While other doctors and their wives were having babies and raising them, the Harringtons were a close, interdependent couple, estranged from the social life of their Pill Hill neighbors.

A blizzard fell upon Rochester the night Jim and Alicia Clagett's first child was born. Snow was a soft, thick blanket over the town. Dr. Harrington that night put on his boots and his black overcoat and scarf, pulled ear flaps down over his ears and trudged in the sub-zero air a mile or so through untracked snow to the small apartment near the Clinic where his young assistant lived.

Jim Clagett opened the door to his chief and invited him in.

"No," Dr. Harrington said. "I just want to shake your hand and congratulate you on the birth of your son."[9]

I think of Dr. Harrington with his thin red hair turning white, living in his big house with his quiet wife and the collie dog Taz. Seeing him in my mind's eye on his lonely trek lit by occasional streetlights, following his own tracks back through the snow after shaking Dr. Clagett's hand, I feel tears moisten my eyes. This man's life was so valuable to the thousands of people he helped back to health. He left an important record in

The 1914 Building and Beyond

the world's history of thoracic surgery. But something essential was missing in his life. He made up for it when he turned his young protégé into one of the most broadly experienced surgeons at the Mayo Clinic during this time of its greatest stress, the World War II years, when many Fellows and staff surgeons were away in military service.

Everything at the Clinic has changed now, in the years since Jimmy Drummond sat at the keyboard in the tower and played "Away in a Manger" on the carillon bells in the middle of summer for a little girl who asked him to. Today the bell tower on the Plummer Building is brightly lit at night, revealing its graceful arches and stonework. Pilots of rescue helicopters, Mayo One and Mayo Two, descend slowly nearby to land at the heliport on top of the Methodist Hospital. No one in 1929 could have dreamed that in twenty-four years another and larger Mayo Clinic building would be in place across the street from Dr. Plummer's dramatically beautiful building with its resonant bells. But space was again needed.

The large new Mayo Building was up and running in 1953. Everywhere the eye turns, there is beauty in and around that building. Flowers, fountains, sculpture and paintings adorn the walls and free space. History is told and on view; some of the carved exterior stone from the 1914 Building has been inlaid in the Mayo Building walls. Dr. Will and Dr. Charlie, "the infrangible brotherhood," would have liked this building, although it would have astonished them that it was needed. They felt that beauty in nature and in its many man-made forms is conducive to mental and physical health for both the creator and the beholder.

Over the years, through the generous gifts of many people, the Mayo Clinic art collection has grown. Large epic murals on one wall of every waiting room depict life and nature, science, history, busy families at home and at work. A pedestal faces each mural with a statement by the artist on the meaning of his or her creation. Especially enchanting to me is the bronze "Boy with Dolphin" at the entrance to the Mayo Building. Two playful creatures seem to be flying above the tranquil pool. David Wynne, the British sculptor of Boy with a Dolphin, wrote of its magnetism, "The boy is being shown that if you trust the world thrills and great happiness are yours."[10]

This gray marble building is the hub of a vastly expanded Mayo Clinic organization. Included under that sponsorship are two new multi-specialty group-practice Clinics: one in Jacksonville, Florida, opened in 1986, and the other opened the following year in Scottsdale, Arizona. Patients at those locations stay in close touch with the Rochester headquarters through an advanced satellite telecommunications system; a Jacksonville doctor can place the records of a Jacksonville patient on a screen before a specialist in Rochester to enable consultation, as if three or four people were conferring in the same room.

In 1938, the year before Dr. Will died, he gave his home on Fourth Street to the Mayo Foundation and he and Mrs. Hattie moved into the smaller home he built beside it. Since then the Foundation House has been a meeting place for many Clinic functions. In addition to banquets and receptions, graduate students gather there at weekly meetings. The Emeritus Staff meet there for dinner the first Monday of every month. Men and women of science from all over the world are entertained at the Foundation House, an extension of the hospitality that was always abundant when Dr. and Mrs. Will Mayo lived there.

An amusing illustration of that homey hospitality is the incident that happened during a visit from the personal physician to the British royal family and his wife. That evening, when the other dinner guests had gone home, Sir Eric and his wife, who had had a busy day at the Clinic, said goodnight and retired to their room. A little later when Dr. Will and Mrs. Hattie went up to bed they saw in the hall outside their guests' bedroom a pair of dusty shoes. Mrs. Hattie wasn't a bit surprised when her husband picked them up. He whispered to her, "Let's not tell him we don't have a shoeshine man." Dr. Will went downstairs to his workroom in the basement, gave the shoes a good "Pullman porter" treatment, and put them back outside Sir Eric's door.

The year 1964 was chosen as a grand year for a Mayo Centennial celebration. A century had passed since the birth of the Clinic's founders, Dr. Will in 1861 and Dr. Charlie in 1865. It was also the fiftieth anniversary of the Mayo Graduate School of Medicine. And in that very year

The 1914 Building and Beyond

the last Dr. Mayo on the surgical staff, former chairman of the Mayo Properties Association and board of regents chairman Dr. Charles William "Chuck" Mayo, retired from active surgery.

When my mother was at Saint Mary's recovering from a hysterectomy, she took an immediate liking to "the dear lad," young Chuck Mayo, who changed her dressings. "He will be as fine a doctor as his Dad," she wrote in her diary.

Dr. Chuck, in his autobiography, *Mayo: The Story of My Family and My Career*, tells of the year-long centennial celebration in Rochester that culminated in Mayo Recognition Day.

Throughout the year 1964 more than fifty medical and scientific groups scheduled meetings and seminars in Rochester, including an international symposium that included the retired NATO commander General Lauris Norstad and Dr. Edward Teller, the nuclear scientist. The post office issued a 5 cent stamp with the likeness of the Mayo brothers, and Rochester installed tablets on Mayo homesites. The *Rochester Post Bulletin* put out a special supplement on Mayo Recognition Day with pictures and history. Dr. Chuck adds this fond comment: "There again were Grandfather, glowering into the sun beside his horse and buggy, and Grandmother's sorrowing, steady gaze...." In the paper that day were Dr. Will's "words for these restless times." He was speaking of the 1930's, but I hear it as if he was alive yesterday. "... With all its advantages, our democracy is often hampered by the appeal of the demagogue to the emotions and prejudices of a public interested in its own affairs and not fully informed as to the merits of the proposition under discussion."[11]

Mayowood, Dr. Charlie's home in the country, has been lived in by three generations of Mayos. In 1965, Dr. Chuck Mayo presented Mayowood to the Olmstead County Historical Society, retaining a cozy part of it for himself and his wife Alice and visiting grandchildren. Bus tours of visitors were always hopeful that some of the younger Mayo generation would be seen on the property.

In 1971, the Plummer Building was designated a national historic landmark. At the ceremony marking the occasion Dr. T. B. Magath, the head of the Mayo Clinic laboratories, compared the Plummer Building with the house referred to in the Bible as built by a wise man on solid rock: "[It] endured the rain of carping criticism, the flood of innovations in medicine, and the winds of changing personnel, and has not fallen. For it was built not only on structural rock, but on the rock of lofty ideals, based on a genuine desire to serve the sick of this and upcoming generations."

"Democracy is safe only so long as culture is in the ascendancy."
—Dr. William J. Mayo, 1924[12]

"The future of any country depends on the proper use
of its most intelligent men."
—Dr. William J. Mayo, 1924[13]

"Probably in the not far distant future we will crawl out of our old
methods of education, as a snake sheds its skin,
and reorganize a new plan."
—Dr. Charles H. Mayo, 1928[14]

❧ 5 ❧

Pill Hill Children

> To children is given the power of readily acquiring languages; later,
> mathematics is acquired with some readiness; but reasoning from
> cause to effect is a development of adolescence. . . .
> Dr. William J. Mayo, 1921 [1]

WE Masson children and our neighborhood friends lived and mingled in years that spanned devastating wars and financial insecurity of which we were only vaguely aware. We were privileged children; we all had bicycles. We were allowed to explore our territory. Feeling safe, we dabbled with danger in a world we trusted.

I grew up in the durable old house built by Dr. Emil H. Beckman. In addition to a clothes chute to the basement laundry room, the house had other newfangled conveniences including a "whistle and talk" pipeline. For us children it was a toy. We could blow through the whistle hole in the big room upstairs, push back a hinged metal cover, and talk to someone in the kitchen. In the basement there was a noisy vacuum motor, a "big old clunker" my brother Stan called it. Pipes went from it to the brass outlets on the upper floors where the vacuum cleaning hose could be connected. We also had a water softener in the basement. The kitchen and bathrooms had separate faucets for drinking water straight from the water tower at Saint Mary's Park.

We had a slipshod way of disposing of clean, empty bottles at our house. We threw them over the top of a large hot water tank that blocked the entrance to some dark space that might once have been a closet. That crash of breaking glass seemed exciting to me, but no thrill could compare with what happened in the furnace room on the days the coal truck came. The driver, smudged from head to foot with coal dust, set up his chute to the basement window and let the coal roar like an earthquake down the slide to the bin in the basement.

One of my earliest memories of living at 724 Fourth Street SW was a spontaneous happening that caught me and my brothers like a grand surprise now and then while we were getting dressed before breakfast. We would hear a sudden tinkley crash on the floor of the big room where my parents dressed. Jay, Stan and I, all younger than seven, would run like young foxes from their burrows to pounce on Dad, who was bent over by his closet door retrieving the pocketful of coins that had hit the floor when he took his trousers off a hanger and the pockets turned wrong side out. Coins bounced and rolled in every direction as we shoved and struggled to get our share of the bounty. The game was finders—keepers, losers—weepers. "By golly, you're cleaning me out," Dad would say as we crawled all over him.

Another delightful privilege from my earliest days was going to the street with Mother to greet the milkman's big black horse. She lifted me up to pat his nose and give him a lump of sugar.

On August 12, 1926, when I was six, a crate arrived at the train station and was brought up to the house. It was addressed:

> To: The Masson Kids
> Rochester, Minnesota
> From: F. P. Knowles
> Highlawn Farm
> Auburn, Mass.

Grandpa Knowles had long since forgiven my father for marrying my mother and taking her off to the Midwest. From the crate came the plaintive bleating of two pygmy goat kids, one brown, one white. We were wild with excitement. We named them Biff and Bang and kept them in a box stall in the "old garage," as we referred to the barn where Dr. Beckman kept his horse. A ramp to an outside pen was quickly assembled by Sylvester, our man of many skills.

Word got around fast on Pill Hill. Suddenly, we Masson kids had friends we'd never met before. At the Edison School pet show, both goats got blue ribbons—Bang for the longest whiskers and Biff for the cleanest animal. I always wished the goats, both female, would have babies. Mother and Dad never explained to us just why they didn't.

Biff and Bang were gourmands. When Sylvester trimmed the elderberry bushes he put the clippings in the goat pen. They ate leaves till their sides rounded out like baskets on a burro. They especially liked bread. Three times a week in the late afternoon, the Star Bread truck came to the Hillside Grocery on Fifth Street. My friends and I waited with the goats on leash in a vacant lot across the street. When the truck appeared we slid down the bank and surrounded the young blond driver whose name, Luke, was sewn in yellow on his uniform pocket. As the goats baa-ed and leaped around he handed down stale bread from the rack on top like the driver of a stage coach at gunpoint. With the bread held high we let go of the leashes and ran for home, up Dr. Dripps's driveway, through the lilac hedge to the old garage. In the goat pen we ripped off the wrappers (unnecessary since the goats also ate waxed paper). Their bushy tails twitched as they feasted.

We did this every delivery day till suddenly a new man was driving the truck. "No, you can't have any bread," he said gruffly. He had to account for all of it.

I often thought about that nice young man, Luke, and felt pangs of remorse, wondering if we had caused him to be fired.

A visit to the Star Bakery Company was a wonderful field trip for all of Rochester's elementary schools. We were shown how the incredible bread machine worked. Then we were each given a loaf of bread to take home, but the bread rarely got home with us. It was either eaten or mutilated. I think it was Dave Bach, whose father owned the Bach Music Company, who first got the bright idea of eating the soft bread in the center and slipping the crust on his forearm like a shield. Mock battles erupted among the boys, each with a bread shield raised in front of his face.

My best friends in those Edison School days were my nearest neighbors, Jeannie Rowntree and Jane and Betty Willius. Jeannie's father, Dr. Leonard G. Rowntree, was Chief of the Department of Medicine at the Mayo Clinic. Next to playing with the goats, I liked playing at the Rowntrees. When Mrs. Rowntree was out, neither the maid nor Jeannie's older sister Alison paid us any attention. A large steamer trunk on the Rowntree's third floor was full of dress-up clothes—scarves, flowered hats, high-heeled shoes and evening gowns. We didn't need a nursemaid to oversee our narcissistic pleasure in draping ourselves with glamour in front of a mirror. Nobody came to make us stop jumping on the bed. And nobody saw us come downstairs, open a drawer in the dining room and help ourselves to milk chocolate wafers, two candles and a few red match folders with "Katherine and Leonard" embossed on them in gold.

Back on the third floor Jeannie and I closed ourselves into our secret clubhouse, a storage closet with racks of winter clothing, hat boxes and Christmas decorations. We lit a few matches, got our candle wicks aflame, made wax puddles in a pine cone holder and stood our candles upright in melted wax. Sometimes the candles toppled over and we blew out the fire and began again. Sprawled on a mattress, we ate the party candy, drew pictures and wrote notes to each other on lined notebook paper. Our hair sometimes snagged on the low wooden beams as we shifted around in the flickering light among scraps of crumpled paper.

I am reminded of some old people named Bamber who lived in a big Victorian house kitty-corner from the Rowntrees' and across from Dr. Will Mayo's side yard. They came from a rural area surrounding the Bamber Valley School district. These old people were packrats. They never threw anything away. Every year or so fire engines with bells clanging would race up Fourth Street to their house where flames and black smoke billowed out the upper windows. Every child in the neighborhood would run over to watch the firemen drag out smoking mattresses, chairs and rugs while jets of water sprayed the flaming roof. Nobody was ever hurt in a Bamber fire that I know of. But even now, to remember those blackened beams and the acrid smell of fire gives me the shivers! I think of Jeannie with the light brown hair, us two under the slanting roof in the storage room at the Rowntrees', reading and writing by candlelight as we knew young Abraham Lincoln did.

At the Willius house we were safe and good. In those days, we walked into our friends' homes and called. Doors weren't locked. Good smells from the Willius kitchen always met me at the door. Mrs. Willius made cookies and casseroles and even potato chips, potatoes thinly sliced and deep fried. She passed them around with pleasure. I would have preferred Mother in the kitchen at my house like Mrs. Willius. Our cook didn't want kids "underfoot."

Bessie Anderson and Stella Lecque were two Swedish women who lived on our third floor. Sometimes when I entered the kitchen they would stop talking and look at me. Then they would start again, in a foreign language. I always wondered what they didn't want me to hear. Perhaps it was Bessie's unhappy love life. She had a boyfriend who worked at the Buick garage. I later learned he had a drinking problem. Sometimes I saw him hunkered over a cup of coffee at our kitchen table, smoking a cigarette.

Bessie was a nurse's assistant on the maternity floor at Saint Mary's Hospital when I was born. Dad hired her to help Mother take care of Jay and me. Then Mother had two more babies and Bessie stayed on. She loved babies. She was fastidious, her blond hair always smoothly marcelled in precise waves around her sharp features. She would come in my room and dust my collection of elephants when I thought they didn't need dusting. I'd find them in unnatural positions instead of in conversational groups or all walking in the same direction as I had left them. My love of elephants began with Buster Crabbe in the Tarzan movies. When Tarzan got in trouble he would let out his stridently musical call characterized by a quavering vocal twitch and the elephants would come to his defense.

One day Bessie was attempting to clean out my closet. I had put a shoebox full of milkweed pods in my sock and underwear drawer. I planned, when they ripened, to take them to school for show-and-tell. Bessie picked up the shoebox and opened it. A cloud of silvery-winged seeds popped out at her, giving her such a fright she dropped the box and spilled the pods, scattering the airborne seeds and whisking them every which way on their silky wings. They sailed through the bathroom and into the bedroom, floated down on my sweaters and skirts, on towels and rugs. It was a beautiful mess. Bessie scolded in Swedish. I thought, "You shouldn't have snooped in that shoebox." But, as I said, she was fastidious; she vacuumed milkweed seeds and silk to her heart's content.

Bessie was with us long after there were no children to take care of. Eventually she became ill with a disease almost impossible to diagnose in those days, cancer of the pancreas. She was cared for till she died at Saint Mary's, visited almost daily by my mother.

In the late 1920's, as the lofty Plummer Building was being built, my friends' fathers were as busy as mine was. But Saturday afternoon and Sunday gave the fathers a little slack time to get to know their children. Often I was at Betty's house when her father, Dr. Fredrick A. Willius, was around in his shirtsleeves. I thought he was wonderful, not because he was a learned heart specialist, the head of the section of cardiology at the Mayo Clinic, but because he was an artist and a craftsman. He was a small, spry man with a large head, big glasses, straight salt-and-pepper hair and always a smile for us children. He did beautiful pen and ink drawings of nature scenes. Even more impressive was what he built with his hands for his three daughters, Jane, Betty and Dorothy, a unique doll house. Not only was it beautifully crafted, it was in every respect a miniature model of their own first house on Seventh Avenue, complete with furniture.

Also, Dr. Willius was the first person I knew who had written a book. Being a "heart man," two of his books were on that subject: *Cardiac Clinics* and, with Dr. Tom Dry, *Heart and Circulation*. In later years he published two more books, *Aphorisms*, a collection of wise statements culled from the writings of Dr. Will and Dr. Charlie Mayo, and a short biography of his close friend and mentor, *Henry Stanley Plummer, A Diversified Genius*.

One summer in the 1970's when I was home to visit Dad with my four children, I stopped in to see Dr. and Mrs. Willius. A lot of memories floated back. Dr. Willius spoke of the goats, Biff and Bang, and we laughed, remembering it was he who dubbed the round black pellets they dropped on his front walk "goat pills." Dr. Willius questioned me, as Uncle Don Balfour always did, about my life. When he learned I was divorced but had started writing and had published four children's books, some poems and an article in *Redbook*, he told me I seemed busy and happy. He went to a bookcase and brought a book down from the shelf.

"I want to read you something written by Dr. Will," he said. "It fits you. This is my favorite of all Dr. Will's wise sayings: "Contented industry is the mainspring of human happiness.'"[2]

He opened Lucy Wilder's book, *The Mayo Clinic*. "That sentence," Dr. Willius told me, "came from a letter Dr. Will wrote dated February 26, 1934, to Dr. L. D. Coffman, the president of the University of Minnesota." Dr. Will was explaining the background leading to a transfer of $500,000 in 1919 from the newly established Mayo Properties Association to the Mayo Foundation for Medical Education and Research for which the University was the trustee.

Dr. Willius read me the rest of the paragraph that contained his favorite (and now it is my favorite) aphorism:

Contented industry is the mainspring of human happiness. Money is so likely to encourage waste of time, changing objectives in life, living under circumstances which put one out of touch with those who have been lifelong friends who perhaps have been less fortunate. How many families have we seen ruined by money which has taken away from the younger members the desire to labor and achieve and has introduced elements into their lives whereby, instead of being useful citizens, they have become wasteful and sometimes profligate.[3]

When Dr. Willius put the book down and looked up I could see his eyes smiling behind the lenses of his black-framed glasses.

"It's true, Helen," he said. "Too much money doesn't make happiness; enthusiasm for work does. The Mayos knew that, which is why they set it up so individuals wouldn't inherit profits earned by the Clinic. Profits were invested in the Foundation."

He put Lucy Wilder's book back in its slot and brought out a copy of his biography of Dr. Henry S. Plummer. "I think you should have this, Helen," he said, and autographed it to me.

What a privilege it is to remember Dr. Willius. As so many of the friends I grew up with have commented, as we talked about our childhoods, we never knew the value of the people we took for granted.

The Williuses' first house was beside a Fifth Street vacant lot, a field of tall grass and trees that ended abruptly at a steep clay bank propped up by a stone wall at the sidewalk's edge. Across the street was a less dramatic hill of sandy soil. We children, a loose bunch of Edison School friends, thought of ourselves as the Clay Bank Gang. I always assumed our leader to be my older brother Jay, now a retired plastic surgeon still living in Rochester and married to his high school sweetheart, Lillian.

In the days of the Clay Bank Gang when Jay was in the sixth grade, his girl was Jane Willius. To impress her he used to lie down in the middle of Seventh Avenue at the foot of the steps leading up to the Willius house. Jane would scream frantically at him, which caused the occasional car on Seventh Avenue to drive around the two of them. Jay was not quite old enough then, as Dr. Will might have observed, "to reason profoundly from cause to effect," but Jay certainly knew that lying in the middle of the street got Jane's attention.

The sandy bank across Fifth Street "belonged" to another group of Edison School kids, the Sand Bank Gang. Sometimes our two groups built shacks together in our back yard, using our tools and lumber furnished by Dave Bach, whose father owned the Bach Music Company and had plenty of wooden boxes and piano crates to give us. But now and then war broke out between our two camps and we fought it out at the vacant lots. We threw hardened clay balls at each other, back and forth across Fifth Street. The Sand Bank Gang dug their ammunition from our clay when we weren't there. But war has no rules, and soon those harmless clay balls that split apart when a target was hit had stones hidden inside. The last battle ever staged there ended when my brother Jay was knocked down by a stone to the back of his head. Blood streamed down his neck and soaked into his shirt. We ran for home, with me bawling my head off, till Jay turned around and yelled at me, "Shut up!"

Mother cleaned up our minor wounds because Dad was usually at the Clinic, Saint Mary's or the Colonial Hospital. She took out slivers with a germ-free needle and removed wood ticks from our hair after picnics in Mr. Butlin's pasture. We had a standing invitation to use that pasture because Mr. Butlin's wife was a patient of Dad's. We children pulled the ticks off dogs. Back then, wood ticks didn't carry the serious disease Rocky Mountain Spotted Fever, for which there is now an effective vaccine. I didn't mind dealing with little brown ticks, but the old bloated ones hiding in the long hair around Barney's or Taffy's ears, big as a pea, gray and ugly, were too repulsive for me to touch. Mother or Dad dispatched those with a drop of rubbing alcohol.

For serious injuries we were lucky if Dad was there when the accident happened. On one Sunday afternoon picnic at Cedar Beach with the Haines family, my brother Stan had a run-in with our heavy wooden rowboat, The Tortoise. The boat, with fateful momentum, rammed the dock, squashing Stan's thumb which was hanging over the edge. His thumbnail instantly turned black as blood surged under it with no outlet. Ten-year-old Stan yelled bloody murder. Dad, knowing it was the pressure behind the nail that caused the pain, did what any carpenter would do if he thought of it. From a tool chest kept at the cottage Dad brought out a small triangular file and, as poor Stan submitted with horror in the strong arms of Dr. Sam Haines, Dad filed an opening in the surface of the nail which let the blood spurt out and ease the pain. It was certainly a relief in emergencies having a father who was calm and knew what to do.

It is the custom everywhere in the world that a doctor doesn't operate on a child without parental consent. However, sometimes the rules had to be bent. Bob New, when he was about fourteen, had an acute attack of appendicitis when his parents, Dr. and Mrs. Gordon New, were at a medical meeting in Chicago. The New's cook, Josie, called Dr. Jim Masson. Dad examined Bob, then took it upon himself to remove the appendix without delay. Gordon and Ethyl New returned from Chicago, relieved that the emergency had been handled promptly. Bob stayed at Saint Mary's Hospital a week and was having such a good time being pampered by the nurses that they let him stay an extra day.

When we were sick with the usual childhood diseases Mother called my favorite pediatrician, tall, dark and handsome Dr. Roger Kennedy. He was Clark Gable with a deep, bass voice. He would sit on the edge of my bed and ask me about the goats and my rat terrier, Taffy, as he counted my pulse, took my temperature and, with a stethoscope, listened to me breathe and to my heart pump. He'd suggest soup for lunch, orange juice, ice cream, ginger ale and a new bottled drink, Coca Cola, with half an aspirin if I had a fever. Mother brought me all those things and straws in my ice water, as well as new crayons and paper from Woolworth's and scissors and magazines to cut up. She gave me back rubs and cold compresses on my hot forehead, and she read to me. *Rikki Tikki Tavi* by Rudyard Kipling was my favorite story.

When Stanley and I had our tonsils out at the same time we shared a room at the Worrall Hospital. Mother brought us toys with wheels which we raced competitively down the sheet drawn tight over our raised knees.

When anyone was sick at the home of Dr. and Mrs. Sam Haines visitors were scared off by a sign on the front door: "No Admittance—Communicable Disease." In the days before television, children read more and invented their own entertainment. Olivia Haines Blackburn said when she and Elizabeth "Piv" Kendall, close neighbors, were sick at the same time, they spelled out notes to each other, displaying large letters of the alphabet at their bedroom windows.

Children's birthdays brought out the creativity of mothers. The Spider Web party, for instance: Eight girls on my eighth birthday. Mother wove yards and yards of string, a ball for each girl, all over the house, between bannister rails upstairs and down the back stairs to the kitchen, under and over chairs and tables, everywhere, till the house was a network of string that ended in some unexpected place with a gift attached.

The rule was: each girl had to wind up the string as she struggled through the web to the prize.

Public school for us in Rochester began at age five with a half day of kindergarten. After that it was an eight-hour day with an hour to go home for lunch. We on Pill Hill went to Edison School, one of about six elementary schools in Rochester at the time. In the coldest months we were bundled up in woolen layers and wore galoshes that buckled over shoes. Our parents never drove us to school or picked us up.

We had fire drills, even in winter. When the bell gonged, shrill and fast, we formed lines and ran outside. In addition to the Three R's (Reading, 'Riting and 'Rithmetic), history and geography they tried to teach us Palmer method penmanship. We learned to be kind to books, to open a new one a few pages at a time so as not to crack the book's spine. We learned how to cover a book with heavy paper or oilcloth, and we were expected to get our mothers to help us cover our new books.

In November when the ground was frozen the Fire Department made the rounds of the schools. Their powerful hoses shot a beautiful arc of water over the baseball fields and slowly a lake would form and freeze within the raised lip around the lot. From then on we often took our skates to school.

The fire department was also willing to make a rink for whoever had a level place for water to freeze, such as Dr. Bumpus' tennis court at Tenth Avenue and Eighth Street and the Helmholz's court at Sixth Street and Eighth Avenue.

Jack Pemberton, who lived next door to the Bumpuses, reminded me of a freakish winter day when nobody played hockey at the Bumpuses' rink. The weather was capricious that day. Sleet rained from the sky, then temperatures dropped. Suddenly ice covered all of Rochester. Cars couldn't move without chains. We children and many grownups skated everywhere up and down the streets, sidewalks and driveways of Pill Hill. It was as if on this one winter's day, as Jack put it, "the streets had all been paved in ice just for our fun."

Sometimes Mother drove us out to the frozen lake at Mayowood, the country home of Dr. and Mrs. Charlie Mayo. If wind hadn't blown the snow off the ice, skaters with snow shovels cleared it off. Once Sally Mayo, the Mayo's youngest adopted child, had a wiener roast by the frozen pond. But most fun, I thought, was skating at the public rink where we could skate as if dancing to the music that went with us around the circle. When we were cold or hungry for a hot dog and cocoa we went into the warming shack and mingled with other kids.

Dog sledding was a challenge undertaken only by the Massons—we had a dog with the "right stuff." With leather straps and rope and Dad's help we made a harness for Barny, our big, brown, part-Gordon Setter. We hitched him to a Flexible Flyer. Eleven-year-old Stan wrote to Mother, who was visiting her parents in Massachusetts, telling her of one foray into the neighborhood:

Dear Mom,

Yesterday I took Barny out with the sled. He went fine. But when we got to the bottom of Hanses [Dr. Sam Haines] hill another dog was down there. He was a great big one. I think it was Jud's [Dr. E. Starr Judd] dog. And he came over and Barny growled at him and they started fighting. The other dog got Barny down and fell right on top of him. He had the advantage on Barny because Barny had on a harness. I got mad too, and I picked up the sled and lamed the other dog across the back good'n hard. But anyway he got up and beat it. He went around the corner, he peeked around it at me. . . ."

A lot of skiers got their start in Rochester. Saint Mary's Park at the top of Fourth Street sloped gently down for beginners. The Country Club hills offered long, smooth ups and downs. But being safe was not enough for the more adventurous skier. Three boys in my high school class yearned for a little risk. They found a shed full of lumber in the woods at Dr. Plummer's beautiful rock house on a hilltop, and they appropriated enough boards and nails to build a ski jump. Those three boys, Jack Crenshaw, Dick Hempsted and Clarence Stearns, all survivors of World War II, are still skiing together in ski territory, Colorado.

The best place for downhill sledding, not counting Ninth Avenue which was too steep to be safe, was on Third Street behind Dr. and Mrs. Will Mayo's yard where the Police Department closed off the cross avenues to cars during school vacations. But Dr. Will's sloping back yard that went all the way to a fence at Third Street was my favorite place to slide. In spite of the cold weather it seemed cozy, the wind blocked by the big house at the top and a small windbreak of trees on each side of the broad, snow-covered hill. Sometimes, when we looked up from our snow-

Pill Hill

men and our sleds, we would see Dr. Will and Mrs. Hattie Mayo watching from the picture window in their castle-like stone home. They smiled and waved, as if we were a troupe of players they were welcoming.

Midway down their hill a path dipped in, like a tight belt around a fat stomach. That dip gave us a thrilling lift when we flew into it, lying flat on our Flexible Flyers. Then we'd trudge uphill and fly down again. It wasn't a big enough thrill for the older boys and girls. They made the jump higher with more snow, packed and hardened with water brought in a bucket from the Mayo's garage. Sometimes dozens of children from the immediate neighborhood and beyond were there at the same time with sleds, aluminum pans, toboggans and skis.

One afternoon a small girl on a sled went over the frozen jump. She flew off course and slammed into a tree. She cried and couldn't stand up until Mary Elizabeth Giffin, a natural leader among us, gave instructions, and the girl was helped onto a toboggan and hauled to the Giffin's house where Giffie, as Mary Elizabeth was known, called Dr. Will at the Clinic. She told him she was sending him a patient to Saint Mary's for emergency treatment. She thought the girl had "a greenstick fracture of the tibia."

Giffie might have been nine or ten at the time. Her father was Dr. Herbert Z. Giffin, a pediatrician and specialist in diseases of the blood and spleen. She had had polio at an early age and wore a leg brace. Dr. Will was her doctor and her very special friend.

About a week after the accident in Dr. Will's back yard, Giffie received the following letter:

Dear Dr. Mary:
I would like to take this opportunity to thank you for referring your patient, Jean, to the Mayo Clinic. Careful examination here confirmed your diagnosis of a greenstick fracture of the tibia.

Surgical procedures included the application of two casts. The latter permitting her to return home five days after your referral. It is anticipated that Jean will have a good result from the procedures.
With kindest personal regards,
Sincerely,
W. J. Mayo[4]

Mary Giffin from an early age had listened to the language of medicine. She thought scientifically. She found it easy to think of herself as a doctor, especially after Dr. Will addressed her as "Dr. Mary."

Pill Hill Children

It isn't surprising that she grew up well ahead of the rest of us Pill Hill children. Most of us had very little struggle in our young lives. For Giffie, struggle began early. At the age of two she was hospitalized with a broken leg. Six months later she contracted polio myelitis and became Dr. Will's special patient. He devised her treatment at a time when nothing much was known about the disease. He talked to her as an equal. He invited her, a half-grown child, to staff meetings, where she sat quietly beside him and listened to the men talk. Frequently she was invited along with visiting doctors and their wives aboard the North Star, the Mayo's yacht on the Mississippi River. On these trips Marlizbeth, as Dr. Will called her, got in her swimming therapy with Carr, the ship's engineer, but her greatest pleasure was listening to the doctors talk shop.

Some of Mary's awkward efforts to master her handicap took place on the sidewalk in front of Dr. Will's stone wall. My mother, seeing this struggle across the street, often spoke of her admiration for her friend Bess Giffin who restrained the impulse to help her daughter stand up when time after time the little girl fell down. Giffie succeeded at most of the activities healthy children want to do. In lieu of a bicycle, she learned to manage a "push-pull" which allowed her to get where she wanted to go in a hurry, such as around Dr. Will's semicircular brick driveway. In her own awkward way she learned to run, to roller skate, ride horseback and swim. At Rochester High School she was elected head of the student government and at Smith College she was senior class president. After graduation from Johns Hopkins Medical School and a fellowship at the Mayo Clinic, she founded the Irene Josselyn Clinic in Northfield, Illinois, which specializes in the psychiatric treatment of young people. She practiced general psychiatry in Winnetka, Illinois.

In her first book, *Her Doctor, Will Mayo*, Giffie reveals how much it meant to her as a youngster that Dr. Will seemed to enjoy her company as much as she enjoyed his.[5]

At Edison School one spring day we Pill Hill children learned one of life's stern lessons—people die. Life is a privilege; it can be taken away. A girl I had hardly noticed lived across from school in a small frame house on Seventh Street. She was shy. She didn't pass notes, whisper in class or race around on the playground. She could play on the swings after we noisy ones had all gone home. One Monday morning in spring, as Betty

Willius and I walked across the baseball field with our books, the playground seemed oddly calm. Kids stood around in groups. The boys weren't playing marbles in the dirt. The girls weren't skipping rope or playing jacks. Then the news caught me and Betty. The girl who lived across the street was dead, smothered by an avalanche of dirt. We shuddered. "What . . . what . . . ?"

No one was laughing; it was true. In the girl's front yard the city had dug a deep hole to fix a broken water pipe. They left it over the weekend, fenced around with an orange ribbon. The girl—I think her name was Clair Webber—climbed to the top of the dirt pile. It shifted, and she slid into the pit and was covered by the heavy spill of loose soil that fell on top of her.

The news sapped our energy. We looked at each other and at the teachers, their arms around some children who were crying. I imagined the panic the girl would have felt, unable to breathe, her face, arms, all of her, covered with dirt. Screaming would fill her mouth with dirt. Where was she now? Where was Heaven? What happened when you died?

Two or three days later Hugh Kendall, a sixth-grader, and his friend, Henry Stark, were returning to school after lunch when they saw a lot of people going in and out of the house where Clair had lived. Curious, they fell in line, thinking it might be a reception, food given away. People whispered. Maybe it was a church service. Suddenly, it was too late to drop out and run to school; the two boys stood in front of an open casket surrounded by roses, their fragrance nauseatingly sweet. There was the girl, Clair, lying on a white satin cushion, wearing a yellow dress. Her eyes were closed, her cheeks pink like the roses.

Hugh was so shocked he was shaking, he told me recently. The horror he felt stayed with him a long time. He went from Edison School to Junior High and he was still experiencing sleepless nights, haunted by the sight of that dead girl. In the eighth grade, he said to himself, "This has to stop!" He devised a plan to get rid of his obsession with death. He made a new friend at school, a boy whose father was the owner of the Vine Funeral Home.

"I forced myself to go with him and look around that place. It was next to the fire house. I went often. I got used to seeing dead people in caskets, and I went to wakes. Finally I stopped having nightmares."

Thoughts of that pit became a frightening memory for many of us.

Pill Hill Children

Accidents happen sometimes, we knew. But the following year we learned that death could come also in the course of an ordinary problem, like a hurt knee. When something ached, grownups said it was "growing pains." How serious was that?

Our friend Ruth Finney had a pain in her knee. She limped home from school one day before the bell rang. The next day the pain was in her hip and she was rushed to the Colonial Hospital. Two days later we were given the bewildering news that Ruth would not be back in school. She had died. How could this be? To us, at age ten, the death of our classmate was unbelievable. It was not caused by an accident, like the one which happened to Clair. It was unresolved, like the uneasiness we feel when not sure if we have been lied to. Perhaps, if someone had explained to us the sad metaphor of Humpty-Dumpty, we would have at least understood the finality of death. Just as all the king's horses and all the king's men couldn't put Humpty-Dumpty together again, so the many superb doctors of the Mayo Clinic and all the medical knowledge of 1930 couldn't bring our friend Ruth back to the playground at Edison School.

Our seventh-grade friend, Mary Giffin, once asked Dr. Will what happens when you die. He told her in his calm, sensible way, "Whatever happens in that future time is a mystery to us now. But I accept it and respect the fact that we don't have answers to everything. When my time comes, I would be glad for my ashes to be thrown from the bluffs at Wabasha into the Mississippi River. I would be proud to be part of that mighty river."

The summer passed, and in September I returned as a fifth-grader to Edison School. Something new on the playground caught my eye, a marvelous geometrical structure made of steel pipes. Before my friends and I knew what it was, we were climbing all over it. Our teachers told us it was a Jungle Gym, the latest in outdoor playground equipment. But more meaningful than knowing its name was learning it was a gift to us from Ruth Finney's parents, Dr. and Mrs. W. P. Finney.

❦ 6 ❧

Kendall's Movies

> We, as parents, must give up our professed right
> to fix our children's thinking.
> Dr. Charles H. Mayo, 1931 [1]

WE who were children in the Pill Hill neighborhood of the early 1930's all will agree there was one unforgettable, stellar weekly event in our childhood. I can safely assume it was one of a kind in the whole world. Adults had nothing to do with it, except for one understanding parent, Mrs. Rebecca Kendall, the wife of biochemist Dr. E. C. Kendall. The idea and execution of the venture came from her son Hugh, a young entrepreneur. Hugh went on to become a research engineer at MIT and director of research at the General Railway Signal Company of Rochester, New York.

Hugh at fourteen was impressive, big for his age, with a voice too stentorian for one so young. He started the Movie King Theatre, a business that captivated the neighborhood. His showings took place twice every Saturday, beginning in March and lasting through June, for several years. The movies he rented and showed on the third floor of the Kendalls' house were mostly the first animated Disney cartoons and old classics starring Laurel and Hardy, Charlie Chaplin and the kids of "Our Gang Comedy," the "Little Rascals" of modern television.

On Friday after school a courier on a bicycle circled the Pill Hill streets yelling, "Kendalls' Movies five cents! Get your ticket here!" That sent us speeding home to the box where we kept our allowance money. We'd track down the courier and buy our ticket. The one-by-two-inch cardboard strip was printed professionally by Hugh's Sunday School teacher, Mr. Rentz, who owned a print shop:

Pill Hill

Kendalls' Movie King Theatre
5 cents
10 a.m. & 2 p.m. Saturday

Long before 10 o'clock on Saturday morning, forty or more kids with tickets converged on the home of Dr. and Mrs. Kendall, a white frame house with a steep driveway. The driveway was parallel to a deeply shaded, jungle-like gulch known as Kendall's Canyon. On the other side of the house the lawn sloped down to the top of a wall that kept the Kendalls' yard and garden from washing downhill. A stone path led past the Keith's rock garden to the Helmholz's tennis court on Eighth Avenue. On those Saturday mornings, bicycles jammed the driveway and lay all over the Kendalls' yard. At five minutes till ten Mrs. Becky Kendall unlocked the kitchen door. Children of all sizes, all chattering, burst into the kitchen and headed for the back stairs. They were stopped at the foot of the stairs, and their tickets were collected by Jack Pemberton, one of Hugh's assistants.

Mrs. Kendall was always awed by this weekly muster generated by her son, Hugh. She stood her ground before the refrigerator and the cookie jar as we thronged up to the loft on the third floor. To the lively strains of "Anchors Away" on the phonograph, we squeezed onto the orange crate/wooden plank bleachers of the Movie King Theatre.

At a signal from Hugh, David Stark, the "curtain man," pulled back the sheets from in front of the screen. The record was changed, and the soothing music of Jesse Crawford's concert organ came on. It was authentic, Hugh said, like the prelude at the Chateau Theatre downtown. It was supposed to settle us down, and it did. From his "projection booth," a table in the doorway to the maid's room, Hugh operated everything, including (after David didn't show up one time) a system of ropes and pulleys that opened and closed the curtains. When he doused the lights, the screen lit up; we cheered and clapped and then hushed. For more than an hour we laughed and hooted at the crazy fun of something new to the world—motion pictures and cartoons made especially for children.

At times the film slipped out of its sprocket holes and the picture flickered noisily. We screamed, "It's skipping, skipping, skipping!"

We battered the floor and the bleacher rails with our feet. Down below, Mrs. Kendall undoubtedly feared for the plaster on the ceilings over

Kendall's Movies

the bedrooms. From the projectionist's chair came Hugh's strident bellow, "Shut up, you dopes, I'm fixing it!"

Between reels, a Master of Ceremonies, perhaps Bob Roesler or Henry Stark, whistled for attention. Kids stood up and made announcements about lost dogs and neighborhood happenings. Compton Broders might read a list of kids who had books overdue from his basement library. A horror story might be told such as the one about what happened to Olivia Haines one day on her way home from Libby Pemberton's house—the Harwick's bulldog attacked her. Woody, the Harwick's yard man, pulled the dog off, picked up Olivia, who was streaming blood, and carried her home. Mrs. Haines opened the door and fainted. The bulldog was tested at the Research Institute. He didn't have rabies, but the Harwicks had him put to sleep anyway.

Barbara Benedict's father, everyone knew, was an eye doctor, an ophthalmologist. She might have told the funny thing little Bobby New, age three, did. He brought his teddy bear to her father and asked if he could fix its eye, which was hanging by a thread. Her father said he thought he could. He did. He returned it the next day, the eye firmly attached.

Sometimes at intermission live music was volunteered by a group calling itself Jimmy Joy's Orchestra. Featured musicians were Dave Bach on the drums, Bob Roesler and his violin, and others, with or without talent, performing with harmonicas, Jew's-harps and combs. Sometimes kids did headstands and backbends on a wrestling mat, and sometimes Barbara Benedict and others could be talked into doing the Charleston.

One Saturday morning at Kendalls' Movies, Hugh no longer had to yell at us to shut up. There was no more "skipping"! He had a new projector. Word had got around among the parents that young Hugh Kendall was showing movies for the neighborhood kids. Dr. Howard K. Gray, who came to the Clinic in 1928 as a surgical fellow, heard of it and called his friend Nick Kendall.

"What projector is your son using?" he asked.

When Dr. Kendall told him it was an obsolete specimen, Dr. Gray said he had a good self-threading 16mm Bell and Howell he wasn't using. He wanted to contribute it to the cause.

This thoughtful gift to an enterprising fourteen-year-old was in keeping with the personality of Dr. Gray, perhaps the most profoundly kind and morally incorruptible man our parents ever knew. He never drank, smoked or passed along an untidy joke. The dean of students at Princeton described their outstanding athlete as "easily the most popular young gentleman in the University."

One Sunday morning at Saint Mary's Hospital a number of patients reported to their doctors that a strange man in a bathrobe and slippers had come into their rooms early that morning, started IVs and done other chores. The "strange man," they were told, was just a friendly surgeon, their eminent colleague Dr. Howdie Gray. He was at Saint Mary's recovering from an appendectomy and had volunteered to take calls for the Fellows who wanted to attend the Fellow's Association picnic at Whitewater Park on Saturday.

At the onset of World War II, Dr. Gray took leave of the Mayo Clinic to enlist in the Medical Corps of the U.S. Navy. He served with distinction in the Pacific. After the war he resumed his busy schedule of surgery at the Clinic, plus additional duties he took on as a member of the Board of Governors. The favorite free-time activity of Dr. Gray, his wife Dewenta and the two children, Howdie and Wendy, as with many Rochester families, was boating on the Mississippi. It was a cruel shock for the city of Rochester and for patients, friends and the family of Dr. Gray to learn that on September 6, 1955, at the age of fifty-four, that fine man was drowned in his favorite river while attempting to retrieve a runaway dinghy.

Hugh Kendall, in 1931, was overwhelmed with appreciation to Dr. Gray for his thoughtful gift of an up-to-date projector. "The cause" was greatly benefitted. "It wasn't much of a money-maker," Hugh said later, "but it was a lot of fun." After paying back his mother for her $2.50 check every week to the Codascope Film Library, he usually cleared $1.50.

In 1913, five years before Hugh was born, young Dr. E. C. [Nick] Kendall, with a Ph.D. in chemistry from Columbia University, had been working as a biochemist under bothersome conditions in a New York hospital. Desperate for a place to work where he would not be fettered by untenable restraints on his time and the lack of equipment and supplies he needed, he submitted a proposal to the two Drs. Mayo. Could they possibly give him space, supplies and assistants to allow him to complete a project to isolate the active hormone of the thyroid gland?

At that time the Mayos and Dr. Plummer were eagerly rushing toward the completion of the first Mayo Clinic building. After some soul-searching, the Mayos invited the young biochemist to bring his work to Rochester. They would build a laboratory for him on the top floor of their new red brick facilities, the 1914 Building.

In the interval necessitated by the move of his laboratory from New York to Rochester, Nick Kendall had some much needed recreation. Family and friends conspired, and he met Becky, an intelligent and attractive graduate of Dana Hall and Wells College in Aurora, New York. She became the perfect wife for the dedicated scientist, Nick Kendall. A permissive mother by nature, she raised her four children—Hugh, Roy, Norman and Elizabeth—in a disciplined household. Hugh grew to be so much like his father, his mother accepted whatever he wanted to do as an important step toward a worthy goal. In the Kendalls' Movie King Theatre days the muddy kitchen floor, the noise of many children traipsing into her house and up to the third floor and the cracked plaster over the bedrooms were aggravations easily balanced out by the pride she felt in Hugh's capacity for carrying through ambitious ideas. She, too, had that capacity; she taught herself to play the piano all on the black keys. Hugh remembers the music she made was beautiful.

Another of Hugh's inspired ideas carried more risk than operating a projector. The Kendalls spent their summer vacations and many weekends at a cottage Dr. Kendall helped build near the village of Oronoco. It faced a lake created by the damming of the Zumbro River; it was thirty feet deep at its center. The Kendalls had seen over the years an uncounted number of boats overturned and sunk in that deep water. Hugh felt the challenge to salvage those boats.

He devised a diving bell which enabled him to explore the bottom of the lake. His contrivance was made from a thirty-gallon hot water tank cut out at the sides and padded with a rubber tire, leaving his arms free and the weight of the bell resting comfortably on his shoulders. He inserted a window pane to look through and attached lead weights to the bottom edge so it wouldn't float up with air inside. In case of emergency, he could throw it off and swim to the surface. Air was supplied through a long hose screwed into a fitting at the top and connected to a bicycle pump. Family and friends in a boat or floating platform pumped a continuous supply of air into the space above Hugh's neck so he could breathe as he walked around on the mucky bottom of the lake.

The salvage operation began after a mishap experienced by a neighbor downriver, Dr. Faucet, a Rochester dentist. In order to build a rock wall on his property, Dr. Faucet had taken his motorboat across the river to where rocks were plentiful and piled it full. The boat was low in the water but all was well when they pushed off from shore and Dr. Faucet started his big fifty-horsepower motor. Slowly and sedately the boat moved through the still water, making hardly a ripple. But suddenly, along came a saucy little Chriscraft, its bow elated as it sliced a path in the water, trailing behind it a slowly heaving wake. Dr. Faucet's heavily laden boat rocked from side to side, dipping water over the gunwales. Then it sank. Dr. Faucet and his helper swam to the Kendalls' cottage.

Jubilantly, Hugh and his family and friends went to retrieve their neighbor's boat. Behind their outboard they towed a swimmers' float, a wooden platform resting on sealed oil drums. At the estimated site of the sinking, Hugh, dressed in his heavy gear with a long coil of hose attached, sank out of sight. As the pumpers pumped, keeping air in the bell, Hugh descended to the murky depths. He had with him one end of a coil of rope and Dr. Faucet's instructions on how to detach the motor from the boat. When finally he found the sunken boat, detaching the motor was easy. He tied the rope to it and surfaced. Dr. Faucet, in another neighbor's boat, dragged the motor to shore. He was overjoyed to get his new motor back. He told Hugh he could keep the boat if he could get it up, and gave him the magnificent sum of forty dollars, two twenty-dollar bills. Because of the boat's cargo, retrieving it was a weighty problem. When the stones were removed, the wooden boat still didn't rise, its hull stuck fast in the muddy bottom. Finally, with ropes attached fore and aft, he was able to wobble it free.

The marina at White Bridge got word of the rescue, and Hugh and his diving bell were in demand. People fishing off the bridge were always losing things, like glasses and tackle boxes. Sometimes, motors not firmly attached to boats flipped off, and once, during a boat race, two boats collided and both went down. Hugh had himself a lucrative business for a fifteen-year-old.

At home on an ordinary day, Dr. Kendall's children knew their father's whereabouts like the face of a clock. His routine never varied. After breakfast he walked quickly to the Clinic, a matter of nine blocks. Drivers learned to watch out for him as he paid no attention to stop signs. He walked home for lunch and straight to the table where his wife and children, on lunch break from school, were assembled and the food was ready to be served. After lunch he took a twenty-minute nap, then walked back to the Clinic. His route home was always the same, past the Helmholz's tennis court and up the stone steps through the Keith's rock garden. He was a prolific reader of scientific magazines and three newspapers: the *New York Times*, the *Minneapolis Tribune* and the *Rochester Post Bulletin*. When he was reading, no one asked for his attention.

Sometimes Dr. Kendall did surprise his family. One day he brought home some white rats for his daughter Elizabeth, "Piv" as she was known. She and her friends formed the "White Rat Club." They went around with the friendly white rats in their jacket pockets or perched on their shoulders.

Year after year, from the day Dr. Kendall moved his project from New York to the Mayo Clinic, he worked doggedly toward his goal. At least one member of the Clinic staff had expressed doubts that anything would ever come of his efforts. Dr. O. T. Clagett, who began his fellowship in 1935, wrote in his autobiography he had heard the rumor soon after his arrival that a certain senior staff member had grumbled to Dr. Will about a waste of time and space in that fifth-floor laboratory. Dr. Will is said to have replied, "Dr. Nick Kendall is a brilliant and honest man, and a very hard worker. We will support him in his efforts."[2]

It was also said that at certain critical stages in Dr. Kendall's work, a person walking the streets of Rochester late at night might look up in surprise to see the windows of the entire top floor of the 1914 Building ablaze with light. Dr. Kendall would be up there keeping an eager eye on things. The first such period of ineffable excitement in that lab came on a snowy December 25th, 1914. On that Christmas day, the exacting process of isolating the active hormone of the thyroid gland yielded a pure crystalline substance. Dr. Kendall named it thyroxin. Helen Clapesattle writes in *The Doctors Mayo* that although Dr. Kendall claimed he wasn't a superstitious type, often in the years after 1914 he dropped in at the lab on Christmas day, "just to see whether anything might turn up."[3]

In Dr. Claggett's first year as a fellow, 1935, he attended a Clinical Pathology Conference every Wednesday evening in the 1914 Building. He always noticed a "terrible odor" that came down the elevator shaft from the top floor. After silently wondering about that, he finally learned that the Hormel Meat Packing Company in Austin, Minnesota, was sending large quantities of adrenal glands to Dr. Kendall's fifth floor lab.[4] In that same year, Dr. Kendall's odorous work culminated triumphantly in the isolation of cortisone. Fifteen years later, after a thorough testing of its effect on human patients with Dr. Philip S. Hench, the whole world, with profound relief, learned what Dr. Kendall went to the Mayo Clinic to do and how well he succeeded. He had found a stunning cure for pain. Cortisone was acclaimed a miracle by many thousands of arthritis sufferers.

On December 10, 1950, Dr. Kendall and Dr. Hench were awarded the Nobel Prize for their work. But I think with sadness of that day. It is the last time my mother wrote in her diary. It must have been an effort for her to write, in pain as she was. She died of a massive heart attack a few days after recording this one line: "Nick Kendall is receiving the Nobel Prize in Stockholm today."

❦{ 7 }❧

Halloween and Belva L. Snodgrass

The great contribution we can make is to prepare the oncoming generations to think that they can and will think for themselves.
Dr. Charles H. Mayo, 1914[1]

I was twelve when the Lindberg baby was kidnapped. Everyone talked of it and parents worried that a ripple effect might bring some copycat criminal to Rochester with a plan to abduct a Mayo grandchild. I thought of that when I saw spotlights come on at dusk trained on the home of Dr. and Mrs. Waltman Walters. Mrs. Walters was Dr. Will's youngest daughter, Phoebe. The five Walters children were all under ten: Phoebe, Joan, Waltman, Mayo (his friends called him Jim) and the baby Carolyn. Their white house all lit up looked like the many newspaper and newsreel pictures we saw of the Lindberg house where the ladder leaned on an upstairs windowsill and the kidnapper we all hated made his escape with the sleeping two-year-old boy. Carolyn Walters, now Mrs. Frederick Brown of Rochester, told me she lived for many years with none of the privacy of freedom available to me to go off on a bicycle with my friends. She said it was a great relief to finally, in her teens, say goodbye to her nanny.

We always felt safe in Rochester, allowed to go anywhere, to hike or ride bikes into the surrounding countryside or across town to visit new friends we met in high school. We were given a lot of freedom, but Pill Hill families had the usual firm schedules: bedtime, mealtimes, time for homework and a few chores. We had a big brass bell mother rang if we weren't home when expected. My chores were everything to do with pets—changing the papers and filling the seed and water cups for our canary bird, Dickie, cleaning the terrarium, washing my dog Taffy in the basement washtub, making my bed and helping Mother get Sunday night supper and do the dishes. It was a soft life. Mother didn't pressure us other than to insist we write thank-you notes, have decent table manners and keep up with our schoolwork. It was a temptation to be unruly, to sneak out at night and go to a spooky movie with a friend, but I never dared. On one day of the year, though, October 31st, we youngsters got away with considerable mischief.

On Halloween we could dress in outlandish getups and run around after bedtime in shadows made by the streetlights glimmering through trees. The neighbors were on the alert for us, offering us all sorts of goodies to avoid being tricked. Today's small Trick-or-Treaters in store-bought costumes make the rounds of a safe neighborhood collecting treats in grocery bags or pillow slips, but their parents are usually on the sidewalk keeping an eye on the polite little beggars.

We on Pill Hill in Rochester, Minnesota, in the 1920's and early '30s were more interested in tricks than treats. We roved the neighborhood looking for piles of raked leaves to scatter, door mats to hurl on the roofs of houses, porch furniture to push into the bushes, doorbells to ring and run away from, car windows to scribble on with Ivory soap.

To thwart this kind of behavior homeowners waited for us and invited us up on the porch or into the house for doughnuts and hot chocolate with marshmallows, or cookies and cider, popcorn balls, candied apples or fudge and punch. Then we were up and off after saying, "Thanks a lot." A few hours of this wildness and we were stuffed and happy.

Some people had Halloween parties. At our house I remember bobbing for apples in the laundry room. Apples floated in a big copper tub full of water. The children, hands behind their backs, knelt by the tub and tried to grab an apple with their teeth. There'd be prizes for quick grabbers, and mother was there with a towel to dry our hair, which inevitably got soaked. At Portia Vinson's house, according to Carol Haines Anderson who was there, everybody screamed their heads off as Dr. Vinson enhanced a ghoulish story with sensory side effects for each child who dared to touch the peeled grapes he said were eyeballs, and gooey spaghetti, the entrails of an unknown specimen run over by a car.

On one particular Halloween Aunt Laura Masson, Uncle Morrie's playful wife, dressed as a witch, took about eight of us small spooks out for an unforgettable, riotous night. First we made a lot of noise and rang doorbells on Fourth Street, beginning with Dr. Will's house across the street from us Massons. Then we paid noisy visits to the Bargens, the Sistruncks, the Gaardes and Hallenbecks. Aunt Laura then led us to a dimly lit little house on Ninth Avenue across from Saint Mary's Park. We rang that bell and ran away. All the lights came on, the front door opened and a man gruffly demanded, "Who's there?" We stayed hidden. He went back in the house. Aunt Laura egged us on and we continued to torment that house. We threw leaves on the porch and tapped on the windows, rang the doorbell repeatedly. Then we discovered the door wasn't locked. We pushed it open and burst into the front hall, yelling bloody murder and throwing armfuls of leaves on the rug. Two young grownups appeared then, looking startled, their hands up as if at gunpoint. When Aunt Laura appeared in her black stockings, black dress, black peaked hat, one blackened front tooth and a toy broom, the two of them burst out laughing. We realized then that these were friends of Aunt Laura and Uncle Morrie and they were expecting our tricks. The man brought in a red tin of chocolate chip cookies and a pitcher of punch with paper cups and we all sat on the floor in the midst of the leaves, and the cookies and punch were passed around. The young couple and Aunt Laura seemed to enjoy the whole thing in spite of the mess we made.

Another year when I was older word went around that on Halloween night an oil drum would be rolled down Ninth Avenue at the Henderson/Adson driveway. We didn't tell our parents, though we must have understood the danger to people and property of a 55-gallon steel drum careening down the steepest hill in the neighborhood. I didn't see the event, but I'm told the drum didn't roll straight. It wobbled from curb to curb, scraped the wall in front of the Adsons and Hendersons, roared past the Lobbs, Crenshaws and Broders going faster and faster, creating a wild thunder as it ricocheted back and forth. At the bottom of the hill it streaked past the Hartmans' and Woltmans' houses and spent its remaining momentum in the vacant field, where, according to Meg Crenshaw Diessner, a white-haired lady bird-watcher used to sit in a chair with her notebook and binoculars.

Somewhat less successful but equally dangerous was the attempt by a gang of our Pill Hill boys to get a manhole cover to roll straight as a hoop down Ninth Avenue. Fortunately, Bob Roesler tells me, it didn't work. Gravity always pulled it off balance.

In winter, that Ninth Avenue descent was an arena for daredevils. Audrey Woltman remembers that after every snowfall Compton Broders, now a doctor at the Scott-White Clinic in Texas, used to shovel mounds of snow which he and his friends iced with buckets of water, creating a course of treacherous jumps for sleds and toboggans. They would race into the first jump on a sled, fly into the air, aim for the next, and the next, and the next till they finished their exhilarating downhill course on the level end of Ninth Avenue. Compton, our intellectual who ran a library in the basement of the Broders' home, named his wild winter creation "The Rocky Road to Dublin."

Halloween was supposed to be merely a fun little holiday from good behavior for kids, but over the years it became more and more of a concern for adults. Mischief turned into crime. The downtown business community, after years of putting up with the destructive pranks of teenagers on Halloween, accepted the inability of the police department to control it and presented their cause to our high school principal, Miss Belva L. Snodgrass. One by one they presented their grievances: storefront windows soaped, windows broken, streetlights shot out by BB guns, trash cans dumped on streets and sidewalks, the popcorn wagon pushed into the middle of Broadway and tipped over, water hydrants turned on full blast. Adding to the worry, broken liquor bottles suggested the kids were getting drunk.

The police confirmed all this. On Halloween night calls lit up their switchboard from all parts of Rochester with complaints of damage to property. The culprits couldn't be caught. They were lithe young boys who knew the back alleys and safe houses.

That session with Miss Snodgrass, who probably looked sternly around the table at each store owner, undoubtedly left some of the men wondering what good it would do, dumping their woes on a female school principal when even the police were stumped. They didn't know Miss Snodgrass. None of us in Rochester High School at the time will ever forget how she handled the challenge dropped in her lap by the business community.

The next year in September Miss Snodgrass announced a Halloween party. Attendance was mandatory. Miss Snodgrass first involved the parents with the following information given to each student to take home for the parents' signature, to be turned in to the principal. Among Dad's papers I found a copy:

Halloween and Belva L. Snodgrass

Halloween 1935

Name of parent _____

Correct address _____

I understand that _____ has
(name of child)
expressed a desire to have an all-high school party on Halloween, and that _____ has promised to do all in _____ power to make the evening a happy occasion for the entire community. The closing hour of the party is 12 o'clock. All pupils are to be at home, at the high school party, or at some place approved by parents during the evening.

_____ understands that any student who in any sense makes Halloween an occasion to insult neighbors and others of the city will be barred from any participation in any phase of the high school extra-curricular activity during the rest of the school year.

_____ understands that the policy of the Police Department will be to require any person doing damage to pay for it and also that the names of those found guilty will be turned in to the high school principal.

_____ understands that the reason for this is to protect and promote the privileges of the great majority.

_____ understands that students are requested to leave cars at home.

Signature of Parent _____

Every student would have a role to fulfill at this party. Any absence would be noted. Each homeroom would plan and sponsor an event such as games, stunts, skits, food preparation, story telling or whatever. A chairman, committee and helpers would be chosen to include all thirty-five or so kids in the homeroom. The event, with or without help from the teacher, would be repeated continuously until midnight, with different teams of pupils taking over at certain times. When a student wasn't busy in his or her homeroom he or she would be free to roam the building and visit other homerooms and the gym, where two bands would provide continuous music for dancing.

Miss Snodgrass stood at one end of the gym. If a couple was dancing cheek-to-cheek she would go up and tap the boy on the shoulder. In spite of Miss Snodgrass's prudent chaperoning of the dance floor, that Halloween party was undoubtedly the most fabulous party ever engineered by a high school principal. The Rochester police had an easy Halloween night, as they did for several more years when the parties were repeated. After that, I am told, the police took over the role of party-giver.

Our junior/senior high school, with its 1800 students, using two buildings joined by a tunnel, needed a strong top sergeant. Even the big boys respected Miss Snodgrass's rules. When the bell rang for classes to change, we formed lines in the hall moving single file in opposite directions. You could drop out at the ladies' room, but there was no loitering in the halls. Student monitors stood at intervals between the lines. We liked being chosen monitor of the week. It got us out of class early.

Along with Latin and other languages we had English lit, math, history, journalism, home economics for girls and manual training for boys, plus gym and swimming classes. In winter, a swimming class late in the day meant that our hair, if it fell out from under our caps, would be frozen when we got home. We walked to school and home for lunch, then back for afternoon classes which ended at four. On really cold days some of us went in the front door of the College Apartments on Fourth Street, down the warm hall and out the back door. After school there were extracurricular activities, including glee club, play rehearsals, Girl Scouts, etc. Boys on football or track teams walked to Soldiers Field in their uniforms and back to the gym to change. They got home about six.

Misconduct of a minor sort, like tardiness, improper dress, drowsiness in class, loud talk or failure to turn in homework would be reported to Miss Mary Whiting, the assistant principal. A few good students were asked to work in Miss Whiting's office during study period. In addition to clerical jobs they delivered notes to delinquent students, summoning them to Miss Whiting's office immediately. Miss Whiting, a little gray-haired lady, presented a stern face to a miscreant standing humbly before her. "You had to know her to like her," said my sister-in-law, Lillian Miller Masson, who, as a student, was one of Miss Whiting's helpers.

A note from Miss Snodgrass herself was something to worry about all day. Typed instructions above her bold signature might read: "Please report to my office this afternoon at four o'clock."

At the fifty-fifth reunion of the class of 1938, a Peanuts cartoon was reproduced in the *Book of Memories*. There is Linus, the little boy with his blanket, sucking his thumb. Lucy, the bossy girl, says, "Stop it or I'll knock your block off." Linus doesn't move. Lucy threatens again. Finally Lucy says, "I'll report you to Snodgrass!" Linus flips off the floor, his blanket flying.

One day Margaret Helmholz Burchell, an excellent student and athlete, a leader in the ninth grade, was handed a note from Miss Snodgrass. She might have expected a request to head a committee or some other honorable assignment, but no. At four o'clock she met a glowering Miss Snodgrass. In a letter Margie reminded me that Miss Snodgrass had added to the dress code the requirement that girls had to wear stockings and garter belts. (Panty hose had not yet been invented.) "I rebelled," Margie wrote, "and I tried to get by with knee highs. She called me in and asked me who I thought I was, 'some special doctor's kid?'"

It was a cruel remark. Margie could not restrain her tears. It was so unfair. "I don't know when I first became aware that there was a feeling about Pill Hill kids," she wrote. "I truly hated it and tried my best to live it down. It is true we had advantages, but it was up to us to make something of them." In her senior year Margie worked in Miss Snodgrass's office and so had a chance to get to know her and her methods of discipline. "We ended up fast friends," Margie wrote.

I, as probably all of us Pill Hill kids, sensed I had something to live up to in our big all-Rochester student body. We were born privileged. It wasn't comfortable being deferred to, being thought snobbish, just because our fathers were doctors at the Clinic.

Margie Helmholz began early wanting to work at the Clinic. When she was only fourteen, in the midst of the Depression, she was finally allowed to volunteer for a summer job in the Orthopedic Department as a sort of general service person for Dr. Tarara, "the foot man." Every day she went to work. She ran errands, folded bandages, and cleaned up the dressing rooms between patients. She loved her job, especially "listening to Dr. Tarara's chatter as he fixed everyone's feet."

My initial encounter with Miss Snodgrass turned into a slapstick scene. I mustered my courage and went to her office to reply to a question she had asked at assembly for us to think about: "How could we make money for new uniforms for the basketball team?" We could sell cookies and punch during the games, I suggested. She, leaning back in her swivel chair, nodded, her chin protruding. Beginning to relax, I noticed on her desk what I thought was a glass paperweight with pink, white and blue marbles in it. Being nearsighted and not wearing my glasses, I wanted a closer look at the pretty object. The instant I picked it up I knew it wasn't a paperweight. It was a small bowl of little flowers. Water spilled into a dish of paperclips and pencils, slid across the glass desktop into a stack of papers and over the edge to the floor. Mortification!

Miss Snodgrass didn't leap up as the water soaked into her lap. No problem, or words to that effect. She put the dripping papers on the radiator and produced a stack of paper towels. Together we cleaned up the mess. The cookie/punch idea was accepted a week or so later and I was appointed chairman.

When Miss Snodgrass realized the problem of acoustics in our assembly hall had to be addressed she called in Hugh Kendall, whose fame as a problem fixer had come to her attention. She asked him to go out and buy whatever equipment was needed for a public address system in the assembly hall. He could charge it to her. He did, and from then on he was her right-hand man till he graduated in the class of 1934.

When our principal strode onto the stage, we hushed. We felt her authority. We stood and faced the flag and recited the pledge of allegiance to the flag of the United States of America. Miss Snodgrass was hefty, big-boned, with short brown hair, probably with a permanent wave that kept it lifted a little, neat but not stylish. She wore dark skirts and print blouses or a dress with a cardigan sweater and heavy brown shoes. Her jaw was square, and when she listened her brows knitted together, her arms folded across her ample chest, her lower lip protruded.

At assemblies she reminded us of our manners, our reputations, our heritage and the meaning of our school motto, *Nulli Secundi*, second to none. Before all sporting events with neighboring cities, including Red Wing, Winona, Austin, Albert Lea, Fairbault, Mankato and Owatonna, she revved up our school spirit with pep talks about fair play and sportsmanship. We had winning teams in those years.

My brother Jay Masson and Roy Kendall always came in first and second in the breast stroke at swimming meets. They swam the first lap and a half under water, which now is common, but in the 1930's that strategy hadn't been discovered by our competitors. Our pool had very little space around it for spectators. The front row always got wet. When the meet was held in Rochester Mother was always there, leaning precipitously close to the edge, cheering for our boys. People often joked about how hilarious it would be "if Mrs. Masson fell in."

"Memory Training" was the phrase Miss Snodgrass coined for her basic discipline. It meant staying after school for an hour. It was imposed for infractions of rules such as passing a note, whispering in class, tripping someone when classes were changing, shoving or getting out of line, muttering a wisecrack, fighting or yelling in the tunnel between buildings where voices bounced off the walls with great reverberation.

Miss Snodgrass had a subtle way of dealing with matters too sensitive to bring up in assembly before the whole student body. Sex, for instance, was never openly discussed in a mixed group of boys and girls. If she heard a rumor that worried her she called in a few influential students and discussed the matter. Then she gave out accurate answers which those students were instructed to pass along to their friends. Isobel Lobb Jones remembers such a session with Miss Snodgrass when there was talk that you could get syphilis from a public drinking fountain.

Eagle-eyed, scrawny Mr. Ralph Nelson oversaw the study hall during after-school Memory Training. He sat at the elevated desk at the front of the hall and we took seats scattered around the room where, without diversion, we did our homework. When boys tested Mr. Nelson's authority he took them out in the hall and shook them physically. We could see that "conversation" through the window in the door. He never laid a hand on the girls.

Weekdays, with Miss Snodgrass and Mr. Nelson at the helm, our lives were unflaggingly monitored. On Saturday we told our mothers where we were going, such as riding our bikes to Cedar Beach, but we didn't tell everything we planned to do, like taking one of Dad's cigars, lighting it and sharing it around. We never told the lesson we learned: smoking cigars is sickening for beginners.

There were many things the boys did in those junior high school years that were never told till now when, for this book, I began asking questions.

{ 8 }

The Dreams of Youth

> Youth has visions of the future which are not shared to an
> equal extent by those of middle and later age: youth
> is a builder of images, a dreamer of dreams.
> Dr. W. J. Mayo, 1936[1]

On an ordinary, hot summer day in 1935 my brother Stanley and his friend Norman Kendall, both about thirteen years old, went down for a close look at the Mayo Clinic. Rochester then was a town of about 20,000 residents with one tall, beautiful building on its skyline, the Mayo Clinic. That elegant skyscraper of my early years was later renamed for the genius who singlemindedly conceived it and oversaw its construction, Dr. Henry S. Plummer. Some of us Pill Hill children were lured by its mysterious beauty. On bicycles we coasted downtown for a closer look at it, inside and out. We came to think of it as part of our territory, like a museum we were free to enter and browse around in. The two boys on that summer day didn't go to the Clinic as tourists, as we girls often did. They went like challengers for a prize, having promised each other, out of some heedless derring-do, that they would touch the light at the top of the Mayo Clinic. It stops my breath just to think of it.

Stan and Norman went straight up in the elevator to the fourteenth floor. The door to the carillon was unlocked. Jimmy Drummond, who played the bells, wasn't there. No one was. The boys went up the steps past Mr. Drummond's console and higher. Stan's memory of the route they took has both clear and fuzzy spots. A perpendicular steel ladder, he remembers, was attached to a marble wall higher than the bells. Through an airy space between Greek columns a brisk wind blew. At other times the music of the bells flowed out to the countryside like goodwill from the Mayo Clinic.

Studying a photograph of the head and shoulders of the Plummer Building, at the summit the boys aspired to reaching, I see the tiny ladder on the flagpole side of the building. Once they had climbed those steel rungs and were over the wall around the slanting sides of the pyramid at the top, it might have seemed safe to them, a wall around and a stone floor under their feet. Stan remembers, though, the terror he felt at knowing they had yet to crawl over roofing tiles to reach the cupola that houses the light. I asked him if Norm was as scared as he was, and he said, "Norm was a better climber, so maybe he wasn't. I just remember that when we got to the top we came immediately down."

An older pair of boys, my brother Jay and Norm's brother Roy Kendall, also went up to the bell tower in search of adventure. They went to the area where griffons and gargoyles embellish the outer walls. Jay said he watched his best friend climb over the enclosure around the bells and down, like a mountaineer without a safety rope, to the back of a stone griffon.

"I couldn't watch," Jay said. "Looking straight down you could see Joe Clinic (the doorman), small as a doll, helping people out of cars, escorting them up steps to the bronze front doors of the Clinic. I was scared to death all the while Roy was out there riding the griffon. But you know Roy; heights didn't scare him. He had perfect balance like some people have perfect pitch."

Yes, we all knew Roy. I remember watching him climb to the top of our tallest pine tree and swing with it, holding on with one hand. Another time he scaled the side of the water tower in Saint Mary's park. Bob Roesler remembers Roy on the unprotected beams of the Willius's house on Eighth Avenue when it was under construction. And Carol Haines Anderson told me she saw Roy from her bedroom window walking on his hands along the ridge of the Kendalls' roof, shortly after he came home from the hospital when his appendix was removed.

To my mind, the most impressive scheme hatched by the boys was the "Drawkcab" language invented by Jay, Roy and Dave Berkman. We knew the code for translating; it was just backward spelling. But they spoke so rapidly we couldn't figure it out. "Stel teg dir fo eht slrig," for

The Dreams of Youth

example, would mean, "Let's get rid of the girls." I thought their invention was uniquely theirs, but, to my surprise, an AP story in the *Charlotte Observer*[2] published a picture of a girl named Kelly Inch, a computer expert in the cardiology department of Duke Medical Center, who had attracted the attention of Garrison Keillor, and was on his "Prairie Home Companion" radio show. Her talent was Drawkcab. He talked her into singing "Jingle Bells" backward.

We young junior high girls didn't seem interesting to the boys, but our presence must have been like a bleachers full of fans to a football team. We probably bolstered their self-esteem. They showed off spectacularly. In addition to speaking Drawkcab, they raced their bikes, making them leap over curbs; rode no-hands and backward, sitting on the handlebars. They whistled louder and shriller than any girl. They handled tools well and built tree houses. Jay and Roy each built a kayak from a kit. Stan and Dick Thorson made a diving bell, a small copy of the big one built by Hugh Kendall. A triumph for my youngest brother Bill was the milkshake mixer he made from a motor found in the city dump. Later he built radios from spare parts.

These boys had a yen to gain acceptance from a beloved and often absent father. This need was acknowledged by Dr. Charles W. Mayo, known as "Chuck," in his autobiography, *Mayo: The Story of My Family and My Career*.[3] Young Charles William Mayo, the son of Dr. Charlie, worked through his awkward years and became a handsome, universally esteemed man like his father and an excellent surgeon. He was one of eight children growing up at Mayowood with Dr. Charlie and his lovely wife Edith. A friend, Dr. William D. Haggard of Nashville, was visiting at Mayowood one day when Dr. Charlie came home from a long, tiring day at work. Dr. Haggard watched the children come running when they heard their father's car on the gravel driveway. They met him with squeals, wrestled him to the floor in a gleeful free-for-all tussle.

Dr. Haggard said to Edith, "That poor man can't get any rest at home. He needs . . . ." Edith pointed to her husband. "Don't worry about Charlie," she said. "Look at him." The children were flopped all over their father. His eyes were closed; he was sound asleep.

Dr. Chuck worked hard to measure up to the standards set by his father and his Uncle Will. It took a few years for him to become his own man, not just the son and nephew of the two world-famous Mayos. In his autobiography, he describes his feelings:

Pill Hill

It wasn't surprising that as a young man I should have felt a wretched sense of my own inferiority. My brother Joe and I eventually had discovered that our father and uncle were world-famous men, not only respected in countries we scarcely could spell, but revered. If one of them was ill halfway across the continent, tracks were cleared so the other could rush to his side and the newspapers would chronicle the trip on their front pages. As a small child, I had an adoring relationship with my genial father but saw little of him. As a teenager I was intimidated by his importance.[4]

Whatever it was that drove the creative engines in the boys who grew up around me on Pill Hill, it affected us young girls differently. We were no longer tomboys. We felt like independent, sophisticated girls, proud of our fathers who worked for the Mayo Clinic. We kept secrets from our parents. With a Girl Scout knife we cut off short sections of grapevine in Bumpus's pasture or Kendall's Canyon. We lit them with matches from Dad's tobacco cabinet and smoked that woody, throat-searing vine. Some girls brought cigarettes from home. Once after a Girl Scout meeting, on our way home through the alley behind Madge Mussey's house on Second Street, we discussed the latest rumor. Madge, in those days, was known as "Squawk." Squawk said she heard you could get drunk by taking an aspirin and drinking a coke at the same time. Ginny Moersch said she would try it, but I wouldn't have taken the risk; if it worked, and I was seen staggering around, my parents would hear of it and be terribly ashamed.

When we were old enough for boyfriends, we discovered kissing a boy was exciting. We kissed a boy when no one was looking, on the walk home from a movie between mouthfuls of popcorn, and at the side door saying goodnight. When "necking" advanced to "petting," fear intervened. A line was drawn. No girl in her right mind, headed for college, would be heedless enough about romance to risk getting pregnant. The boys as well as the girls of our generation understood this. Fear kept us straight. A date to us meant singing, dancing, skating, bowling, bike riding, going to movies, running barefoot in the rain on the golf course. Silly, fun things. We drank root beer, milk shakes or cherry-flavored Coca-Cola at the drug store. Most of the Pill Hill parents that I knew didn't drink at home or serve alcohol at parties. Drugs were unheard of.

The Dreams of Youth

So, we weren't swept into unintended, oblivious sexual activity. I didn't know anyone, even in the expanded neighborhood of Rochester High School, who dropped out of school to get married and have a baby. Having a baby without a husband would have been unthinkable to my peers. After all, we knew the contemptuous "B" word for the innocent child of an unmarried woman.

But we young girls *did* know a grim Pill Hill scandal. None of us spoke of it to our parents; they learned of it through the grapevine of their friends. It happened in the late 1920's in Kendall's Canyon.

Kendall's Canyon was a deep and verdant ravine, a split in the crust of the Pill Hill neighborhood so unmanageable as part of a safe, orderly neighborhood that to this day, it remains an interruption of Seventh Street between Eighth and Ninth Avenues. When it rained, water gushed down the gutters of Ninth Avenue and into a culvert. It spewed like a waterfall into Kendall's Canyon. We loved that wild jungle. On hot summer days its leafy canopy gave us a cool place to play. A wall on one side propped up Dr. Fred Moersch's driveway. A dirt path on the other side went downhill from Ninth Avenue to Eighth Avenue with access through a hedge to the driveways of the Kendalls, the Keiths and the Helmholzes.

Dominating the Moersch side of the canyon was a granddaddy of the cottonwood family of trees and some huge gray boulders. The tree had been there so long the grape vines that grew up its trunk had branched and tangled into its upper limbs and hung over the ravine as tough as Tarzan's vines. Older children would swing on the vines, sweeping across the gulch and back to the smooth boulder as if to the back of an elephant.

Late in the afternoon of the day I have in mind, a group of Edison School boys were digging a cave into the bank at the lower end of the canyon. With shovels and trowels they scooped out a pile of sandy soil, creating a hole in the bank big enough for a hibernating bear and her cubs. Then the streetlights came on, the signal for the boys to go home. A few days later they gathered at the canyon again to continue their excavation. It had rained in the meantime. The usual torrent had dashed through the canyon, washing away most of the loose soil the boys had scraped out of their cave.

One jab with a trowel exposed the top of a cardboard box. Among the boys who dug up the box were Roy and Hugh Kendall, Henry Stark, Ed Meyerding and Bob Roesler. Bob, now retired from his career at the Clinic in many administrative capacities, remembers the excitement they all felt as they dug the box out of the ground. It was a letdown when they pulled back the flaps and saw only a doll in the box. Someone reached for it and jerked his hand back. It was not a doll; it was a dead baby. The children ran home, terrified, and told their parents.

The next day the dark news spread among the children of the neighborhood, and presumably also among the parents: a dead baby, one or two days old, was found buried in Kendall's Canyon. Whose baby? What hideous secret was buried in that wet ground?

That event remains as hearsay for most of my younger Rochester contemporaries. But the boys who discovered that cardboard box will never forget the drama they were drawn into.

The parents immediately called the police. One can only surmise how the identity of the baby's mother became known. She was a live-in maid at the Finney's house. Did Mrs. Finney, after getting the Finney children off to school, knock on the door to the girl's room and find her weak, tearful and bleeding? When the boys discovered the evidence a day later, the police and the doctors must have exchanged information, uncovering the truth.

The following morning an early phone call to the Kendalls' house informed Dr. Kendall that his son, Hugh, was required at the county courthouse as a material witness to a crime. "No," Dr. Kendall said into the telephone, "I don't want Hugh to testify in this matter." He said goodbye and hung up.

The other boys were also summoned as witnesses. The boys would be paid five dollars for their testimony.

The next day a police car drove into the Kendalls' driveway as the Kendalls were having breakfast. A polite policeman handed Mrs. Kendall an official document demanding the presence of ten-year-old Hugh as a material witness at the inquest.

When Dr. Kendall read the order he let out a roar that could be heard next door at the Keiths'. He strode into the yard after the retreating policeman. "I thought I made myself clear on the telephone!" he yelled. "I won't allow my son to be used in this way!"

"I'm sorry, Sir, but this summons is issued on the order of . . . ."

"I don't give a damn whose order it is! I am the father and this is my son we're talking about!"

The argument didn't go any further. The policeman left, refusing to take back the summons.

The Dreams of Youth

Never in his life had Hugh seen his father so angry. Red-faced with righteousness, he stormed around the house muttering, defending his right as a father to protect his son from hearing a sordid story of sex and sin. The poor girl on the stand would be forced to tell the circumstances of her pregnancy, who the father was, and was the baby born dead, or did she bury it alive?

Dr. Kendall called his friend Judge Burt Eaton and sputtered out his fury. The judge said, "Calm down, Nick. I'll fix it." And he did. The name Hugh Kendall was crossed off the list of witnesses.

This horror story would be today's ordinary soap opera. All its lurid details would be on television and in newspapers. But in those days, publishers and the press were more discreet; the story was never released to the public.

We children knew our mothers went to the hospital to have a baby and stayed there for ten days at least. What agony it would have been for that unfortunate girl living at the Finneys' to feel so afraid and friendless she had to go through delivery all by herself. Did she come from the country, a farmer's daughter who got a job in Rochester hoping to have a happier life in a bigger world? If she had trusted her parents she'd have gone home with her trouble. Mother, trying to foster communication with her distant young daughter, once said there was nothing I could do she wouldn't understand and want to help me with. If we girls thought of the Finneys' maid now and then, she must have served richly as a parable of the wanton girl.

We will always grieve to remember the brief, heedless romance in the life of one of our own, lovely Anne Louise Meyerding. Her friends were awed and envious when she said she had a date. She told them all—Meg Crenshaw, Carol Haines, Helen Keith, Janet Stark, Portia Vinson and others—but she didn't tell her parents, Dr. and Mrs. Henry W. Meyerding. They wouldn't approve; fourteen, they thought, was too young. She told the boy to come when her parents had left for the graduation exercises of their son, Ed, from Rochester High School's class of 1936.

Down Sixth Street the two on a bicycle sped. Anne Louise probably whispered, "Where are we going?" and he might have said, "Would you like a root beer float?"

They rode like the wind, downhill. She on his handlebars leaned against him, liking his speed, his style, the fact that he was older, a junior. Her hair streamed across his face, and her warm shoulder pressed his chest, her feet and slender legs out straight, her hands beside his on the handlebars, gripping. It was a glorious moment.

At the corner of Sixth Street and Eighth Avenue they were hit by a car driven by a responsible young driver. No one could have stopped in time to avoid the bicycle in the dusk as it raced into the intersection. Carol Haines and Helen Keith at the top of the hill heard the squeal of brakes, the terrible crash. They ran down the stone steps, past the Helmholz's tennis court. Jack Hempstead, a passenger in the car, sat on its running board, his head in his hands.

"That was the tragedy of my young life, what we found there," Carol Haines Anderson told me. Anne Louise was killed instantly and her date seriously injured.

Mother recorded in her diary on June 4, 1936: "Jay's graduation at 8 pm. Exercises went off without a hitch and I was so proud of dear Jay. For 18 years he has been a joy to us!"

The following day, Mother learned the dreadful news. For many days afterwards she wrote of Henry and Lura Meyerding and the small things friends did for friends at such a time: "Took Mrs. Stinchfield and Mother Meyerding to ride, kept Ed here for meals. They are all so pathetic. Poor Lura! My heart aches for her."

"Youth has visions of the future which are not shared . . . by those of middle and later age. Youth is a builder of images, a dreamer of dreams."[5]

Dr. Will wrote these words in 1936 in a paper for an audience of medical educators. There is something capricious in human nature that sometimes squanders the dreams of youth.

{ 9 }

Exploring the Mayo Clinic

[Study within these buildings] does not make brains but merely molds them and equips them for more and greater work.
Dr. Charles H. Mayo, 1926[1]

EXPLORING the Mayo Clinic was a pleasant way for us girls to have some fun on a slow summer day. But on one breezy spring day my friend Jean Davis (now Mrs. Charles Warman of Wichita Falls, Texas) and I walked to the Clinic after school with something special in mind. We went up on the elevator to the eleventh floor, dropped our books in the lounge of the Ladies' Room and opened a window. We were ready to test the power of wind, a science project we hadn't discussed with our teacher. Air currents always hit the sheer limestone wall at the front of the Clinic building and slid along it to the southwest corner where pedestrians on the Second Street sidewalk were buffeted by a wind that often blew their hats off. How long a strand of toilet paper, Jean and I wondered, would the wind support when released from a window this high up? How long would it stay airborne?

We dangled a few feet of a full roll out the window. It fluttered in the breeze till it tore loose and slowly staggered down to the street. We were littering, of course, but our excitement overcame guilt as we tried different launching techniques. After some experimentation we stayed with the best. Taking turns, we reached out over the windowsill with a roll of toilet paper loosely unwinding over a pencil which we held at each end. A long streamer reeled out, buoyed up on a steady horizontal current of wind. When it broke off, we started another. Soon we had two long white streamers floating high above cars, people on the sidewalk and Joe Fritsch. Joe was the Clinic's official greeter, known fondly by all of us as Joe

Clinic. Always jovial, he opened the doors of cars and taxis and escorted people who needed help up the steps and through the bronze front doors to the lobby of the Clinic. In a later upgrading to benefit patients unsteady on their feet, the street was raised to the level of the first floor, making the front entrance wheelchair friendly.

One blustery zero-degree day, Joe Clinic in his fur-lined mittens, boots, long navy blue great coat and beaver hat with ear muffs was at the front door of the Clinic greeting patients arriving in cars and taxies when Dr. Philip S. Hench joined him for a chat. Dr. Hench was chief of the Clinic's department of rheumatic diseases. He worked with Dr. E. C. (Nick) Kendall in the testing of the pain killer cortisone, which Dr. Kendall had isolated from many tons of adrenal glands provided by the Hormel Meat Packing Company of Austin, Minnesota. Together, the two Clinic doctors and a Swiss chemist, Tadeus Reichstein, were awarded the 1950 Nobel Prize for physiology and medicine. Dr. Hench, like Joe Clinic, was an amiable man. He usually had lots to say on many subjects and was often invited to speak at medical meetings in spite of the fact that he was hard to understand. He didn't speak with a foreign accent; he had a cleft palate, but it wasn't evident. There was no cleft in his upper lip. His speech was like a punctuated hum that humped over the S's and resonated in his nasal cavities.

On this particular day, a man with a cleft palate and also a cleft upper lip came up to Dr. Hench as he and Joe Clinic were talking and asked in hollow nasal syllables how to get to the Clinic Library. Dr. Hench turned to Joe and shrugged. Joe gave the visitor directions.

When the man had left, Joe turned to Dr. Hench and demanded, "Why didn't you answer the man?"

Dr. Hench in his humming voice replied indignantly, "Do you think I want my block knocked off?"

Only twice did Joe Fritsch not come to work. On those days the beautiful, sculptured bronze front doors of the Plummer Building were closed. Those were the sad days in April and July of 1939 when the two Doctors Mayo died, Dr. Charlie of pneumonia and then Dr. Will of cancer of the stomach. Everything in Rochester closed on those two days. Flags flew at half-staff and everyone stayed home. All over the world the deaths of those two great men, once described as "the infrangible brotherhood," were noted with sorrow.

On that windy day in my youth the best efforts of my friend Jean and me at testing the power of wind could not have met a more spectacular denouement. Our fragile streamer fluttered across the intersection of Second Street and Second Avenue, lost its drive and settled decorously into the branches of a tree in front of the Congregational Church. One floor below us Jean's father, Dr. Austin C. Davis, in his office on the tenth floor, went to his window to discover the source of the phenomenon of the floating ribbons. Jean, in a letter to me recently, wrote, "Do you remember, Lena [a name they called me]? I was leaning out with a very successful streamer, and there was my father looking straight into my eyes!" Dr. Davis was a likeable blue-eyed diagnostician with a special interest in exophthalmic goiter, or Graves disease. He never told on us. His wife, Helen Davis, might have been less respectful of our inspired experiment.

That mysteriously decorated tree in front of the church caused quite a stir among adults as well as children. How, people wondered, could anyone throw a roll of toilet paper in a way that would cause it to drape its length so expertly in the very top of that tree? Perhaps the firemen with a ladder pulled off an April Fool joke in the middle of the night? Jean and I enjoyed all the talk.

Several years before Dr. Davis reached age sixty-five, the Clinic's age for retirement, his vision was severely impaired by macular degeneration in both eyes. He was unable to see patients or write reports. To think of himself as a man without a job, without value to the Clinic, would have been a devastating blow to him. Rather than let this happen to Dr. Davis, the Clinic created a need for his talents. Calls from patients wanting a conference over the phone were relayed to his office, where he would listen to their problems and ask the right questions. Then he set up an appointment with an appropriate specialist.

An ordinary Saturday exploration of the Clinic for us junior high girls always began on bicycles. We coasted down Fourth Street, went over a block to Third and into an alley beside the Worrall Hospital. We leaned our bikes against the wall, entered the side door of the hospital and went down a flight of steps to the white-tiled tunnel lit by two rows of overhead lights. Our tour began here in the subway system. One-and-a-half miles of heated and, in later years, cooled underground walkways were built in the 1930's. The tunnels are a great advantage to patients and their companions in Minnesota's snowy winters and often 90-degree August heat. They connect the Mayo Clinic with hotels and all parts of its service except Saint Mary's Hospital, which was more than one straight mile down Second Street.

We heard rumors that some of the Pill Hill boys had sneaked their bikes down those stairs and raced around the tunnels. It was probably true.

We girls usually had the place to ourselves since patients, at least in good weather, preferred to be outdoors between appointments. If there were wheelchairs by the elevator, we borrowed one. We took turns being the pusher or the pushee, the girl with a sprained ankle. At intersections arrows pointed in several directions: to the Mayo Clinic, the hospitals (Damon, Worrall, Kahler and Colonial), the Diet Kitchen, three hotels (Kahler, Zumbro and Damon) and the Franklin Heating Station. We headed for the latter. From the doorway looking in, this furnace room seemed like a science fiction movie set for the comic strip "Buck Rogers in the 21st Century," a neat arrangement of big, clean, colorful machines with pipes, wheels and dials like clock faces. Today it does more than warm the Plummer Building, the Worrall Hospital and the Kahler Hotel. Greatly expanded, it now supplies cold drinking water from two deep wells; hot, softened water for laundry; and steam, electricity and refrigeration for the sixteen or more buildings of the Mayo Rochester campus.

But, there's a sad chapter in the early history of the Franklin Heating Station. A year or two after a group of us girls lingered in that warm doorway, an explosion ripped the room asunder, caused by a leak in the gas line. That weekend a convention of the High Y Clubs of Minnesota met in Rochester, sponsored by the YMCA. High school boys from all over the state were in town staying with Rochester families. Mother wrote in her diary, November 2, 1932, "... We have two nice lads from Albert Lea as house guests. Both are Eagle Scouts." The boys were exploring the Clinic's tunnels when the accident happened. Mother reported the following day, "... a terrible gas explosion in the Clinic power plant at noon. Two persons were killed and eight injured. Curtis Keller, one of the boys we had last night, was badly hurt and is in the Colonial."

It is fortunate that Dr. Henry Plummer insisted, when the plant was in the planning stage, that it should be housed in its own building since it might need to be expanded in the future. Had the explosion occurred in a hospital basement, as some of the building committee advised, the devastation might have been comparable to Rochester's worst disaster, the tornado of 1883.

Distant footsteps echoed in these underground walkways. Sometimes we passed a person with a bandage at the bend of his or her elbow, indicating they had had a blood test at the hematology lab. We said hello to anyone we met, and we planned that if somebody needed a wheelchair we'd give them ours and push them up the ramp to the Clinic where somebody at General Service would take them where they needed to go.

Next on our tour was the Diet Kitchen. We stood in the doorway getting hungry watching people eat. Patients went there to learn how to prepare special diets when they returned home. Today the tunnels are bright, colorful arcades lined with shops selling fine clothes, beaded deerskin jackets, gloves and moccasins, luggage, crafts, toys and delicacies from everywhere. Weber & Judd is still in business to fill prescriptions, independently operated like all the shops.

At the broad entrance to the Clinic we left our wheelchair with the others parked like grocery carts at the A&P. We drank from the fountain, the "bubbler" we called it, and walked up one flight of stairs to the lobby with its beautiful marble floor of many colors. Next, we took the elevator to my father's floor. The desk girls told us if he was there. If not, he was operating at Saint Mary's or the Colonial, and we'd say hello to his secretary, Miss Predmore. If he was there with a patient and the door was closed, we sat and waited till he came out. When he did, he'd be happy to see us and would introduce us to his patient, who usually said something nice. We felt like very special children.

This unquestioned acceptance of us as worthy of notice by adults in their place of business gave us, myself at least, a flawed impression of the world beyond our town. I had to unlearn the notion that I could walk into the boss's office if the door was open, and that he would welcome me with a smile and introduce me to anyone else in the room. Once in 1944, as a junior-grade chemist at the National Institutes of Health in Bethesda, Maryland, during World War II, I dropped in on my boss, Dr. Fairhall, with a simple question to ask. He was talking with Dr. Neal, another department head. Both men turned stony faces to me in my white technician's uniform. In the excruciating pause I caught on, said, "Excuse me," in barely a whisper, and retreated.

Pill Hill

We children in the 1930's felt at home in the Mayo Clinic's beautiful skycraper. We enjoyed looking at people from all over the world. Some were very fit. They walked briskly and smiled at us. Some of the ladies wore floor-length costumes, bright shawls and dangling jeweled earrings. They chattered in a foreign language and scolded their children who wiggled on the leather seat cushions. These dark-eyed children watched with envy our freedom to weigh ourselves on the tall scale, to drink and dabble at the fountain, to push the elevator button and disappear.

Other patients looked drab and gray, leaning together like sacks of mail at the post office. We felt sorry for them. They were too fat or too skinny, lame and old. When their names were called they rose slowly, one helping the other shuffle across the rug to the smiling girl who had called their name.

I asked Dad about people like that and he said, "I wish they had come sooner. We could have helped more."

"Maybe they couldn't afford it," I said.

"That wouldn't matter," he said. "They'd be cared for the same as anyone else."

That philosophy has been Mayo Clinic policy from the beginning. Before the Mayos even had a building of their own, Dr. Will Mayo wrote, "The best interest of the patient is the only interest to be considered."

Before we returned to our bicycles we had a few more doors to open. We got off the elevator at the fourteenth floor, the top of the building, not counting the carillon. We opened the heavy door to Plummer Hall and flipped the light switch. Our fingers traced the intricate carving on the oak wall panels, touched the velvety backs of chairs as we passed behind them. Red velvet drapes fell to the floor beside stained glass windows. Facing the auditorium was a magnificent mantelpiece. Lucy Wilder, the wife of Dr. R. M. Wilder and owner of Rochester's best little bookstore west of the Mississippi, refers to this mantelpiece in her book, *The Mayo Clinic*, as "composed of violet Formosa marble from Germany."[2] Above it in an elaborate gold frame hung the stern face of the old patriarch, the horse and buggy doctor, William Worrall Mayo. He looked like the man he was said to be, one who never left an argument in limbo. Superstition and flimsy thinking were anathema to Dr. W. W. Mayo. When he found a serious infection under a slathering of goose grease he firmly rebuked whoever had applied that loathsome, pestiferous, virulent, old-fashioned goo.

Louise Abigail, his wife, described her husband as a forward-looking man. She said that looking backward is not a good thing for one's soul. But one Sunday morning everyone in church knew the doctor's wife was not listening to the sermon, she was looking backward. Helen Clapesattle records that Mrs. Mayo rose suddenly from the pew and said in a loud voice, "God Almighty! I left my bread in the oven!"[3]

The old doctor looked down from his portrait on us young girls with a quizzical expression, as if he expected us to answer a question he had asked. His portrait is not there now; it is displayed in some other building on the expanded Mayo campus. On my most recent visit to Plummer Hall three gold-framed portraits of three other forward-looking, admirable men faced the seats in the auditorium, men I remember as they were at the height of their careers: Dr. Will Mayo, Dr. Charles Mayo and Dr. Henry Plummer.

Plummer Hall seemed to me a more sacred place than the Congregational Church where I attended Sunday School. Graceful ghosts of profoundly moral men and women seemed present here. We young preteens listened to the silence as if expecting a voice to come out of it. Important matters had been raised here, issues had been resolved or left for more study. Young doctors not yet self-confident learned to speak in their own voices here.

Dr. O. C. Clagett in his autobiography described meetings in Plummer Hall after Wednesday evening pathology conferences.[4] Dr. Will and Dr. Charlie always sat in the front row if they were in town. Any fellowship student or member of the staff could ask for a place on the program to present a paper of scientific interest. He might describe a series of patients with a common problem or report on what he had learned on a trip to another medical center. Dr. Clagett declared he had never been so frightened in his life as when he first delivered a paper to the august group meeting in that room. His topic was tuberculosis of the stomach. In the front row sat four of the world's authorities on the subject: Dr. Will, Dr. Charlie, Dr. Plummer and Dr. Donald Balfour. What made that evening's reading a fulfilling experience for young Dr. Clagett was receiving a note from Dr. Will, congratulating him for giving a fine presentation.

The door to the carillon tower was locked, so we girls couldn't get up to see the huge bells that lofted their majestic clanging over the Zumbro River Valley. Once, when the bells were new, my father had led me up the steep steps to see them being played by that bell-ringing specialist, Mr. Jimmy Drummond.

Jack Pemberton recalls that once he and a friend, exploring the Clinic, were lucky enough to find the door to the tower open. Jimmy Drummond invited them in for his five o'clock recital. "He had an electric keyboard inside and a manual one out among the bells," Jack wrote in a letter to me. He remembers watching Mr. Drummond "work up a sweat in sub-zero weather, putting all the energy he had into the manual keyboard."

I, thinking of piano keys, didn't understand why it would take such energy to play a keyboard. Then, Carol Haines Anderson added some new information. She once saw Mr. Drummond playing the bells wearing boxing gloves!

We young explorers of the Clinic often saved for last a visit to the Mayo Foundation Museum of Hygiene and Medicine. I remember especially a lifelike wax model sculpted by the museum director, Dr. Arthur H. Bulbulian, the torso of an actual case, a farmer who had fallen off a hay wagon onto the prongs of a pitchfork. The tines entered his chest and protruded from his back. We were relieved to read in the description of how the accident was treated that the man made a good recovery. We also inspected the world's first transparent man. All his inner parts were visible as he rotated on a pedestal, arms uplifted. In 1933 the transparent man was displayed at the Century of Progress Exposition in Chicago. Another interesting display in the museum was a series of colored wax models of an appendix operation, also sent to Chicago for the Century of Progress Exposition.

As we made ourselves at home in the Clinic we often saw grownups who knew us. Once on an elevator somebody's grandmother in a blue straw hat with a short polka dot veil said, "Hello, Helen. How are the goats?"

I told her Biff had chewed Bang's leather collar off so Sylvester made them new collars out of chain. Later I asked my friend, "Who was that lady?"

"I thought you knew," she said. "That was Mrs. Hattie Mayo, Dr. Will's wife."

10

Sunday Picnics

> Probably in the not far distant future we will crawl out of our
> old methods of education, as a snake sheds its skin,
> and reorganize a new plan.
> Dr. Charles H. Mayo[1]

SUNDAYS were slow days for most of us in the '20's and '30's. A lingering morality left over from the Blue Laws imposed on colonial New England made many of the things we liked to do taboo on Sunday. In the South, I am told, if you weren't in church, you visited Grandma, still in your Sunday clothes. In Canada, according to Cousin Allan, "you couldn't even play Parchisi." In Rochester the stores and both movie theaters were closed on Sunday, and few people worked. Doctors with patients in the hospitals, of course, made rounds while most of the mothers and children attended one of several denominations of church and/or Sunday School. After that we had a big Sunday dinner.

We Massons then, if it wasn't raining, went for a ride in the car. We had a dark blue, seven-passenger Packard with folding jump seats and running boards. Seat belts hadn't been invented, so there was constant motion among us children in the back.

Mother, with Billy on her lap, tried to direct our energies in peaceful channels. Bouncing was not all right, and neither was throwing paper out the windows. It would spoil the looks of the roadside. We were not litterbugs. We pleaded with mother, "Not even a scrap *this* little?" Well... Mother could be talked into things if we made sensible points. She had to admit that newspaper or a paper napkin torn in tiny pieces and given to the wind, one by one, over a series of miles, would not litter the landscape. So, for our entertainment, one Sunday we tore up the

Pill Hill

entire *Rochester Post Bulletin,* letting loose little half-inch petals of newsprint over miles of country roads.

 Sometimes we came upon a string of Burma Shave signs, advertisements for a new shaving cream competing against the old-fashioned shaving brush and soap. Bouncing and giggling, we avidly read aloud and memorized those witty shaving cream ads that appeared on three, four or five wooden signs planted in the ground, one phrase per sign, about forty yards apart along the shoulder of the highway:

> Pity all
> the mighty caesars
> they pulled each whisker out
> with tweezers.

> Beneath this stone
> lies Elmer Gush
> tickled to death
> by his shaving brush.

> A peach looks good
> with lots of fuzz
> but man's no peach
> and never was.

> Said Juliet to Romeo
> If you won't shave
> go homeo.

> Don't stick your elbow
> out too far
> It might go home
> in another car.

 We got loud and competitive playing "Cats, Dogs and Horses," with two extra points for goats. Cows didn't count; there were so many of them. Dad had excellent distance vision. You were lucky to be on his team, the left side of the car.

Sunday Picnics

Sometimes we hung things out the windows to watch them flap. If it was Billy's favorite bunny rabbit or my sweater the tease didn't last long; Mother intervened. Sometimes a toy, like an airplane with a whirling propeller, escaped into the wind and we screamed, "Stop, stop!" Dad would put on the brakes, and we were eagerly out of the car and racing down the road to find the lost item. On those country roads we rarely saw a car, and, since it was Sunday, not even a man plowing a field. I always liked the route that had a little stream to ford. Once, however, the water was high; the underbelly of the car got wet and the motor conked out midstream. A farmer with a horse finally pulled us out and we got going again. That farmer and his kids were probably glad they had something interesting to do that Sunday afternoon.

Sometimes on that ride in the country we sang songs together, and sometimes we tried to drown each other out with a different song. One day after we finished Old MacDonald's noisy farm animals, Mother began singing a funny song we didn't know, like the barroom song from some opera. I can't remember the words, but its verses were followed by laughter: "Ha ha ha, ho ho hee, ha ha ho ho, hee hee hee." It was so contagious we three in the back seat joined in with wild laughter till Billy put his hands over Mother's mouth and she put a stop to the ruckus.

Some days those Sunday rides must have driven our poor mother batty. One day when the weather was wet and blustery and we all had friends in and were running all over the house, she wrote in her diary, "How could a woman in a tenement with nine children on a rainy day keep her sanity!"

I remember with sorrow one of those Sunday afternoon rides in the country when our heedless energy was too much for Mother. We begged her to sing the laughing song again. She didn't want to. We were oblivious to how she felt and pushed her into it. Some deep grief welled up in her and the jolly song put her in tears. My brothers and I had never seen our mother cry before. Dad reached over and patted her, but we kids were just stunned, silent in the back seat.

Perhaps Mother's sudden sobbing that Sunday was triggered by a tragedy that hit the Sistrunk family who lived two houses up the street from us. Their oldest son David was riding his bike in front of their house when he was hit by a car. A strong, healthy boy, he lived four weeks in a coma before he died. Mother grieved for friends. Her diary records her daily thoughts of her close friend Celia Sistrunk. When the Sistrunks left Rochester to return to their roots in Texas, Mother wrote, September 10, 1929: "It makes me sick to see the Sistrunk's house all empty. They're at the Kahler [hotel] and will leave tomorrow for good. Dallas is so far!"

Often in those years we had picnics at the Butlin's farm, about ten miles southeast of Rochester. Mrs. Butlin, an elderly patient of Dad's, and her husband gave us a standing invitation to come to the farm for picnics in their pasture on Sunday afternoons. By then the cows on their rounds of the pasture would have gone past our favorite picnic spot where the Root River was shady, the shore sandy and the stream shallow. We went there often on Sunday with our picnic blankets, a basket of food, a thermos of lemonade and my fox terrier, Taffy. In the Butlin's pasture Taffy had one objective, to dig gophers out of their holes.

Many a picnic at Butlin's pasture ended with Taffy refusing to come when called. Her constant yipping, though, let us know she had found a gopher hole with a gopher in it and was oblivious to everything but the exotic scent from the underground tunnel she was excavating. Behind her was a big pile of dirt, getting higher as she dug deeper, her short black tail wagging with frantic hope. One time I found her with a poor little gopher in her mouth. Full of pride, she let me have it; it was motionless, a little bloody. Tears rolled down my cheeks as I ran back to the mothers and smaller children on the picnic blanket, the warm little thing in my cupped hands. They clustered around me. "Is it dead?" they asked. Mother wrote in her diary, "Helen said, 'He's kinda dead.'"

One of the families who used to join us on picnics in the Butlin's pasture was Ethyl and Gordon New and their three children, Marion, Bud and Bob. Aunt Ethyl's father, a dour Canadian, didn't approve of higher education for women, so Ethyl had left home to take a nursing course in Boston. She came to the Clinic for further training in anesthesiology, met the attractive young fellow-Canadian, Dr. Gordon B. New, and married him.

On those Sunday picnics, we younger kids liked playing in the stream, damming the flow of water and floating toy boats. My brother Jay, about ten years old, preferred to follow Dad and Uncle Gordon downstream with their rifles. They'd shoot at a selected target across the river. Dad

Sunday Picnics

was a stickler for the proper handling of a gun, and his rules applied even to the pop guns that shot corks. If you pointed a gun at anybody, it would be taken away from you for a period of time. Jay and Stan, looking back on our childhood, are amazed at the casual way they and their friends carried BB guns around from the age of twelve on up.

Dr. Gordon New, who came as a fellow to the Clinic from Canada in 1910, became one of three plastic surgeons known as the best in the world. He credited his skill to the unprecedented number and variety of burns and facial wounds he treated in England during World War II when London was being ravaged by Nazi air raids. Dr. New was innovative in caring for injuries never before described in medical literature. During the evacuation of London he invited one of his British colleagues in plastic surgery, Dr. Archibald McIndoe, to send his family to Rochester. Dr. New's youngest son, Bob, remembers how enthusiastically all of Rochester welcomed the McIndoes with a place to live, a school for their children and the everyday necessities. Their eldest daughter Adonia, with her charming British accent, was a popular student in Bob's school.

Very little cosmetic surgery was being done at the Mayo Clinic when Dr. New was head of the section in plastic surgery. My brother Jay was trained by him and became Dr. New's first assistant after he returned from service in the Korean War. Jay remembers his chief's strict cosmetic surgery parameters. He was willing to nip up droopy eyelids that interfered with a patient's vision to the point where she had to tilt her head back to read. If he thought surgery would relieve a psychological problem, Dr. New would reshape a bulbous nose. But he disapproved of "frivolous" surgery; if a patient looked good to him, he wouldn't be talked into rearranging her face. His specialty was reconstructive procedures to correct serious distortions caused by cancer or accidental injury.

"It's a funny thing about Uncle Gordon," Jay once said. "When I was assigned to his section in plastic surgery, I was introduced as 'Dr. Masson.' Ever after that, it was as if we had never met before. Never once did he call me 'Jay' or ask about my family, or even meet my eyes and smile. He seemed to have forgotten the picnics at Butlin's pasture and the old close family connection. He was a wonderful teacher, but it surprised me, how tight his professional personality was."

Pill Hill

When Uncle Morrie, Dad's youngest brother, came to the Clinic on a fellowship, he began dating a nurse; I think her name was Alice. Alice's mother came to visit, and Uncle Morrie suggested a picnic lunch. They headed for Butlin's pasture with a blanket, a folding chair for Alice's mother, who was stout, and the usual basket of food and lemonade.

It was early in the day and the cows were midway in their grazing route back to the barn. Uncle Morrie spread the blanket under the shade tree and Alice got out paper plates and cups. She served the potato salad, ham sandwiches, grapes, ginger ale and brownies. After lunch the two women lay on the blanket for a nap and Uncle Morrie walked upstream with his rifle. Suddenly, he heard screams from Alice and her mother. Fearing a skunk attracted by the smell of food had waddled into their picnic site, he quickly ran back along the edge of the stream. He would not shoot any peaceful little skunk, only shoo it away. If it was a snake, he'd shoo it away too, with stones. Where were the women? He could hear their high, quivering voices, then a loud scream from Alice, "Morris, help, help!"

He saw them then, almost hidden in the lower limbs of the shade tree. Simultaneously, he saw the Butlin's Jersey bull, a broad-chested monster with vicious-looking horns. It was trampling the Scottish plaid picnic blanket and nosing the remains of the picnic in the overturned basket. The bull swung his head up to look at the screaming women and caught sight of Uncle Morrie. He snorted, trotted a few steps toward Uncle Morrie, stopped, pawed the ground and again looked at the women in the tree, as if confused by this unexpected annoyance in his territory. At a trot, his head high, he headed for Uncle Morrie.

Uncle Morrie shot his rifle in the air. The loud bang stopped the bull short. When he came again toward Uncle Morrie, another shot stopped him. Uncle Morrie dashed beside the stream until his car was between him and the bull. He ran to it, honked the horn to distract the bull, and drove to the tree. Somehow he got those women, disheveled and tangled in their long skirts, out of the tree and into the car.

Hearing the story, as told by Uncle Morrie, we children didn't ask how he got the women down; Uncle Morrie, who had been a soldier in World War I, could do anything, we thought. What we wanted to know was how in the world did Alice and her heavy mother get up in that tree? Uncle Morrie laughed. It baffled him too. "It must have been a big surge of adrenalin," he said.

Sunday Picnics

One Sunday on a picnic with two other families, we were the last to leave. The sun had sunk low to the tops of the trees as we children climbed on the running boards, a privilege always allowed for the ride uphill. Jay opened the gate and closed it after the car went through. We were tired as usual after a picnic, willing to settle down for a quiet ride home.

We had just passed the Butlin's mailbox when Dad slammed on the brakes. "We ran over a snake," he said. "It was a rattler!"

"Oh, Jimsie, don't stop!" Mother said.

We kids were instantly revived. We hung out the windows, and so did Mother and Billy in the front seat. The snake had slid off the road into the ditch. Dad regretted using up his bullets on target practice; he couldn't leave a wounded animal.

"Besides," he said, "a wounded rattler could be dangerous. Don't open the doors," he said to the back seat and ran to Mr. Butlin's barn.

We kids climbed out the windows to the running boards for a closer look into the ditch. Then, here came Dad with a pitchfork, followed by old Mr. Butlin. We were wild with excitement. Jay jumped off the running board and ran to meet Dad. Stan and I followed and were ordered back to the car. We obeyed, but only to the running board. Stanley was about five then. Suddenly he leaped to the road and into the tall, dusty stalks of ragweed in the ditch, pointing and shrieking, "I see him, I see him, there he is!"

Just below his piping little voice, we heard the ominous rattle, like dry seeds in a gourd.

Many times after that moment I have viewed again, like slow-motion film, a replay of a split-second maneuver, like a frog's tongue unfurling to zap a dragonfly. I see Dad with one hand snatching the straps of Stan's overalls, lifting him out of the ditch and onto the road as if he weighed no more than a rabbit. Then, with both hands on the handle of the pitchfork, he thrust the tines into the weeds.

"It's dead," Dad said, as he tied the body of the snake with twine to the rear bumper. "Snakes keep on moving for a long time after they're dead."

It was still moving when we got home, a macabre sight from its big grinning head with a hole pierced by the tines of the pitchfork to the rattles at the end of its geometrically patterned body, all sinuously in motion.

Dad and Jay skinned it the next day. That snake skin with its nine rattles was displayed in our basement "museum" along with a buffalo head over the fireplace, deer antlers, a stuffed trout, a golden pheasant, a turtle shell, a lot of seed pods and other curios brought in from the woods. The walls were hung with framed pictures from *National Geographic* and photographs of Dad and his friends in hunting clothes.

In July of 1995 when that grand old house my brothers and I grew up in was emptied down to its bones, there in the basement in a scroll tied with string was the skin of the snake we ran over late that Sunday afternoon at Mr. Butlin's farm. By killing the injured snake Dad might have saved Mr. Butlin from crossing its path at a later date. Poor Mr. Butlin, though, met a fate even worse than snakebite. He was gored to death by his brown Jersey bull.

⊰{ 11 }⊱

In Hunting Season

> One of the signs of a truly educated people, and a broadly educated nation, is lack of prejudice.
> Dr. Charles H. Mayo, 1926[1]

WHEN the weather turned nippy in October, Mother and a lot of her friends became "duck widows."

Their husbands drove off on overnight duck hunting trips to one of a number of camps, cabins or hunting lodges on the shores of one of Minnesota's ten thousand lakes. Once I asked Dad, as he was laying out provisions for his hunting weekend, why he needed a coil of rope. He probably wouldn't need it, he said, but it might come in handy. In the old lodges in Canada, he said, they kept a coil of rope by the window in the upstairs rooms, one end attached to a leg of the bed, in case the place caught fire. Dad and his friends had never used his rope to escape a burning building, but it had been used to pull many a car out of mud.

Dad's hunting and fishing buddies were mostly Mayo Clinic doctors: Gordon New, Ad Adson, Mel Henderson, George Eusterman, Waltman Walters, Herman Moersch, Henry Meyerding, Dave Berkman, John Crenshaw, Starr Judd, Pete Lillie, Bob Mussey, Harry Harwick, Hasty Wood, Compton Broders, M. C. Piper, G. S. Baker, Jim Waugh and Fred Figi. Two of my father's comrades in hunting season who were not Mayo doctors were Art Osman and Doc Bailey. Mr. Osman owned a sporting goods store in Rochester and a number of fine hunting dogs. Dad outlived most of his old friends, but Art Osman remained a caring friend until the end of Dad's life at age ninety-four. Doc Bailey and his brother Dick owned a lumber company in Virginia, Minnesota. Doc Bailey attended a few years of medical school, but dropped out to take a job in a saw mill. Much of his time at the mill was spent ministering to the troubles and ailments of the tough white men and the Native Americans who worked there. When a Native American was cut by an ax, Doc was his surgeon. But when Doc's only son, nineteen-year-old Brud, developed severe headaches and vertigo, Doc brought him to the Mayo Clinic.

I was a child of ten or so when I met Brud and his father. That was a sorrowful time in our house. Brud was hospitalized with a brain tumor. Dr. Alfred W. Adson, then head of the neurologic surgery section at the Mayo Clinic, removed it. Brud lived for several days, then died. Sometimes during those dreadful days of waiting, Dad and his friend Doc would be together at our house in the library with the door closed. Mother let us children know it was a sad time and we were to stay out of the way. Doctors suffer with the relatives when they lose a patient. Dr. Adson, who also knew Doc Bailey as a hunting friend, was especially pained by the death of his young patient.

Dr. Adson had learned his specialty as assistant to Dr. Emil H. Beckman, the first neurosurgeon at the Mayo Clinic. Dr. Beckman had earned an international reputation for success in the delicate techniques of locating and removing tumors of the brain and spinal cord. It was a cruel blow to the Mayo Clinic when Dr. Beckman died of an infection he contracted during an operation on a severely infected patient. And it must have seemed a calamity to young Dr. Adson to find himself the neurosurgeon next in line to be assigned the neurologic cases. He didn't feel ready, and he couldn't have *looked* ready, having the smooth, round baby-face of a college freshman. He asked for and received from Dr. Will permission to take a leave of absence from the Mayo Clinic to study for several months under one of the world's greatest neurosurgeons, Dr. Harvey Cushing. When he returned to the Clinic he felt more prepared to carry on Dr. Beckman's work, if not to fill his shoes.

One day when young Dr. Adson was getting ready to operate on a patient with a spinal cord tumor, he was almost sure of its exact location. The patient lay anesthetized on the table, when into the operating room walked Dr. Will, Dr. Charlie and a guest referred to by Mayo biographer Helen Clapesattle as "the Great Moynihan of Leeds."[2] Dr. Adson began to perspire and stall for time. Dr. Charlie sensed his uneasiness and suggested they move on, but their guest insisted on staying. Dr. Adson proceeded then, under the eyes of his bosses and the English surgeon Lord

In Hunting Season

Berkeley Moyhihan, who had been knighted by the queen and was said to be one of the greatest surgeons of the century. After he found the tumor exactly where he thought it would be, Dr. Adson relaxed and finished the operation. Lord Berkeley Moynihan returned to England and is said to have remarked with awe that what he saw in Rochester was "a high school boy operating for spinal tumor!"

That "high school boy" earned the confidence of his peers and his patients. The young doctors working with Dr. Adson on a fellowship learned to be on their toes with their chief. His nervousness before and during a difficult case was sometimes accompanied by colorful bursts of profanity. His congenial self was always revived by those fall-of-the-year weekend retreats with his hunting friends.

When Dad returned from such an outing, we children rushed out to see the game or the fish he had brought back. But in deer season mother and I didn't rush out with the boys. We didn't want to look at the lovely buck lying loose over the front fender of the car, its tongue out, belly red and empty. But we were all glad to have Dad home, energized by a weekend of outdoor camaraderie with men and dogs in the crisp, red-leaf days of autumn. He smelled of campfire smoke in his black-and-white wool checkered shirt and his red Hudson's Bay hat, rumpled pants and boots. We wished we could go along with him. Occasionally, when my brothers were older, they were included in that man's world with Dad.

Near the end of World War II, my brother Stanley, a captain in the Army Rangers, went on a pheasant hunt with Dad and his friends. Stan had been severely wounded on the shores of Sicily, was patched up at a field hospital in North Africa and sent home to Ashford General Hospital, the former Greenbriar Hotel in White Sulphur Springs, West Virginia. There his festering right arm had to be amputated. On his first leave from Ashford General he was thrilled to get in on a pheasant hunt with Dad and a group of his hunting buddies. They left Rochester before dawn, drove to a hotel in Huron, South Dakota, spent the afternoon tramping the fields in crisp October weather, got their limit of birds and returned to have drinks, dinner and a good night's sleep at the Huron Hotel. A local veteran, a wheelchair-bound amputee, was invited to join them for drinks.

Conversation in their hotel suite, Stan said, centered on the war in Europe, topics like the faint-hearted Neville Chamberlain, the passionate message of Winston Churchill, FDR's fireside chats, the valorous French

Resistance and the treatment of prisoners of war. Stan said German prisoners "had it easy." Some of them were tending the grounds at Ashford General Hospital, raking leaves so vigorously the grass was getting thin. Spirits were mellow in the Huron Hotel suite. Ice clinked in glasses and drinks were refilled. Then, in some unremembered context, George Eusterman made a reference to "the Goddamn British."

Dad, red-faced with anger at this slur on his ancestors, our allies, put down his glass of Scotch and rose to his feet, glowering at his friend. Dr. Eusterman stood up too, and Stan, and so would have the man in the wheelchair if he'd had legs to stand on. I can feel the fury Dad felt at this insult to the British. His usual restraint seemed gone. He couldn't put in words the surge of loyalty he felt for the city of London and its people who had courageously, and alone, defended their homeland. Stan thinks if he hadn't put himself between Dad and Dr. Eusterman, there'd have been a struggle. It is an exhilarating thought to both Stan and me that our usually temperate and reasonable Canadian father, who was now an American citizen, could be so roused to righteous anger. It was a part of him we had never known.

In the early 1940's I met one of Dad's former first assistants, a Mayo Fellow whom Dad had invited to one of those bird hunts. He told me he felt extremely privileged to have been asked along by his chief, a man so highly respected. Their hunting cabin, he said, was furnished with five double bedrooms, and he was to share a room and bed with my father. He felt nervous about the arrangement.

Dad, however, as he sat on the edge of the bed taking off his boots, said, "Look, Bill, you've been saying, 'Dr. Masson this and Dr. Masson that,' all day. Don't you think, if we're going to sleep in the same bed, you ought to call me 'Jim'?"

That was the ice breaker that gave the young Fellow a good laugh and an easy night's sleep.

One of Dad's favorite hunting dogs was named Trigger, a yellow Labrador retriever, a gift from a patient. Trigger was a litter mate of a puppy that was given to President Eisenhower. Never trained as a field dog, he became Dad's faithful companion, a good, mannerly house dog, though on occasion his tail swept things off the coffee table. As an all-

In Hunting Season

around intelligent pet for children, one with no temperamental hangups, Dad always recommended a mixed breed, like Famous Dog Garby.

Before there were children in the Masson household, there was Garby, a brown mixed-shepherd puppy Jim Masson brought home to his bride in 1915. His name came from his propensity for examining other people's garbage. But his fame was due to his many tricks, both useful and useless, taught to him by his Mistress Marion. Garby could do all the usual things dogs do to show off, and he was photographed doing them—shaking hands, rolling over, playing dead, jumping over an obstacle or balancing a cookie on his nose while sitting rigidly on his hind quarters, paws folded, until instructions were given to toss it up and catch it. Garby had his own pipe, an old one of Dad's. Even as an old dog he would go find his pipe when Mother asked him to and, with it clenched between his teeth, would hop up on the window seat in the library and look toward the driveway when Dad was on his way home.

Garby was also a delivery dog. At the sound of a brown paper bag being crinkled he would, with a wildly swishing tail, prepare to deliver packages at high speed within the neighborhood. He would take the bag in his mouth and race up the block toward the borrowing neighbor, one of Mother's friends—Carrie Balfour, Ethyl Lemon or Mabel Henderson—who would whistle or sing out, "Here, Garby!" from her front porch. The bag might contain a can of baking powder, a cup of sugar in a jar, or a couple of apples, and would be delivered with enthusiasm. Then Garby would race back home for praise and a reward.

Only once, I am told, did Garby fail in his mission. He was asked to deliver a T-bone steak. Its aroma slid out of its wax paper wrappings, past the twisted neck of the brown paper sack. Suddenly, its tantalizing breath seized the poor dog. Mother found him lying at the roadside, deaf to calls and whistles, the T-bone between his teeth. To be fair, Garby might have tried to carry it as gently as a mother dog carries her pup, but, having punctured the wax paper, his *canis lupus* instincts were intractable. Even Rin Tin Tin might have failed.

Our canine pets were numerous. Mine was Taffy, the passionate hunter of gophers. Stan's was Barny, who learned how to pull a sled; Jay had a Boston bull named Skipper. Skipper didn't do any tricks, but a trick was repeatedly played on him. When Jay was studying, Skipper was right there on his desk with the books and papers. He often fell sound asleep on his back. Jay then gently lifted Skipper's upper lip and put things under it: five or six pencils, a few crayons, an eraser, paper clips, more pencils, a key, a tongue depressor, a scroll of paper that looked like a cigarette, whatever was handy. Then Jay would come and get me or someone else to watch the prank unfold. There lay Skipper, breathing peacefully; his Boston bulldog mouth bristled with the assortment of things under his lip. Then Jay would say, "Hey, Skip!" Skipper would leap to his feet, the pencils, et cetera, stuck on the gumline of his upper teeth. He'd shake his head vigorously and we'd laugh ourselves silly as the things in his mouth flew all over the room.

My brother Bill brought home his own dog, a sweet, long-legged brown pup he found on the campus at the University of Minnesota. I was away from home then and didn't get to know that dog. That didn't matter; what did matter was not getting to know my youngest brother as I wish I had. He went through high school like an only child with the three of us older siblings off at college and beyond.

Those dogs of my childhood were smart, healthy mongrel puppies that came from the Institute for Experimental Medicine built on Dr. Charlie's farm property. The animals here were used for testing new surgical tools and chemical products.

When the need for animal research was first realized by the Mayo brothers, Dr. Will had a problem with it; he was more cautious than Dr. Charlie, a sympathetic "people" person. To make a patient with an imagined stomach ailment feel better, Dr. Charlie recommended half a bag of popcorn; it couldn't hurt, and it seemed to help. He looked into the future more quickly than his elder brother. He was the first man in Rochester to buy a car and learn to drive. But no disagreement ever broke apart the friendship of those brothers. As Dr. William D. Haggard of Nashville once said, their great success was not just as surgeons. It was as brothers. It was unique in history.[3]

Dr. Will accepted the idea of experimentation on animals as long as the research was related to a specific surgical or clinical problem, such as testing Dr. Clagett's clamps on dogs' arteries before trying them on human blood vessels. Then he was brought around to a broader view by a persuasive Dr. Plummer and his staunch supporter, Dr. Louis B. Wilson. Their position was that the Mayo Clinic's goals were not those merely of a medical practice. The scope of their work, as the Clinic kept on growing, needed a hands-on approach to research where results could be verified.

In Hunting Season

At first the animals were kept in the basement of Saint Mary's Hospital, but Dr. Wilson soon discovered that the sentimental sisters, not understanding the rigor of scientific research, were prone to slipping little treats to the animals. In 1908 Dr. Wilson offered space for the animals in the barn on his property. That was one of several intermediate solutions to the problem of housing the animals. Dr. Will vetoed the next plan, having animal runs on the roof of the 1914 Building. With hotels in Rochester growing taller every year, Dr. Will thought Rochester visitors would soon be dismayed as they looked out their hotel windows to see dogs in their pens and hear them barking. The perfect solution was Dr. Charlie's offer of part of his Mayowood farmland.

Dr. Charlie's nineteen-year-old daughter Louise used to help her father with his correspondence. Most of it was fan mail, but an occasional "crank" letter had her in tears, like the one from an anti-vivisectionist who asked, "How can you look a little dog in the face and then slit its throat?"[4] Being a kind-hearted man, that letter was hard on Dr. Charlie too.

As the Clinic continued to grow, more and better research became an important part of innovations in surgery, biophysics, bacteriology and physiology. Under the high standards of the U.S. Public Health Service Animal Welfare Policy, fifteen different kinds of animals have been maintained at the Institute, known to Pill Hill kids as "the dog farm." Because of the research done there, major advances were made in the treatment of a host of the major killers and cripplers of human beings: heart disease, multiple sclerosis, organ transplants, cancer, Alzheimer's, diabetes, leprosy, poliomyelitis and small pox.

The chance of a lifetime for an outdoorsman like my father came along in 1919. Under the sponsorship of Kansas University and their Museum of Natural History, he was invited to join a group of six on a big game hunt to Alaska.

At the time, my mother was happily at home with her first child, six-month-old James Knowles Masson. She had had an earlier pregnancy, carried full term, that ended in tragedy when the little boy died at birth. Now, she was blissfully happy and glad for Dad to take an overdue vacation. He hadn't had a vacation in four years, since his marriage and honeymoon in October 1914. In those strenuous days at the Mayo Clinic the surgeons were especially shorthanded. Routinely he handled ten to fourteen surgical cases two or three days a week, plus regular hours for seeing new patients and the daily rounds of his hospital patients. If he needed an excuse for taking time off, the invitation from Dr. John H. Outland of Kansas City was it.

Mother didn't know about the hardships Jim and his companions would endure on that trip—the raging river, upstream and down, the risk of smashing their heavily loaded canoes on rocks, the exhausting portages, the almost daily rain and cold and the possibility of being lost in wild, unmapped grizzly bear territory.

Dr. Outland, whom Dad had met at a medical meeting, organized the trip. Raymond J. DeLano, the self-proclaimed scribe of the group, described Dr. Outland as "the wheelhorse, the wit, the wag, the surgical-cutup...." Also on hand, adding mission and urgency to the adventure, was C. D. Bunker, curator and collector of specimens for the Museum of Natural History, Kansas University. It was Bunker's hope that the trip would provide the rare, taxidermal additions needed by his museum. DeLano's 23-page log is typed double-spaced on legal-size paper, now tattered and crackly. He describes in his rollicking style the wild majesty of that perilous voyage; twenty exhausting, exhilarating, harmonious days from August 22 to September 11, 1919.

The group departed Juneau, Alaska, on a tourist ship, the *S.S. Alameda*. They were dropped off the next day at Kusselof, a small fishing village where they met their Norwegian guide and six native packers, including a cook who kept the party well fed. Their pancake breakfasts were served up with selections such as sirloin of bear, mountain sheep liver, lamb chops, or rib and tenderloin of moose.

Jim Masson would never be thought by his friends as a ladies' man, in the sense of the wandering eye, but women loved him. He made them feel comfortable. This quality was quickly discovered by Raymond DeLano on the leisurely first leg of the trip and he wrote about it:

> Dr. James Masson, a member of the Mayo's staff in Rochester, Minnesota: His round, blushing, Falstaffian face and retiring manner belie the Emersonian statement that "the loud-talking fellow is usually the female favorite." Jim knew every lady on the *Alameda*, and was confidently calling her by her first name before we were two hours adrift.

In Hunting Season

DeLano writes like a poet of a land where nature turns mysterious, beguiling and dangerous:

And so we approached and reached Alaska, the land where Nature turns anomalous and eccentric; the mystic country where the Northern Lights play tag with the 'ghost gleams'; where the flowers and the snow are seatmates, where the clouds come down from the sky and roll on the water's edge; where there are islands, moss-covered, tree-clad, of every size, on every side, while just beyond are rock cliffs breaking sheer into the sea. We saw Tacu Glacier, with its mountains of ice which break, and, with a crash like thunder, fall into the water to make icebergs for us to sail among.

Hunting was a hobby that took my father back to his boyhood, to the satisfaction of the pioneer bringing home Sunday dinner. Most men of my father's generation grew up in towns separated by wide stretches of wilderness where game birds were plentiful all year around. Every man and boy took pride in being a good shot, a provider of meat for the family table. Hunting today is strictly regulated to assure the survival of wild game. Even the farmer tramping his own fields must buy a license to shoot game, in limited numbers at specified times of the year.

On the walls of our basement playroom hung memorabilia from Dad's hunting and fishing trips: A mounted ringneck pheasant perched on a rock. Antlers of deer and elk, discarded in the woods after the season of rut, became doorway decorations in our basement. The Alaskan brown bear rug was upstairs in front of the fireplace until we children wore it out and wiggled its teeth loose. The noble head of the bighorn sheep was mounted on the wall in the sunroom.

DeLano's diary ends with the line, "On another and a harder trip I would ask no better mates." It must have saddened my father in 1930 to hear the news of the death of his friend Ray DeLano. He died in the crash of a small plane en route to a fishing camp in Canada.

Shooting clay pigeons was a pretty tame sport, Dad once said, but trap-shooting was a popular sport for the men every day on board the Swedish ship *Gripsholm* in the summer of 1936. The *Gripsholm* was the sister ship of the *S.S. Kungsholm*, which had been converted for use as a troop ship during World War II and was, after much gallant service, sunk by a German submarine. Jay, Mother and I accompanied Dad and a group of American and Canadian surgeons and their families that summer on a tour of medical centers in England, Scotland, Norway, Sweden and Denmark. The only way to get across the ocean in those days was on board a ship. Transatlantic air passenger service didn't begin till 1939 when Pan American Airways established regular flights from New York to Southampton, England.

For six days we, on the *Gripsholm*, had much to explore, not to mention to eat. Tempting Swedish pastries were offered twice a day with bouillon, tea or coffee, plus three hefty meals and a midnight smorgasbord fit for the Swedish king. Swimming Swedish-style in the salt water pool was available at separate hours for women and men. Elevator access to the pool was strictly monitored. It was a shock, but fun, to roast in the sauna then leap into the chilly ocean water. It was also a shock, and a surprise, following Swedish custom, to skinny-dip with grownup ladies.

Mother and I made new friends, played shuffleboard and lazed around, while Dad and Jay entered the daily trapshooting contest. On the last night of the voyage, Dad modestly accepted an elaborately illustrated Grand Champion Trapshooter Certificate presented at dinner by the ship's captain. I thought it would be a trophy for the basement, but I never saw it again.

We had a shooting range at home in the basement. Its target was four steel squirrels hinged on a metal platform in front of a thick wooden block to protect the plaster wall. The object was to topple the squirrels with a rifle or BB gun. Dad taught the boys the rules and ethics of carrying a gun. His first rule was that he didn't allow cowboy shootouts, even with an unloaded gun or cap pistol. Rule Two: a hunter must never shoot a bird or animal he can't use as food. That didn't apply to shooting rats in a dump. In addition to venison, Dad had a jacket and gloves made from the tanned skin of the deer he shot. It pleased him to give his friends some of the game birds he brought home, all plucked and cleaned by our versatile Sylvester.

Mrs. Hattie Mayo always enjoyed receiving some of Dad's ducks. She served them with an orange marmalade glaze. Once, two of Dad's roasted ducks were in the oven at the Mayo's, waiting for Dr. Will to come home for lunch. When Dr. Will walked in the door with two guests, Mrs. Hattie's mind flew with a jolt to the kitchen and Jim Masson's two ducks. She was used to unexpected guests, but was a little flustered to realize that two ducks were hardly enough for four people. Naturally, though, she smiled and said quite calmly, "Oh yes, do stay for lunch. We're having wild duck."

Mrs. Hattie always assumed the job of carving when her husband brought visiting doctors home for a meal. The men always had much to say to each other. Half a breast and a leg with plenty of vegetables and rolls was enough. No second helpings. She picked up the carving knife and fork and unwittingly caught the full attention of the men. One of the ducks nudged the other off the platter onto the napkin on Mrs. Hattie's lap. She twitched inadvertently and the duck rolled down to the rug. She must have blushed as she rang for the maid, but Mrs. Hattie was a quick thinker. She also must have winked at the maid when she asked the girl please to bring in another duck. The girl scooped the bird off the rug and took it to the kitchen where she probably inspected it for any telltale lint. She put it on a plate, dribbled orange sauce over it, tucked a sprig of parsley into its cavity, and went back to the dining room. She might have exchanged a knowing smile with Mrs. Hattie as she transferred it to the platter beside the other duck.

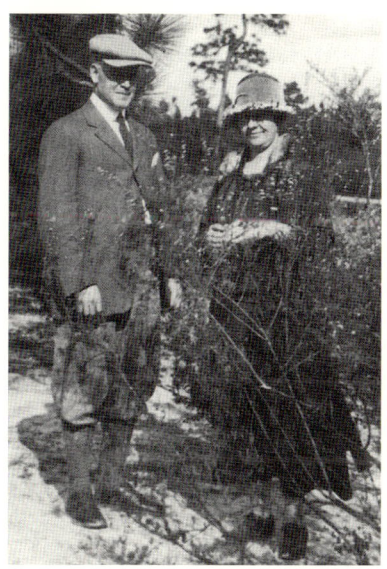

Jim and Marion Masson, 1927

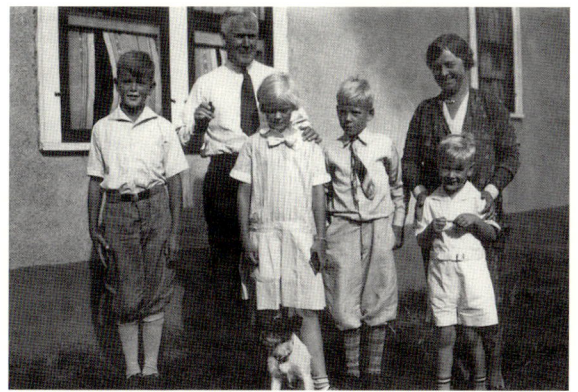

*Jim and Marion with their children:
Jamie, Helen, Stan and Bill*

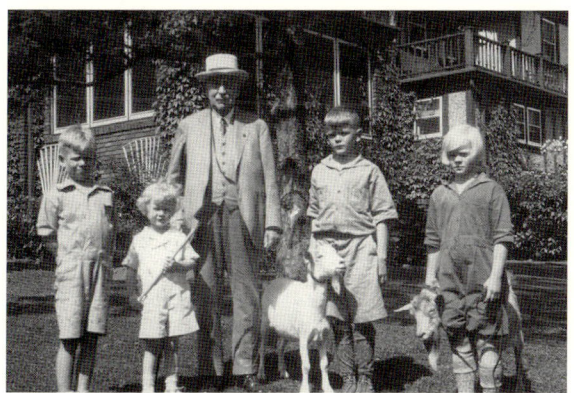

*Uncle Edmund Bigelow with Stanley, Billy, Jamie, Helen
and the goats, Biff and Bang, 1928*

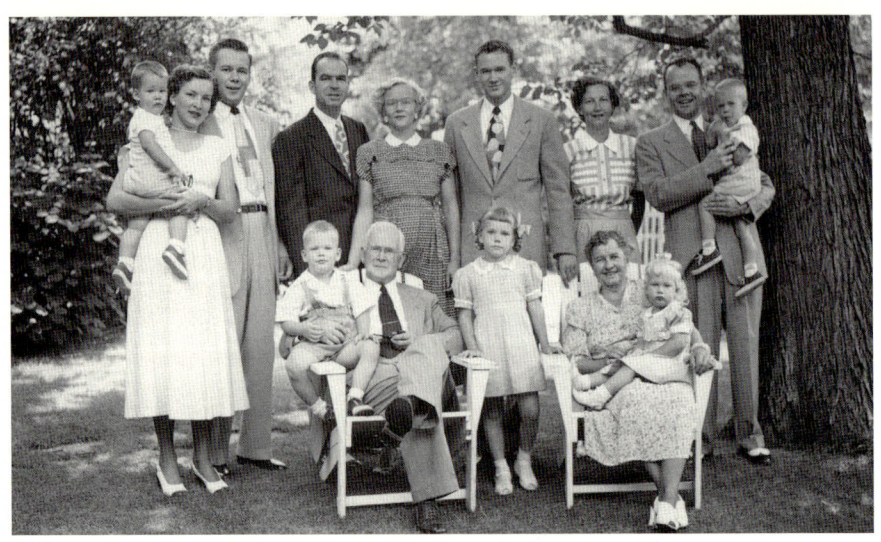

The Masson Clan
Back row: Frank, Gini, Stan, Herb, Helen, Bill, Lillian, Jay and Jimmy;
Front row: Howard, Grandpa, Lindy, Granny and Marion

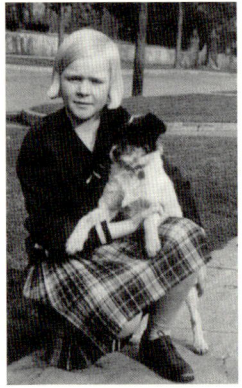

Helen and Taffy

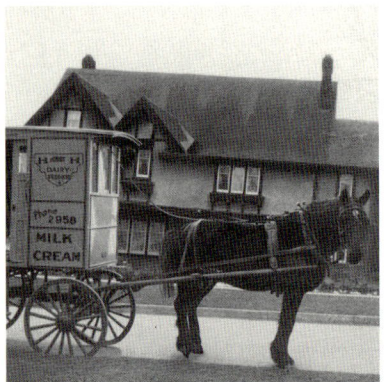

Helen's friend, the milk wagon horse

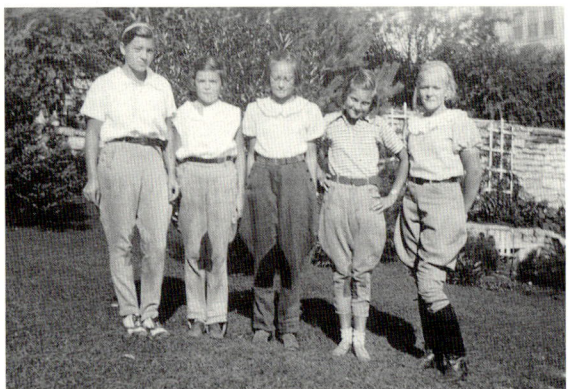

To the horses at the fairgrounds: Jane and Betty Willius,
Barbara Benedict, Peg Plummer and Helen Masson

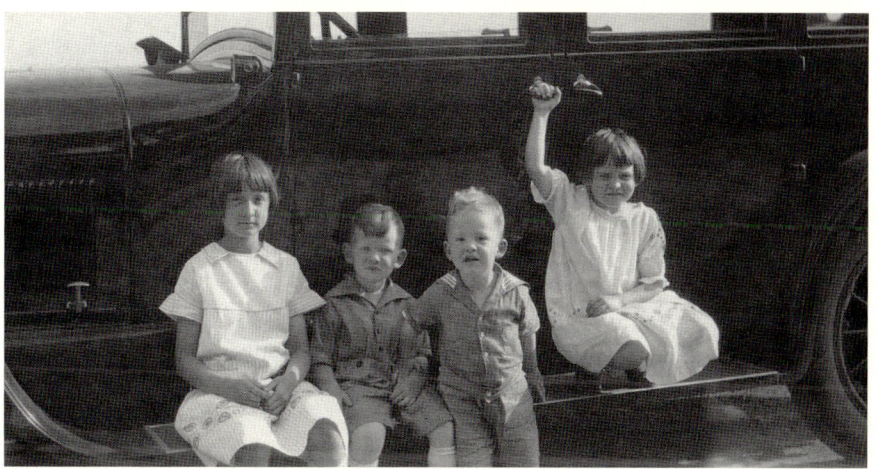

Four Benedicts: Virginia, Walter, John and Barbara

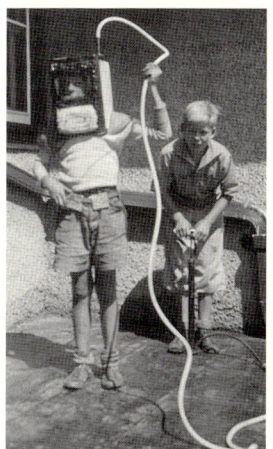

Dick Thorson and Stanley Masson demonstrating the diving bell

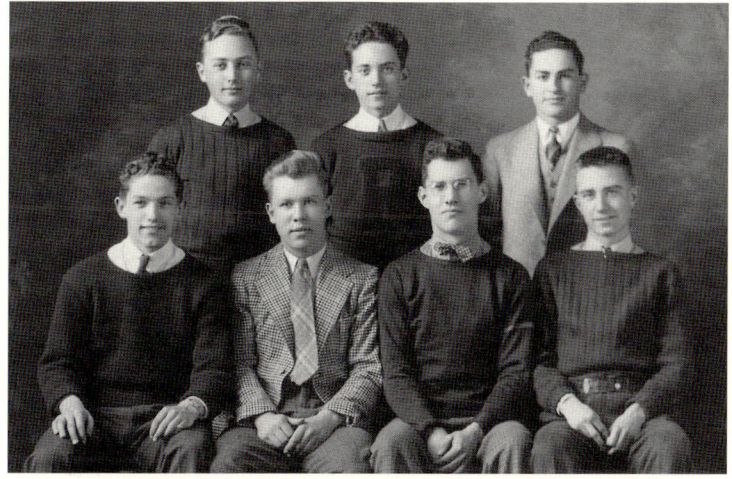

Miss Snodgrass's sports team captains – Back row: Cornie Judd, Henry Mourning, Milt Shapiro; Front row: Lawrence Derksen, Dick Hempstead, Kenneth Denzin, Jack Kamholz

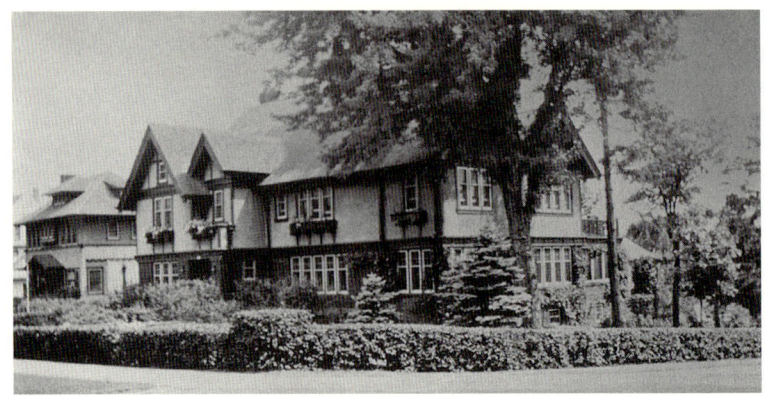
Masson home – 724 4th Street SW

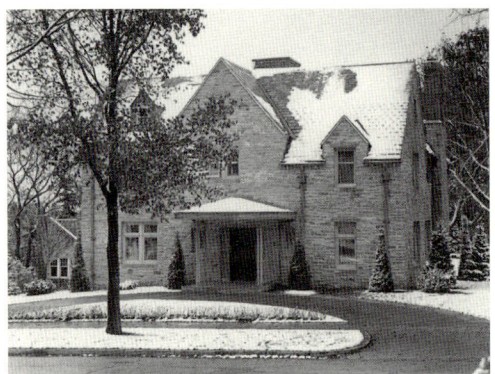
Dr. Will's home – 8th Avenue at 4th Street SW

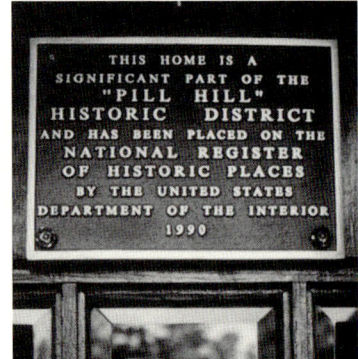
Plaque attached to early Pill Hill homes

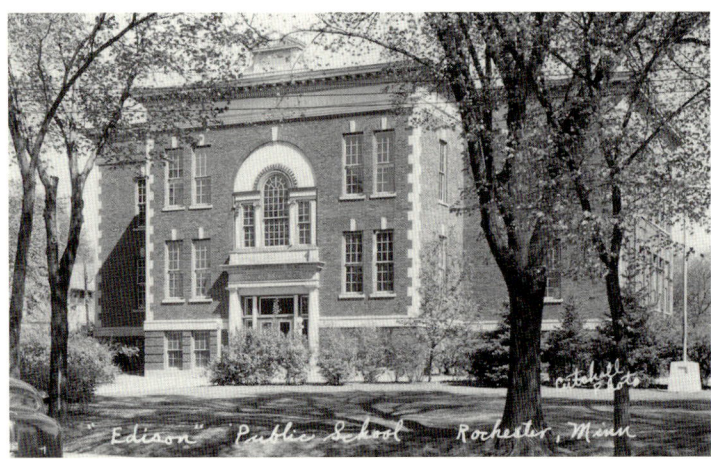
Edison School

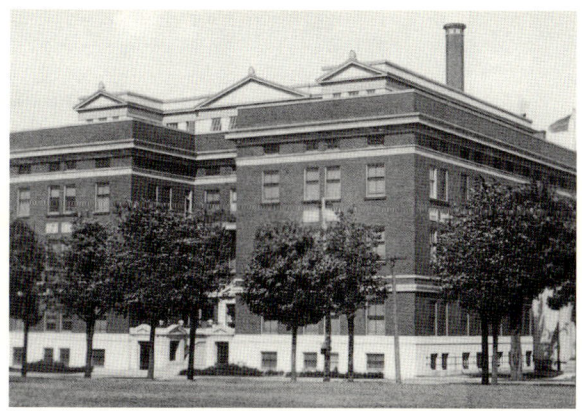

The 1914 Building (first Mayo Clinic)

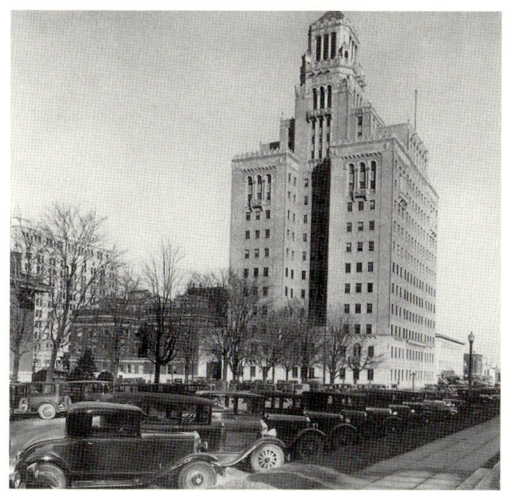

The second Mayo Clinic building, now the Plummer Building
BY PERMISSION OF MAYO FOUNDATION

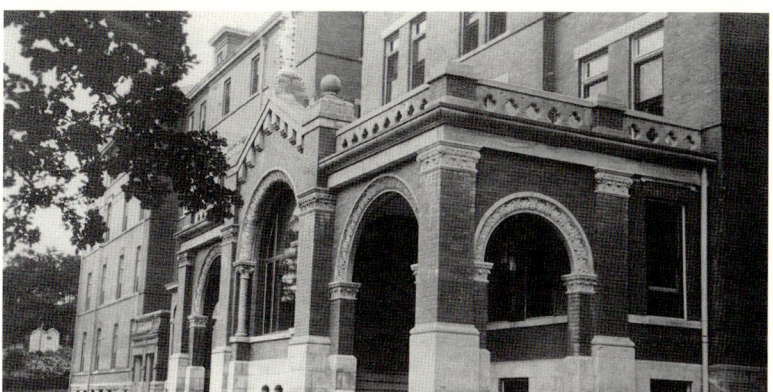

Saint Mary's Hospital

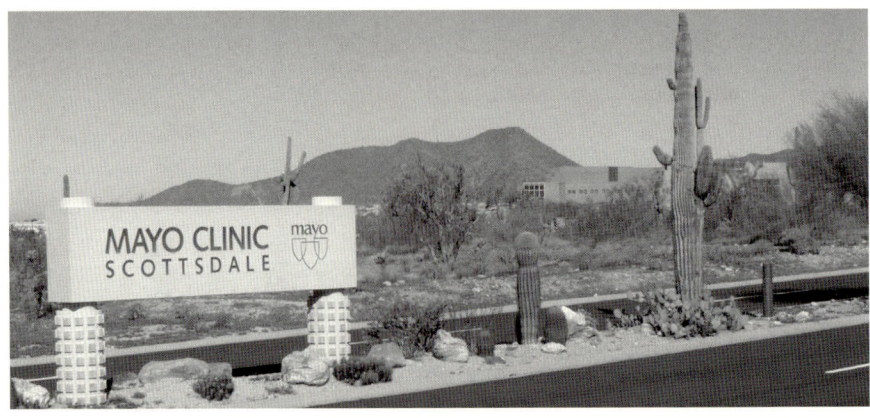
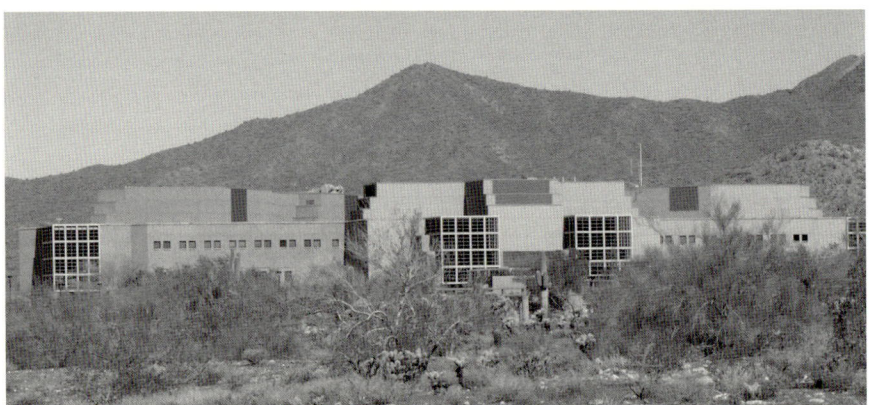

The Mayo Clinic in Scottsdale, Arizona
BY PERMISSION OF MAYO FOUNDATION

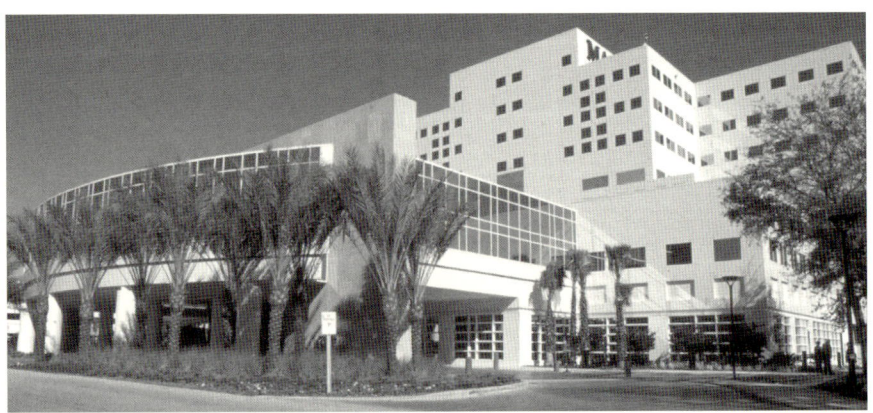

The Mayo Clinic in Jacksonville, Florida
BY PERMISSION OF MAYO FOUNDATION

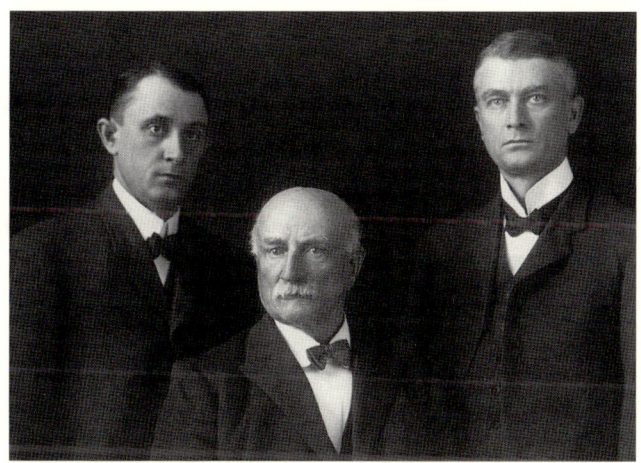

Father and sons: Dr. William W. Mayo (center), with Dr. Charles H. Mayo and Dr. William J. Mayo, ca. 1890

BY PERMISSION OF MAYO FOUNDATION

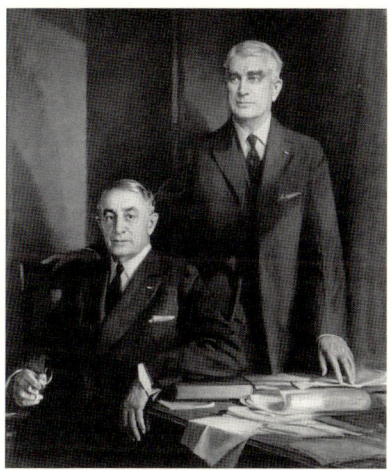

The brothers, Dr. Charles H. and Dr. William J. Mayo

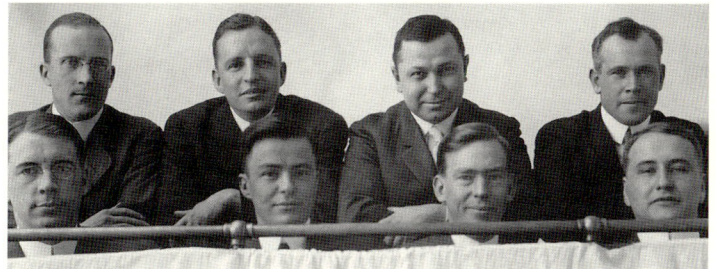

House staff at Saint Mary's Hospital, December 1913
Top row: Dr. Ralph L. Kirch, Dr. Harold M. Rice, Dr. Earnest V. Smith, Dr. James C. Masson; Bottom row: Dr. William C. Carroll, Dr. M. Joseph Henry, Dr. John de J. Pemberton, Dr. Percival K. Menzies

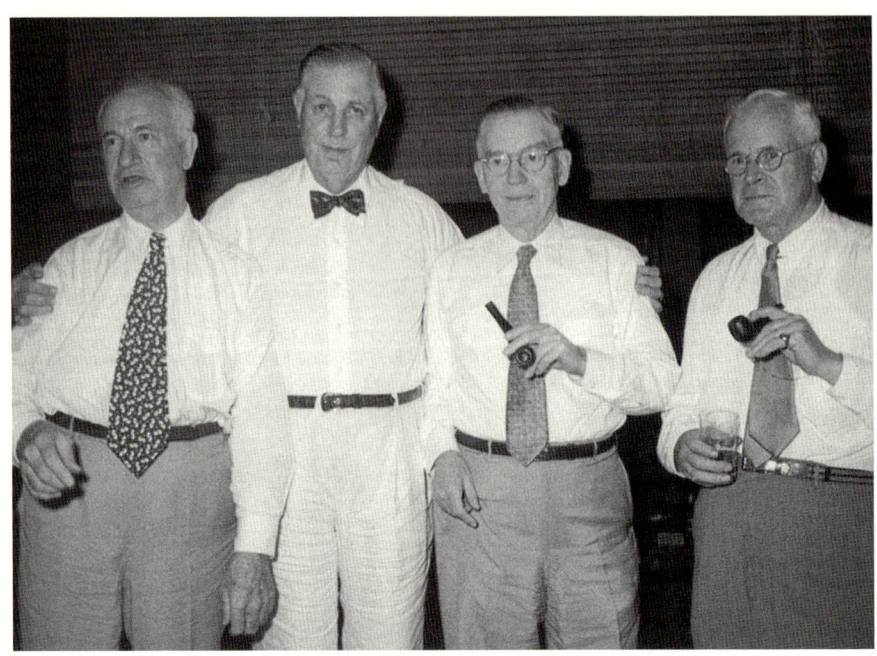

Left to right: Dr. Donald C. Balfour, Harry Harwick, Dr. John Pemberton and Dr. Jim Masson

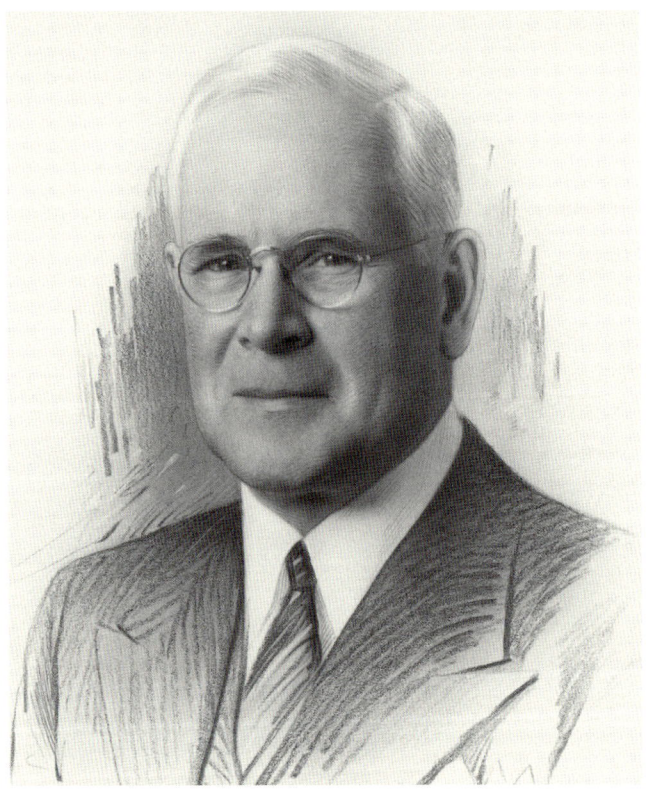

Dr. James C. Masson

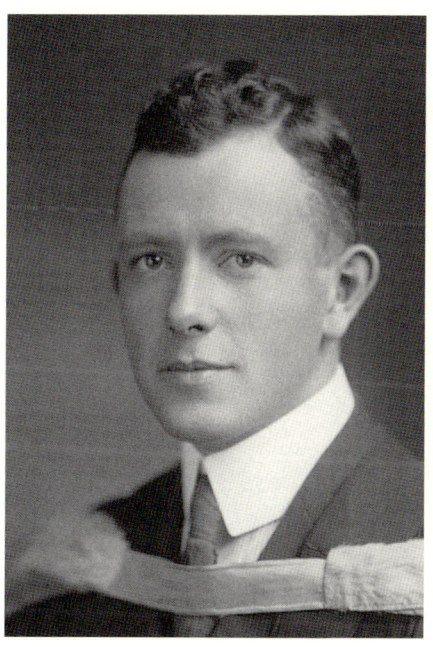

Dr. Duncan M. Masson

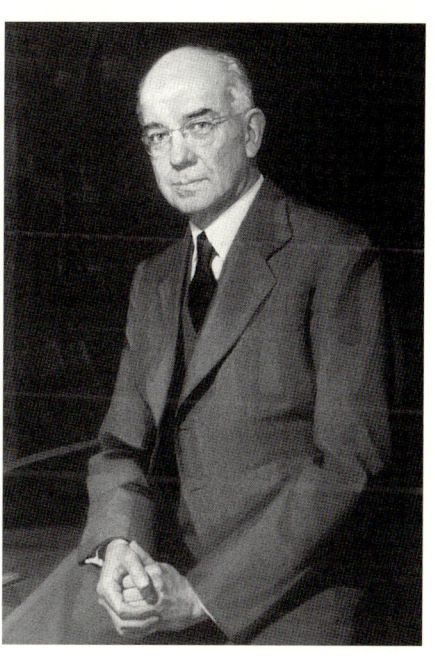

Dr. E. C. Kendall

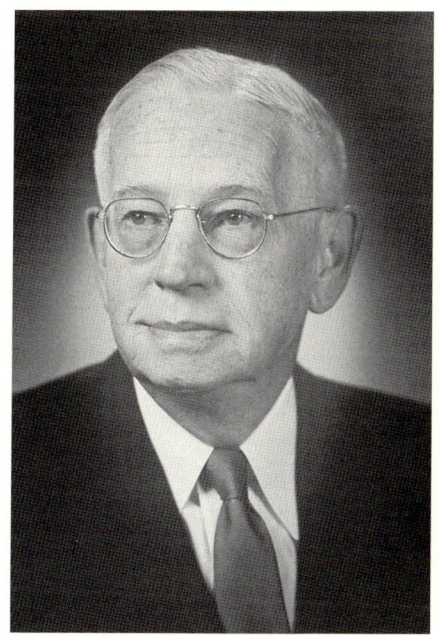

Dr. Fredrick A. Willius

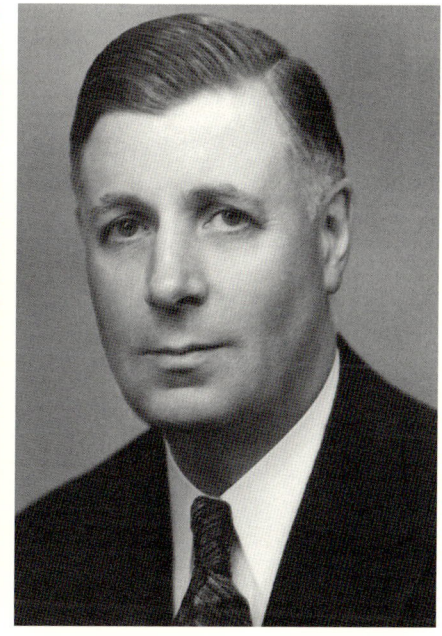

Harry Harwick, the Clinic's
administrator for 44 years, 1908 - 1952

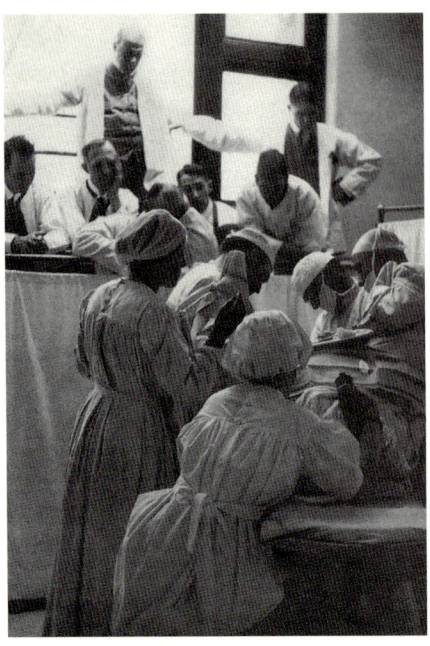
Dr. William J. Mayo (second masked person on the right), 1913
BY PERMISSION OF MAYO FOUNDATION

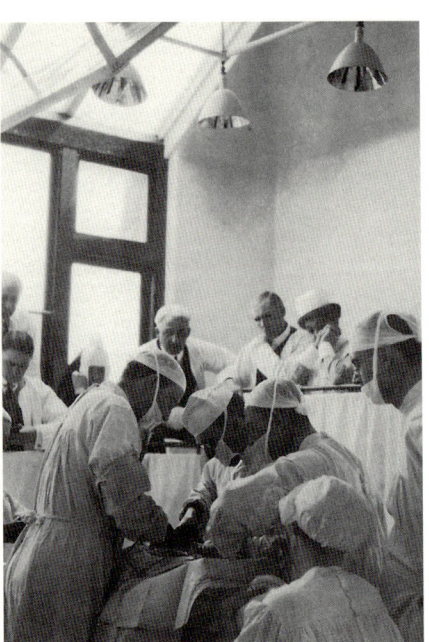
Dr. Charlie Mayo at work

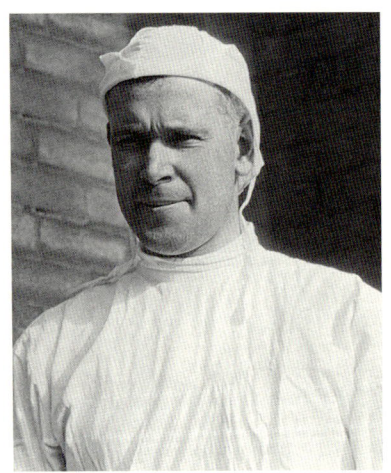
Dr. James C. Masson

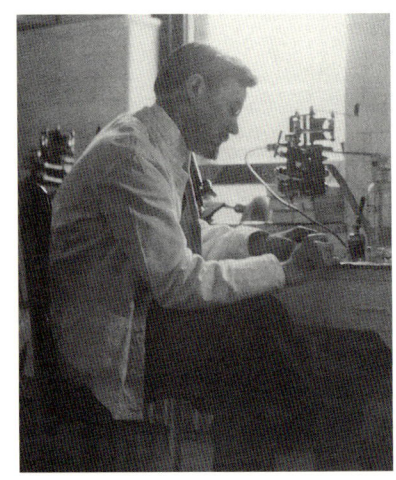
Dr. W. C. (Billy) MacCarty

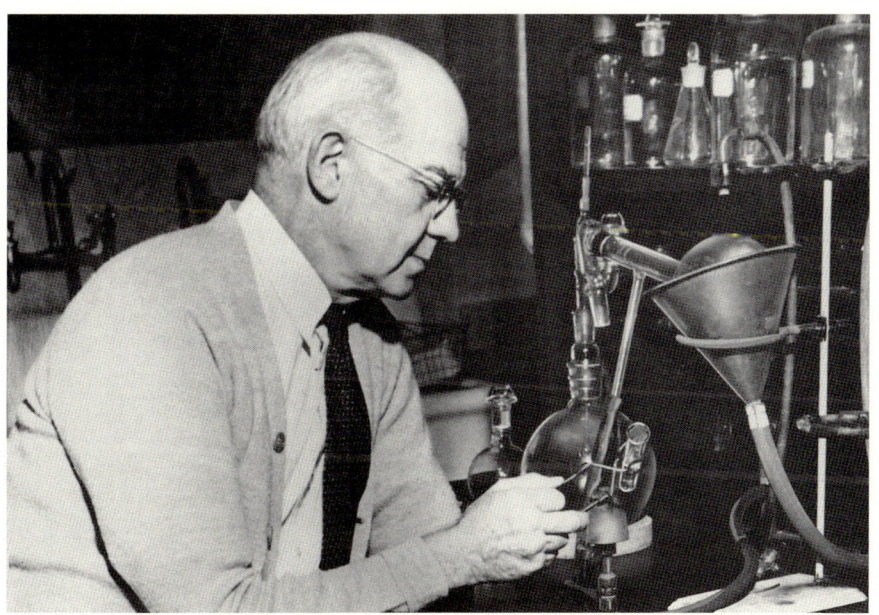

Dr. E. C. Kendall

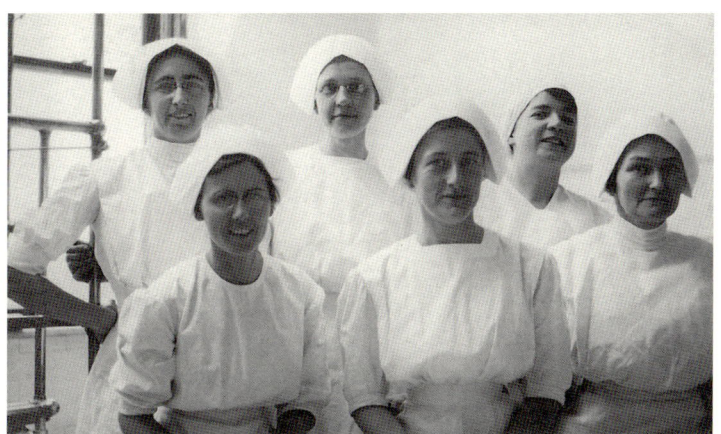

Shortie, Andy, [unknown], Ethyl, Ann and Miss Hines

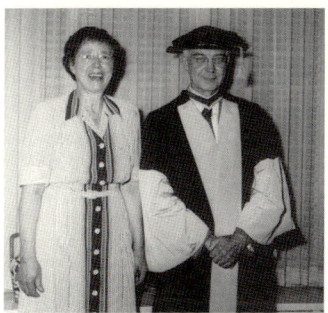

Rebecca and Dr. E. C. (Nick) Kendall in his 1950 Nobel Prize recipient robes

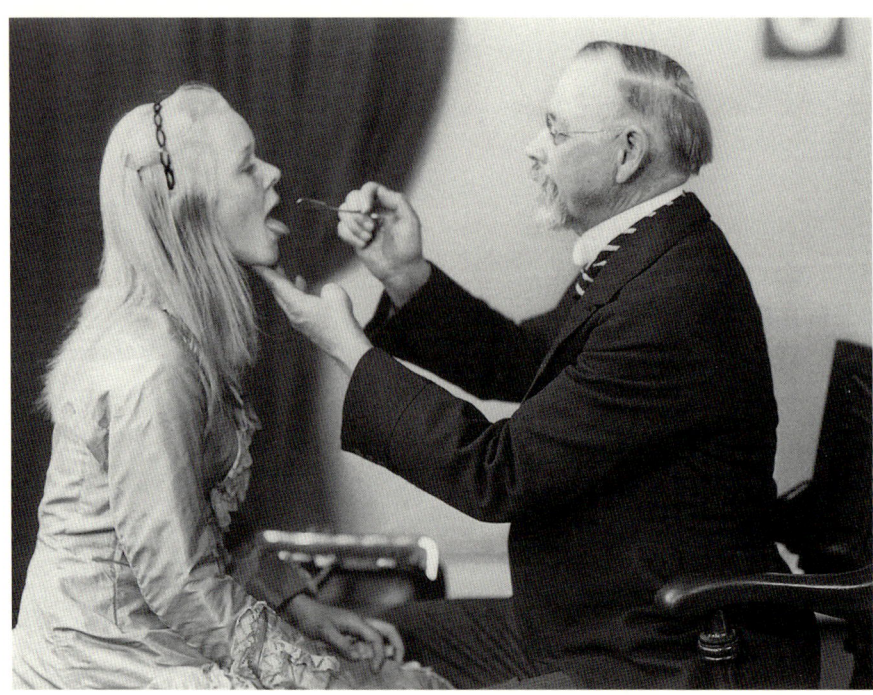

Chicago Century of Progress exhibit, old-fashioned doctor and patient (Helen)

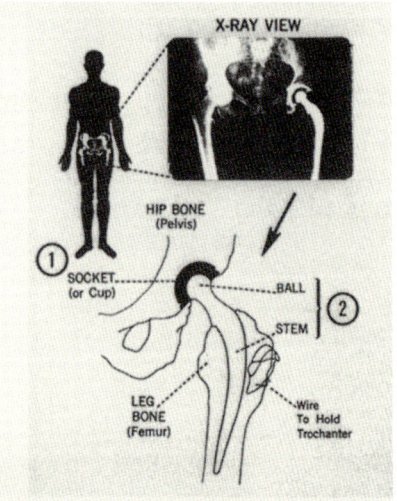

TOTAL HIP IMPLANT

The two-piece prosthetic device is shown (top right) as it appears in a typical X-ray view. Details of this device are illustrated in the drawing at lower right.

The socket or cup portion is made of polyethylene. The stem ranges from 5-7 inches in length with a 1½-2 inch diameter ball made of a highly polished metal. Both pieces are positioned in the bones and held in place with a special cement called "methyl methacrylate."

Once in position, the prosthetic device is considered a permanent assembly.

Mayo hip card, carried by hip implant patients to inform airline security why the bell rang as they passed through the metal detector

FROM THE MAYO ALUMNUS, JULY 1973

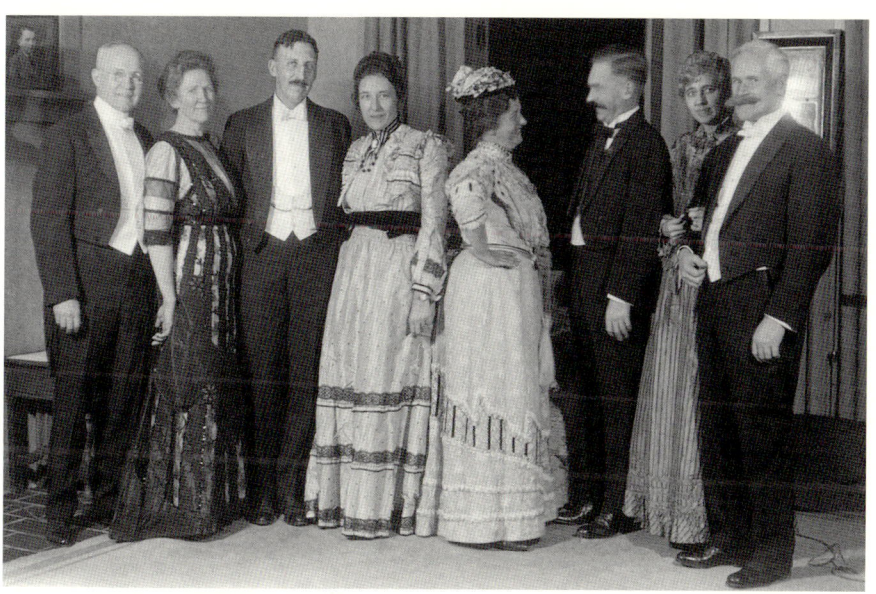

Mayowood's Gay Nineties party – December 17, 1932
Bob and Madge Mussey, Sam and Emily Haines, Marion Masson,
John Pemberton, Ann Pemberton and Jim Masson

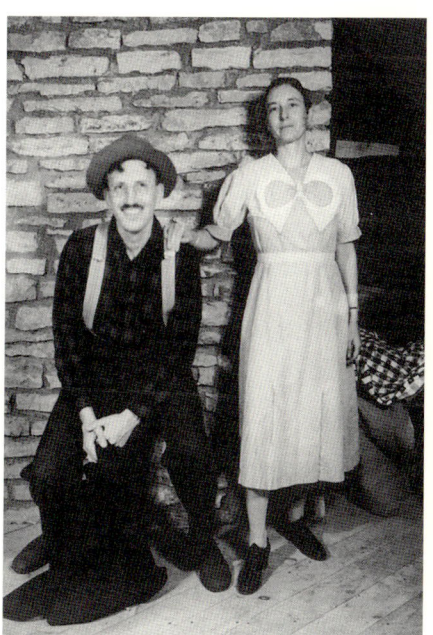

Sam and Emily Haines
Mayowood Barn Dance
September 18, 1937

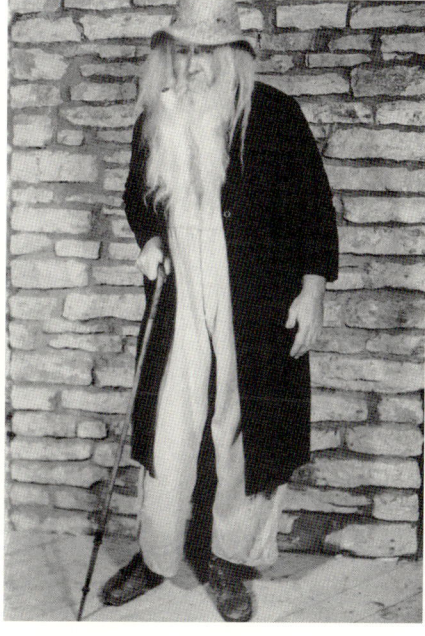

Dr. Duncan Morrison Masson, winner with
his wife Laura of a huge turkey for best costumes.
Mayowood Barn Dance

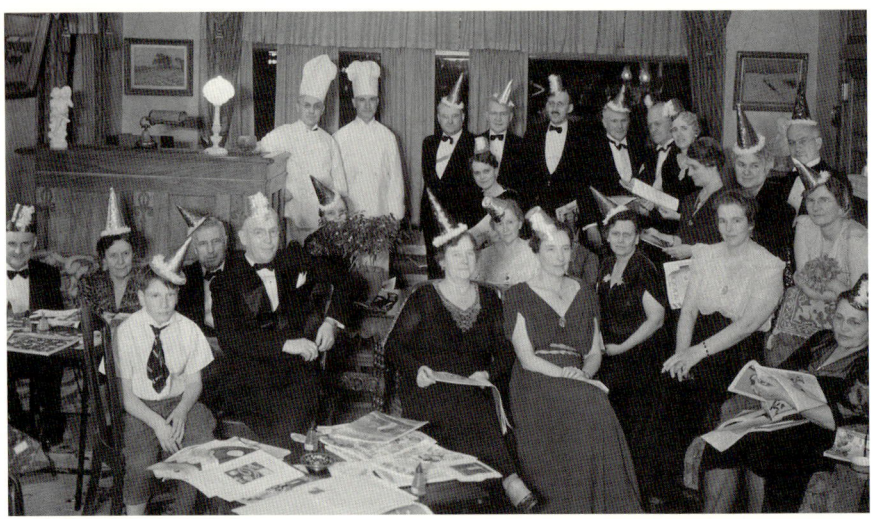

Chez Don and Carrie Balfour – the host is Chef No. 2

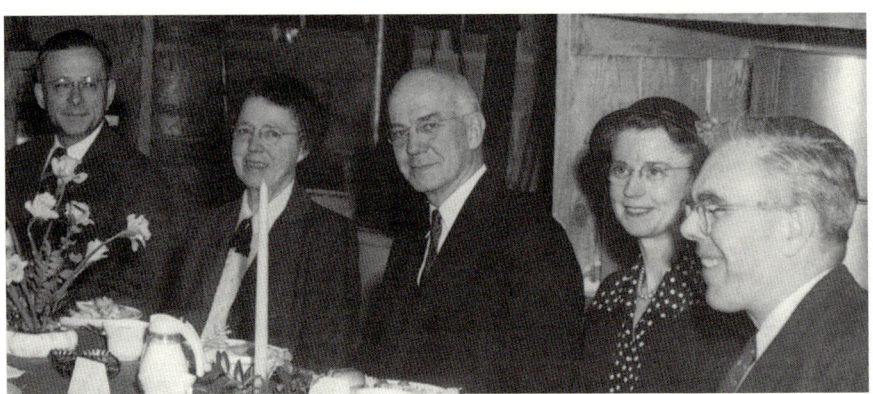

Becky and Nick Kendall (second and third from left), dining in the laboratory

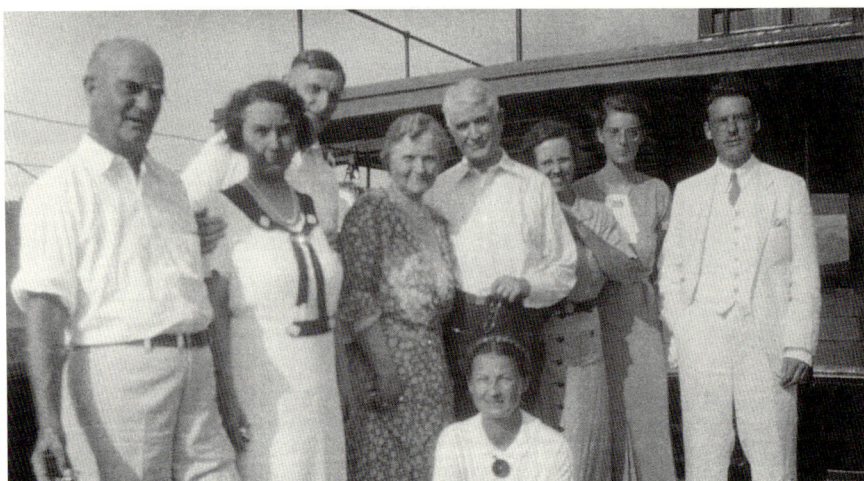

Dr. and Mrs. Will Mayo, at center, on the North Star *with Neal and Winnie Judd, Gordon and Ethyl New, Marion New and guests*

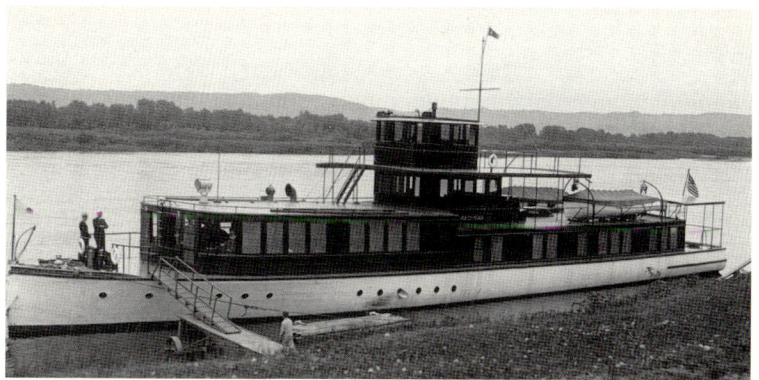
The North Star, *Dr. Will's boat*

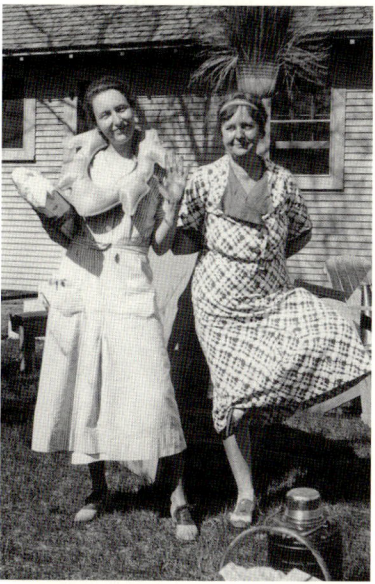
Emily Haines and Marion Masson

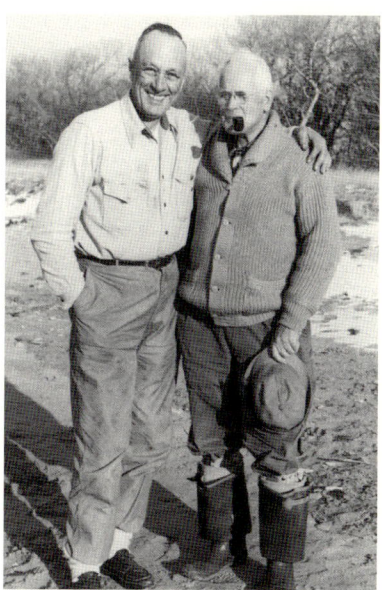
Art Osman and Jim Masson, good buddies

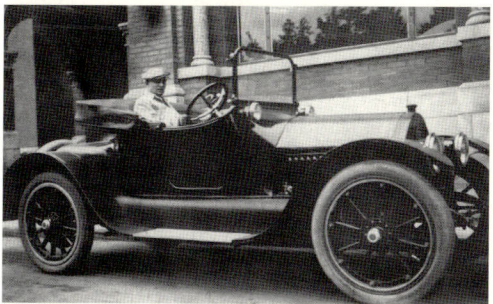
Dr. E. Starr Judd

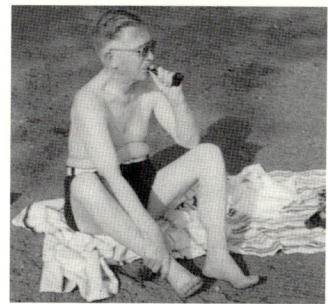
Dr. John Pemberton, relaxing

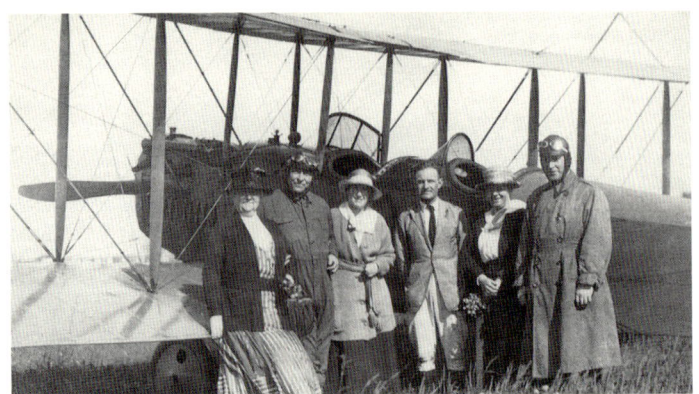

Tex (fourth from left) and his flying machine with Grandmother Knowles (Monty), Dr. Outland, Lou Masson, Marion and Jim Masson

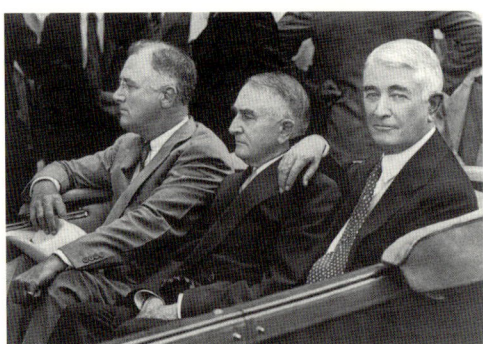

Franklin D. Roosevelt (U.S. President 1933-1945), with Dr. C. H. Mayo and Dr. W. J. Mayo, 1934

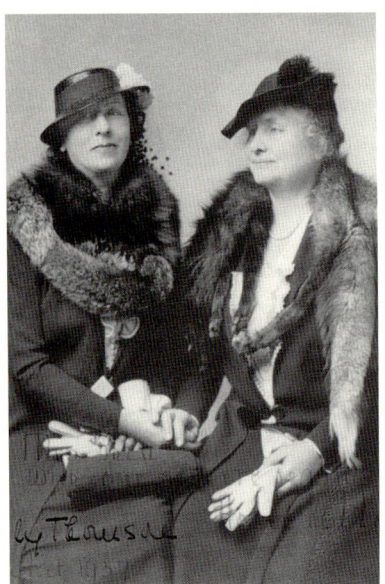

Helen Keller and her speech and sign language teacher, Mary Agnes (Polly) Tomson

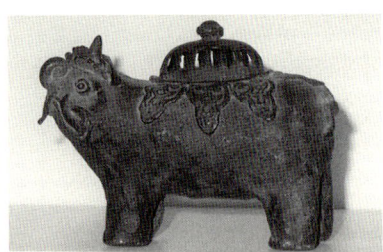

An ancient artifact that caught the attention of Dr. Henry Plummer at dinner

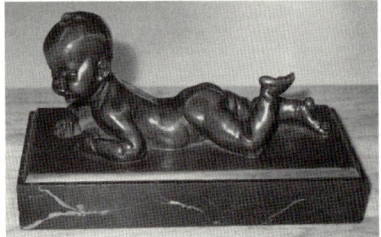

"Billy," by Gutzon Borglum, creator of Mount Rushmore Memorial

❦ 12 ❧

Grateful Patients

> Good health is an essential to happiness, and happiness
> is essential to good citizenship.
> Dr. Charles H. Mayo, 1919[1]

THE Clinic has a policy that the doctors, who are all on salary, should not accept gifts from patients. That must apply only to gifts of exceptional value. How else could a doctor, without hurting the feelings of the giver, return to sender pears from Oregon, Texas pink grapefruit, dates from the desert and Georgia's papershell pecans? Such delightful things arrived at Pill Hill homes frequently. We called these "G.P. gifts" —gifts from grateful patients. When the gift was a box of pungent Cuban cigars we Masson children argued over whose turn it was to get the paper band that encircled the cigar Dad put in his pocket.

Salmon were leaping their way up the rapids in Alaskan rivers when Mrs. Fred Moersch opened her door to a beaming young delivery man carrying a heavy styrofoam container marked "Air Mail Special Delivery, Packed in Ice." "Oh, what a whopper!" Mrs. Moersch said when she opened the box and scooped back the ice, and there lay a beautiful pink salmon. Agnes Moersch didn't know the patient who sent it, but she was terribly glad to see it. Mrs. Moersch was an excellent cook. She immediately whipped up a party for that very evening, the sooner the better to enjoy the lovely fresh salmon.

Guests were invited, the table set, champagne in a cooler, vegetables and rice ready to cook, a fruit salad tossed, bread in the upper oven and the fish in the steamer. The doorbell rang. Early arrivals? No, it was the same delivery man, but this time with a crestfallen face. He was so sorry;

he had made a mistake. His contrition was profound. The Alaskan salmon was supposed to go to Dr. Herman F. Moersch, not his brother, Dr. Fred Moersch. Could he have it back, please?

"Too late," Agnes Moersch said. "The fish is in the oven. I'll invite them over."

So, the Herman Moersches were added to the guest list and my friend Ginny and her brother Bob were given hamburgers in the kitchen.

Bob New wrote that a patient of his father, a Mr. Uhlein (pronounced "Ee-line") from Milwaukee, a member of the Schlitz beer family, regularly presented Dr. New with cases of beer, wine and hard liquor. Mr. Uhlein never knew the facts about his surgeon, Dr. Gordon B. New. Uncle Gordon came from a family of Canadian Baptists who didn't approve of baking a cake on Sunday, let alone drinking alcoholic beverages any day of the week. Bob, now a retired Episcopalian priest in Richmond, Virginia, who is not a teetotaler, wrote that as he and his brother Bud came of age their father occasionally released a case of Schlitz beer to them, but the rest he carried upstairs to a locked attic closet where he kept his hunting guns and ammunition. At parties where drinks were served he would toy with a cocktail to be polite, but set it down somewhere, untouched. "But Mother would have a drink or two and enjoy it," Bob said.

A day came when a messenger delivered a pinch bottle of Haig and Haig Scotch to the News' house, a G.P. gift to *Mrs.* Ethyl B. New. Aunt Ethyl, as I called her, was the former Miss Ethyl Baily who came to the Clinic in 1910 as a post-graduate student in anesthesiology. The giver of the fancy bottle of Haig and Haig must have been an old acquaintance or a patient from those years when Ethyl assisted Dr. Charlie Mayo in the operating room. She left her gift on the front hall table and when her husband came in she proudly showed it to him with the card addressed to Ethyl Bailey New. Uncle Gordon commented on its attractive shape, picked it up and was on his way to the attic when she grabbed it. "Hey, this one's mine!" she said.

Dad's G.P. gifts sometimes came with clever sentiments attached. An exceedingly attention-grabbing necktie for "Dear Doctor Masson" was sent from Felix P. Miller, M.D., of El Paso, Texas. The poem accompanying the gift, "Give Me a Wild Tie, Brother," made us all wish to meet the anonymous author:

Some men long for the soothing touch
of lavender, cream or mauve,
But the ties I wear must possess the glare
Of a red-hot kitchen stove.
The books I read and the life I lead
Are sensible, sane and mild;
I just hate spats, I wear calm hats,
But I want my neckties wild.
>Give me a wild tie, brother,
>One with a cosmic urge.
>A tie that will swear, and rip and tear
>When it sees my old blue serge.
Some folks say that a man's cravat
Should only be seen, not heard;
But I want a tie that will make men cry
And render their vision blurred.
I yearn, I long for a tie so strong,
It will take two men to tie it.
If such there be, show it to me—
Whatever the price I'll buy it.
>Give me a wild tie, brother,
>One with a lot of sins,
>A tie that will blaze in a hectic haze
>Down where the vest begins.

A newly invented boon to the housewife, a Bendix washing machine, was brought to our house in a crate before any of my friends had heard of a washing machine. Doing the laundry once a week was an all-day job for several people at our house. It involved a water softener, tubs, a wringer, clothes baskets and ropes to string back and forth over the driveway from the garage to hooks on the brick wall above the parsley bed. The Bendix was some help to Mrs. Whitley, the laundress; but the other women who came with her on Mondays felt more comfortable with the familiar but risky tub-wringer method. The dryer hadn't yet been invented. On rainy Mondays, the ropes were strung in the basement laundry room and a coal stove was lit to dry out the soggy air. On sunny days, Sylvester Robinson, our super handyman, put up the lines outside. In winter the sheets, pajamas and shirts froze and flapped in the wind with crisp clacking sounds. The next day the folded sheets and tablecloths were fed between the hot rollers of the mangle and came out neat and smooth.

Sometime after the arrival of the Bendix, another state-of-the-art gift arrived. It was made of semi-gloss aluminum, the size of a brick, with four ball feet as if it might roll along like a small robot. An electric cord hung from its underbelly. We plugged it in. Four numbered cubes and two dots were framed behind glass. One number moved—12:32 became 12:33. Of course! A digital clock.

In her diary on November 13, 1933, Mother mentioned another technological innovation: "A Grateful Patient gave Jim a radio for the car. Some swank!"

Another gift for Dad seemed to me very old-fashioned, as if it was created in a Victorian house by a little old lady in a lace cap. It came in a beribboned box, a dozen white linen handkerchiefs with Dad's own personal signature embroidered on each one with baby blue thread. I, who had embroidered one thing in my life, a lumpy "Dad" on the pocket of my father's workshop smock, marveled that some devoted lady patient had put in countless tedious hours with needle and thread and probably a thimble and magnifying glass, pouring gratitude to my father into the tiny stitches that cursively spelled his name. After a few years, I came to realize this fantastically fine work could not have been achieved by the lady herself, but by a clever machine with a computer brain.

Of the G.P. gifts we received, the most tangible, enduring and unique had to be the buffalo head, mounted to hang. It arrived by boxcar at the train station, along with a hundred pounds of frozen buffalo meat. The shaggy-maned monster with black glass eyes and curving black horns was a gift from the forest ranger in charge of thinning herds in the Black Hills of South Dakota. The atmosphere in our basement playroom was vastly enhanced when the head of the beast was hung over the fireplace.

That playroom was called the Billiard Room, even after the billiard table, balls and cues were gone. The table was installed there by Dr. Emil H. Beckman when the house was built. It must have weighed a ton. There was no way, I thought, to get rid of it; but one day it was gone, taken apart and carried off to make room for us children to play. Recently I learned that the slate below its smooth, green, felt-covered top was used by my brother Jay when he was in high school to make bottoms for his tropical fish aquaria. How typical of my Scottish Dad to save any part of that table that might one day be useful. Now the buffalo head is also gone, bought for $300 (as he insisted) by John Kreusel, a likeable fellow, my brother Jay said, who loved that buffalo and collects many things to keep or to sell in his General Merchandise Store.

What did we do with the hundred pounds of frozen buffalo meat that came with the head and hide? Rochester had cold storage lockers to serve the needs of farmers and hunters. Dad rented a locker. The meat was brought out in frozen hunks as needed, once for a children's Christmas party. It had to be spiced, Dad said, to take the toughness out. He did the spicing himself, a lot of rubbing over a period of weeks. Then it was baked, sliced thinly and served in buns, embellished according to personal taste with horseradish, mustard, sweet pickles or catsup. We called them Buffalo Buns.

At my fiftieth Rochester High School reunion, a classmate, Walter Rommel, reminded me of that party and those Buffalo Buns. And there was something more he wanted to tell me. He had met my mother for the first time at that party, though he had often seen her at the Congregational Church. About a year after the party he saw her coming out of Lucy Wilder's Bookstore.

"She called my name," he said. "We talked for quite a while, standing on the sidewalk. It made my day, that she would remember a kid like me. She was a gracious lady."

It was like Mother to pay attention to people, whether it was a shy boy or a famous sculptor. Gutzon Borglum, a renowned Danish-American sculptor born in Idaho, was a patient of Dad's in 1926. He was in the hospital at the same time Mother was there with a new baby, William Bigelow Masson, our Billy. One day during Mr. Borglum's recovery from surgery, he, in his bathrobe and slippers, dropped in to see his doctor's wife and baby. Mother had a great interest in sculpture, a subject she had studied in Art History at Wellesley and in 1911 on a European trip including Egypt and Greece. Her meeting with Mr. Borglum, she said, was the high point of her stay in the hospital, next to having Billy. He spent much of the afternoon in her room full of flowers. He told her about his major work that was scheduled to begin the following year in the Black Hills of South Dakota.

Mother apparently didn't know the nationality of Gutzon Borglum. She wrote in her diary three months later on October 26 when he was back in town, "Jim's Italian sculptor came to the house and took pictures of three-month-old Billy." A year or so later, Mother received in the mail a small, heavy package, a bronze sculpture of Billy which Gutzon Borglum had modeled from his photos. It is mounted on a block of green and black marble. What a treasure!

And what a brave man Gutzon Borglum was, to have taken on so colossal a project as the Mount Rushmore National Monument. He designed and supervised the carving, on a granite cliff of Mount Rushmore, of the faces of our four greatest presidents: George Washington, Thomas Jefferson, Abraham Lincoln and Theodore Roosevelt. They represent the founding, the philosophy, the expansion and the unity of the United States. The head of Washington is as high as a five-story building. The four gigantic heads rise 500 feet above the valley floor, taller than the Great Pyramid of Egypt. Mr. Borglum made models on a scale of one inch to one foot for the workmen to take measurements from. Gradually, over a period of fourteen years, with dynamite, jack hammers and chisels, the likenesses of those four great men slowly emerged.

The work at Mount Rushmore was well underway when Mr. Borglum returned to the Clinic for a checkup. He invited Dad to bring the whole family to the Black Hills to see what was going on with his work-in-progress. That summer, we all drove out to inspect the sculptor's ongoing work. Never could we have imagined the reception we were to receive and the breath-stopping tour that lay ahead.

As we approached the site in our dusty Packard, we saw men on scaffolding crawling like ants over the clearly recognizable faces of the four presidents. A tiny ant-like man moved inside the cup of George Washington's eye socket; one stood on the moustache of Teddy Roosevelt and massaged inside his nostril with a long-handled brush; another with a wheelbarrow walked under Teddy Roosevelt's chin. Ropes dangled from the eyebrow of President Lincoln. On the top of Thomas Jefferson's flat hairdo, we saw a tiny open conveyance, like a roller coaster car. It hung from a cable that spanned the gorge.

Mr. Borglum gave us a robust greeting, and we kids grinned and shook his hand. We followed to an elevator shaft and crowded onto the skimpily enclosed platform. Our host pressed the button; gears grumbled; we were jerked off the ground. How Mother stood it, I don't know, with all four of us to watch over, no sides on the lift, just railings. We rose to a dizzying height, magnificent scenery on all sides. Then we stepped through a doorway to Mr. Borglum's office. I don't know what supported it, if it was land-based or at the top of a steel column, like an enormous erector set structure, but it was a secure room with walls, ceiling, windows and floor.

The sculptor told us the story of his creation. We looked at his drawings and charts and across the gorge to the sheer granite wall topped by the faces of our four honored past presidents. At the base of Mt. Rushmore, a river of whitewater flashed, twisted and churned among boulders. Then, here came the cable car across the canyon. It came for us. This small, fragile-looking gondola would carry us to the top of Thomas Jefferson's head. Mr. Borglum went to the dock and opened the door to his vehicle. We had no chance to say "no thanks." This fearless sculptor didn't seem to realize what courage it took to be his guest.

We sat on wooden benches facing each other. We breathed deeply as the motor growled and we sailed majestically into shimmering space. We were tapped by a playful breeze that rocked our little boat. Mr. Borglum chatted with Dad. Mother, as thrilled and flustered as we bug-eyed children, did well to maintain her poise. She said something like, "My, it's a nice cool breeze," but, with her eye on all of us, her heart was sure to have been pounding desperately.

The four famous faces came nearer and nearer as we swept smoothly along, 500 feet above the jagged terrain below. Then suddenly we arrived at a rock shore; the door was opened by a man with a clipboard, and we stepped out on top of Thomas Jefferson's noble head. Of all the G.P. gifts we Massons received, undoubtedly the generosity of Mr. Borglum's hospitality in the Black Hills of South Dakota gave me the most stimulating and enduring memories.

The other most familiar of Mr. Borglum's works is the Rodin-like head of Abraham Lincoln in the rotunda of the Capitol Building in Washington, D.C. It was carved from a six-ton block of marble. He also made a statue of Lincoln seated on a bench in Newark, New Jersey. It must have made him happy to have a son and name him Lincoln, a son who worked with him all his life. After Gutzon's death in 1941, Lincoln Borglum finished his father's grandest achievement, the Mount Rushmore National Monument.

My favorite of Gutzon Borglum's works is, of course, "Billy," the little naked baby lying on his stomach, one leg bent, toes spread, head up to look around at the big world. Bill Masson lived for thirty-four years, tall, slim and good-looking. He was a graduate in engineering from the University of Minnesota. Intensely curious about many things, a daredevil, he was capable manually and intellectually of building and fixing most anything. An excellent swimmer, his death was an irony. He drowned in 1960 in the Pacific Ocean when the kayak he had built capsized in a sudden squall. His loss is a hole in my life, and in the lives of my brothers and his friends, Mayo "Jim" Walters, Jim Maytum and especially Gloria Hoversten, the lovely Los Angeles girl he would have married.

On another summer trip we took during my high school years, a spontaneous event occurred quite unexpectedly. We encountered a former patient of Dad's whose appearance shocked us as much as we shocked him. The purpose of the trip was to visit our Canadian relatives. Dad wanted to show us some of his boyhood haunts around Owen Sound and Goderich, Ontario. We drove through New England and Maine and around the mountainous coast of the Gaspe Peninsula. We seemed to be driving backward in time, to a century when bridges had roofs and dogs and oxen pulled homemade carts and people's kitchens and bathrooms were outdoors. The motels we stayed in were primitive and had picturesque names like Noah's Ark Inn and Peak O' Dawn Cabins.

The beautiful blue Gulf of St. Lawrence was ever in sight as we approached Quebec City. We had dinner and spent the night at a modest motel. Quebec was renowned for its historic old Chateau Frontenac, a dramatic 16th-century French Renaissance castle, now a hotel. It was perched high on a bluff like the fabled palace in Dr. Seuss's book, *The 500 Hats of Bartholomew Cubbins*, where King Derwin of Didd could look down from his balcony "over the spires of the noblemen's castles, across the broad roofs of the rich men's mansions, then over the little houses of the townsfolk, to the huts of the farmers far off in the fields."[2]

Primarily constructed of red brick with towers and turrets and steep copper roofs, the Chateau Frontenac flew the flags of France and England

and the maple leaf of Canada. It was the most awesome building I had ever seen. And, according to Mother, its reputation for serving luscious and beautiful meals was unsurpassed in the world, which is why we decided to splurge on an elegant breakfast.

Here we were at 8 a.m. at the opulent, red-carpeted dining room of the Chateau Frontenac, a motley crew in our traveling clothes, the boys in shorts, Mother and I in rumpled dresses and Dad in his only clean white shirt and blue cardigan sweater. Were we kempt enough for this sumptuous place? No other stop on our travels had offered so vast a dining room with crystal chandeliers and bowls of flowers on every white tablecloth.

Suddenly, we heard a moan of what seemed to be intense dismay from an extremely tall, silver-haired man in a tuxedo who pressed his hands together, then threw them up as if releasing a dove. He loped away from a huddle of waiters in the dining room and came directly toward us. Dad was talking to Mother, proud, undoubtedly, to be showing her this majestic Canadian edifice. He didn't see the man until he was upon us. From seven feet up or more, he looked down on our little group. I shriveled with embarrassment. Were we too shoddy? Should the boys and Dad be wearing neckties? The man in his black formal attire stood before us, erect and thin as a flagpole, on his face an expression of open-mouthed astonishment.

Then his knees bent, his hands again spread apart at shoulder height. My heart throbbed in fear and confusion as he stooped, crumpling down from the posture of the major-domo. Almost in tears, it seemed, he put out his hand to my father's sleeve. "Can I believe my eyes? It is Dr. Masson!"

We children could breathe again. We were introduced, I suppose, but I didn't remember this magnificent tall man's name till recently I found it written in Mother's diary: Hubert Massarelli, head waiter. I remember his lined face, his intense, bright, black eyes, his extreme height, his elegant gestures, his emotional gladness at seeing my father, who had cured him of whatever his trouble was.

We were shown to a round table with fresh flowers and a window with a view of the blue St. Lawrence as it flowed south toward Lake Ontario. A bevy of alert and smiling waiters and waitresses were on hand to bring us whatever our hearts desired. Without being asked, we were brought melon balls and berries, grapes and fresh pineapple. A tiny orange sticky bun, warm and fragrant, was delivered by silver tongs to our butter plates, beside a butter ball. The boys and Dad ordered French crepes with maple syrup, scrambled eggs, crisp bacon and slivers of ham. Mother had a coddled egg in a Wedgewood ramekin and an English muffin with an assortment of jams and marmalade. My strawberry scone with whipped cream was utterly delicious.

A waiter came by with tea. "Yes, please," I said. I didn't have tea at home. When another waiter came around, I put sugar and lemon in my tea. A waitress with a pitcher of milk almost passed me by, but I caught her eye, and said, "Yes, please," again.

She watched me pour a tad of milk in my lemon-and-sugared tea. It curdled; little white clumps separated out like cirrocumulus clouds. The solicitous young girl offered to bring me a fresh cup of tea. "No, thanks," I said, undoubtedly blushing pinkly, "I like it this way."

No bill was brought to our table, and when Dad looked around for a waiter, his tall former patient came quickly. "Indeed no," he said, and his hands again seemed to throw up a dove. Our breakfast had been his pleasure to give, a small token of his gratitude to his doctor.

It seemed miraculous to me to have, by pure chance, come upon this elegant, emotional man, M. Hubert Massarelli, who was so joyful that he could serve us. It was not a miracle, though; it was serendipity, one of life's happy unforeseen offerings.

We left Quebec well filled and happy and drove on to meet Dad's relatives and visit the sites of his boyhood. We liked our cousins, aunts and uncles, their dogs, their beds and their food. The roast beef was medium rare and Yorkshire pudding went with it. Strawberry shortcake was the old-fashioned biscuit kind and the whipped cream was beaten up to stiff peaks. Water still flowed briskly over rocks to a pool in Mr. Naftel's pasture. Moss clung to the wet rocks and ferns hung over the pond, which still had fish fanning themselves in the clear deeps. Everything Dad showed us was just as he remembered it until he took a nostalgic side-trip to Dunnville.

Dunnville was the little community where he first practiced medicine, first owned a house, a barn, a horse and buggy. He wanted to show Mother his snug, white-painted house with a veranda and bushes and a beautiful sheltering oak tree. It was a place he was proud to have his mother, his sisters and brothers and cousins come visit. Dunnville was a town where the farmers and townsfolk paid their bills if they could, but if money was short, they brought their doctor eggs, baked goods, apples, or a load of cut wood.

The car drew up slowly in front of a drab little house. Its screen door hung open, the screen ripped as if a fist had gone through it. Dad told us to stay in the car. He got out, knocked on the door, then on the window. Unable to rouse anyone, he came back to the car, huge disappointment written all over his face.

"Something bad must have happened here," he said.

Mother probably laid her hand on his knee and said, "I can imagine how lovely it was, Jimsie, and the oak tree is still beautiful."

Later, Dad learned what had happened there, but he didn't tell us children. The story of the doctor who bought Dad's Dunnville practice in 1913 was told to me by my cousin Allan of Oakville, Ontario. "The fellow married an actress from Buffalo," Allan said. "They were high livers, got into booze and dope, and the practice went to pot."

It was discovered early on by the Mayos that a large flow of patients from every state in the union and many countries was causing their little partnership to expand many times over, and the money received for their treatment was accumulating beyond anyone's expectations. In their zeal to preserve the usefulness of their prosperous endeavour the Mayo brothers established in 1915 the rock-solid legal documentation of their wishes for the future, The Mayo Foundation for Medical Education and Research. It mandated that the Clinic continue in perpetuity as a provider of medical care for all who came, and that any money earned or given in excess of expenses and salaried staff be used for scientific research and the postgraduate training of doctors in a specialty.

In the early years, from the Clinic's abundant profits, many gifts were given to the city of Rochester: parks were given, a swimming pool, a baseball diamond, a new public library, a civic auditorium with art gallery, a theatre and arena that could be adapted to any kind of show from a prize fight to a symphony concert. Those available funds built new roads and worked with bus and rail services to extend routes and lower rates for patients coming to Rochester. The "Joseph Lister" coach was put on tracks, adapted for easy side access to stretchers and wheelchairs.

In 1919 a deed of gift was signed by Dr. Will and Dr. Charlie Mayo conveying all the assets of the Mayo Clinic to the Mayo Foundation, a self-perpetuating charitable trust legally bound to aid and advance the study of human health and illness. Nine trustees, who serve without compensation, were responsible for administering the trust. What had been known as a "partnership" of two Mayo brothers was changed in 1923 to "a voluntary association." Salaries to the staff were held to a comfortable living and security in old age. As Dr. Will put it, they didn't want anyone to receive enough wealth from the Clinic "to keep his children on the beach at Miami when they ought to be working."

This plan is still in force; there is no profit-sharing. All gifts and earnings above salaries and expenses go to the Mayo Properties Association. It is true what Dr. Charlie said of himself and his brother, "If we excel in anything, it is our capacity to translate idealism into action."

As a young assistant in the accounts office, still learning the ways of Dr. Charlie and Dr. Will, Harry Harwick sent out a bill of $10,000, a very steep bill in the year 1909.[3] Dr. Will, checking up on the billing of young Harry Harwick, saw the bill marked "Paid." "This is outrageous!" he said, and sent a check for four thousand dollars to the man, with a letter of apology for the "overcharge." The man sent the check back, saying the bill was not too much to pay for his wife's recovery. Many people continue to give to the Clinic in the same spirit as those who give to their religious institutions.

The name "Mayo Clinic," which I as a child thought of as designating solely the beautiful Plummer Building, now refers to a medical complex of buildings given to the Mayo Foundation by families, corporations and thousands of individual G.P.'s. The list includes:

    The Mayo Building
    The Conrad N. Hilton Medical Laboratory Building
    The Medical Science Building
    The Murry and Leonie Guggenheim Building
    The Eisenburg Building of Rochester Methodist Hospital
    The Harwick Building
    The Ruth and Frederick Mitchell Student Center
    The Charlton Building
    The Harold W. Seibens Medical Education Building
    The Damon Building
    The Baldwin Building for Community Medicine
    The Colonial Buiding of Rochester Methodist Hospital

Grateful Patients

    The Gonda Building
    The Stabile Building

Buildings on the Mayo campuses at Jacksonville and Scottsdale are also named for their benefactors.

    All those who gave so generously to the enactment of the Mayo Clinic's long-range goals are no more grateful than one perky little ninety-eight-pound former New Yorker, Natalie Nelson, who many years ago managed Lucy Wilder's Bookstore in Rochester. With age and retirement Natalie's fortunes dwindled, and she moved to be near her only living relative, a cousin, Dorothy Sargent, and her family in Charlotte, North Carolina. Now and then I used to pick up Natalie at the Shawn Apartments, a high-rise public housing development, and we went out for lunch. She loved to talk about her life in Rochester. There, as she once put it, she "knew everybody in town." One day, when I picked her up, she was brimming with exceptional happiness. Her Mayo Clinic doctor had called; he just wanted to chat, to know how she was doing since her last checkup. He had missed her; she hadn't been in for a few years. The fact that he remembered her, missed her and wanted to talk to her brought tears to her eyes and a flood of happy memories.

⚜ 13 ⚜

Cedar Beach

In the study of some apparently new problems we often make progress by reading the work of the great men of the past . . . .
Dr. Charles H. Mayo, 1932[1]

ONE Sunday afternoon in 1929, as Mother stood by with a grin, Dad said, "Let's go for a drive to Cedar Beach."

"Oh, wow!" We had friends who had cottages there. We ran to put on bathing suits under our clothes.

We headed north on the highway, which was not yet paved all the way to Minneapolis, and turned off on a gravel road that passed between furrowed fields sprouting rows of corn. We drove through Oronoco, a town with wooden sidewalks in front of a few stores, then onto a narrow dirt road that followed a fence and utility poles. Suddenly we were in the midst of a flock of barnyard birds who squawked and flapped to get out of our way. We waved at the farmer in overalls. "That's Mr. King," Dad said. Around a few curves and downhill we passed the cottages of our friends. Between them we caught glimpses of the lake.

Many years earlier the Zumbro River changed shape when a dam was built to create electric power. The rushing river, reviled by French fur trappers as the river of obstruction that upset their canoes, was tamed to a long, broad body of water with very little current.

A hill loomed ahead and Dad stepped on the gas, but not soon enough. Our poor car coughed and conked out. We weren't surprised. Cars in those days, on dirt roads that strictly followed the ups and downs of the land, often had to take off a few hundred pounds and make a run for it to get to the top of a hill. After a rain our black soil made slippery mud.

Pill Hill

This road was rutted with fresh tire tracks, a good sign. Other cars had preceded us up the hill.

We all got out and Dad released the brake. The car rolled back to level ground. On the second try, the motor roaring, the car raced to the top and we climbed back aboard. The trail ended at the beautiful man-made Lake Zumbro bordered by densely forested hills. Cars were parked under the trees and we saw kids at the shore skipping stones on the surface of the water.

What excitement! The secret came out. This point of land was ours now, owned in common by four families who bought it from Mr. King, the farmer who waved. Chester King had owned all these hills and riverside property and was selling off lots to Rochester families. Now we learned that the three other families in this grand alliance were: Uncle John and Aunt Anne Pemberton and their five children, Uncle Sam and Aunt Emily Haines and their four children, and Dr. Berkely Stark, his wife Grace and four children. The Starks, a Canadian couple, later returned to their roots after about fifteen years with the Mayo Clinic.

In no more than a couple of weeks a cottage materialized on our land, a picnic cottage: no bedrooms. Of its four rooms two were dressing rooms with black-and-white metal signs, like license plates, nailed over the doors, one marked "Girls" and the other, "Boys." A middle room had a fireplace, cabinets for storage and supplies, shelves for extra clothing for kids who got wet or muddy and a dumbwaiter, a chest that moved up and down on pulleys into a dry well deep underground for keeping food cold. A screened porch faced the lake and the sunset. Two big tables with folding legs were set up on the porch with benches and canvas chairs. Overhead, under the peaked roof, were rafters, unpainted two-by-sixes, which made a sort of play area where the gymnasts could swing from rafter to rafter and hang by their knees. Girls in the dressing room getting in or out of bathing suits were vigilant, lest any sneaky boys on the rafters intended to spy.

Soon after the cottage was built, probably by some Oronoco carpenters, I got a sliver in my hand from a piece of rough lumber. Dr. Sam Haines was first to hear my wobbly voice and see my tearful face as I cradled my hand.

"I know it hurts," he said. "Let me see it."

He brought the first aid kit from the cupboard and we sat on a bench, my hand in his on the red-and-white checkered tablecloth. He named the things in the first aid box, all the while probing gently for the sliver with a needle. When the sliver was out and my hands washed clean, he put on a Band-Aid. I must have asked what "infection" meant, or what did bacteria do, because his entertaining metaphor about the corpuscles in the blood was unforgettable.

After telling me that the bloodstream has two kinds of corpuscles floating in it, red ones and white ones, he picked up the salt shaker and sprinkled salt on the tablecloth. The salt represented the white corpuscles; they were the policemen in the blood. Their job was to protect the red corpuscles, which were too small to be seen, and couldn't protect themselves. They had a big job, carrying oxygen and carbon dioxide around the body to keep us healthy.

"If you cut your finger and don't wash it with soap," he said, "bacteria will get in there and attempt to eat up the little red corpuscles. Bacteria are the bad guys." He sprinkled pepper in a pile beside the salt and stirred them together with his finger. "This is a battle between the white corpuscles and the bacteria," he said. "The white corpuscles eat up the bacteria and the battle ends, leaving a lot of dead bodies that make a scab over the cut."

I thought everything about Uncle Sam Haines was perfect, even his crooked nose. He was a tall, slim, soft-talking man with black, straight hair and a friendly smile. According to his daughter Olivia, one time her father and Dr. Berkely Stark were carrying a canoe over their heads up the hill when her father slipped, and the bow thwart caught him on the nose. It bled, but he didn't think he needed plastic surgery, so for the rest of his life Dr. Sam Haines went around with a distinctively asymmetrical nose.

Dr. Haines' interest in medicine began with hero worship in high school. A football injury sent him limping into Dr. Charlie Mayo's office, which then was over the drug store. Dr. Charlie himself x-rayed Sam's leg. Those two had a long conversation that made Sam Haines's football injury seem worth the pain. Summers, during his Rochester High School years and his four years at the University of Michigan, and even after his admission to Harvard Medical School, Sam Haines worked at the Mayo Clinic, beginning as a gofer before there was a General Service Department.

His wife, Aunt Emily Haines, was also a favorite of mine. As a young woman who had lived in Cambridge, Massachusetts, in love with a medical student from Minnesota, she had much in common with my mother, whose "Papa" attempted to manage her love life. Emily, in her teens, met lots of suitable Harvard boys, but the one she fell for was a medical student eight years older than she. Worse still, her mother thought, the young man came from some little cow town in Minnesota and spoke with a deplorably flat midwestern accent. Emily was whisked off on an extended trip to Europe with her mother, then enrolled at Vassar. Dormitory life didn't cool Emily's ardor for young Dr. Haines, who was then an intern at Massachusetts General Hospital. Finally, at the age of twenty, with her parents' reluctant blessing, they were married.

Some years after his retirement from the Clinic, which is required at age sixty-five, Dr. Haines was interviewed by a writer for the Mayo Alumni Association's anecdotal history of the years 1915–1992. In his charmingly relaxed way, Dr. Haines said, "No, I never applied for a Fellowship at the Clinic." After a pause, he added, "But my mother did." His mother had gone to high school with Dr. Will.

When Sam Haines' Fellowship came to an end, he was working with Dr. Henry Plummer. He was having such a good time and, since no one told him to leave or asked him to stay, he just kept on doing what he was doing, getting his small monthly check. I don't know when Harry Harwick's business office caught up with him, but he stayed for forty years! That's an example of how casually the Clinic acquired most of its early staff physicians. Invitations to stay were verbal. No contract was written, signed and witnessed.

One of the first things needed at our Masson-Haines-Pemberton-Stark property at Cedar Beach was running water. A well was dug about twenty-five feet deep at the bottom of the hill and a lift pump installed and bolted to a concrete platform. To start the flow of water, the pump had to be primed. A quart of water was poured down its gullet to wet the valve and create an airtight seal. Then the handle was strenuously pumped up and down, causing good, clean, cold water to gush forth from an underground source. By closing a spigot, water was shunted into an underground pipe that went up the hill and opened into a steel livestock watering trough which rested on the rafters over the two dressing rooms. A communal shower head for rinsing off after swimming was attached to the back of the cottage. Each of the lavatories was equipped with hooks, shelves, a sink, a medicine chest with a mirror, benches and a flush toilet.

Cedar Beach

That latter was apparently a ritzy thing to have at the river in the late 1920's. My friend, Jean Davis Warman, told me recently the plumber who lived in Oronoco and serviced the chemical toilets in the other Cedar Beach cottages had told her the place at the end of the road had two "slushers."

Keeping water in the tank was the job of fathers and kids. We lined up to prove we were strong enough till the novelty wore off, and then "volunteers" had to be coerced. A screen over the tank kept most of the bugs out of the water, but not all. Therefore, our water to drink and boil corn came straight from the pump.

Mother and Aunt Anne Pemberton dignified the cottage with the name *Deauville*, in memory of an elegant place they had visited in the south of France on a 1928 surgeon's tour of hospitals in Europe. Since Deauville wasn't part of our experience, we children just called it "the cottage." Mother though, in her diary, always referred to it fondly as "Deauville."

My father had one serious complaint about Cedar Beach: chiggers. Those almost invisible mites burrowed into our tender waistlines and other soft parts, causing itchy red welts. Chiggers loved Dad. A surgeon has to stand for long periods of time in one place doing delicate work with both hands. It was torture for Dad to have chigger bites. In hot summer weather before air conditioning there was always a nurse in the operating room whose job included mopping the doctor's brow, lest sweat drip into the sterile field. But how could my modest father ask a nurse to soothe his chigger bites? Mother rigged up what she called "Jim's romper suit" to wear to Cedar Beach, pants and shirt with elastic at wrist and ankle. Under that he sprinkled yellow flowers of sulphur powder which dispatched any chigger that might sneak through the weave of a sock and travel up to bite more sensitive territory.

Because of the age span within our four-family Cedar Beach picnics plus the extra friends we often brought along, three separate suppers were served on the two tables on the porch: first the youngest, who fussed when hungry. To summon the children of middle and upper years someone would call through a megaphone, "Come to supper!" The echo, "supper," would float back from the hill across the lake, and was heard by kids up and down the waterfront.

The food was always wonderful. Most often, there would be a wide-mouth thermos of stewed chicken and gravy, good bread and butter, sliced ham, cottage cheese, tomatoes, cucumbers, deviled eggs, cookies and always, when in season, corn on the cob. Minnesota was famous for its Golden Bantam corn. Dozens and dozens of ears were boiled on the outdoor grate in a large black iron pot over a wood fire. Our most frequent dessert was delicious and entertaining. Eskimo Pies in tinfoil wrappers came packed in cartons with several slabs of dry ice. When the chocolate-covered ice cream was gone we got to play with the dry ice.

We were warned, of course, that dry ice can burn, but after a few kids got hurt by the hot ice, everyone knew those steaming slabs had to be carried on paper plates. We took them outside and slid them off on a rock where they split into hundreds of pieces. Dropped in the lake or in the toilet, dry ice bubbled like the hot springs of Yellowstone Park. But that was only briefly fun. The real fun was to put small pieces in a Coke or gingerale bottle, add water and stopper it with a cork from a fishing tackle box. Pressure in the bottle built quickly from the carbon dioxide released by the mix of dry ice and water. With a *pop!* the cork would fly off. Cork play fights lasted till the dry ice was gone.

It was a relief for the parents when we were all dispersed to our various games and they could sit down to a peaceful meal.

We learned to swim from a short, bald, muscular man, Mr. Batz, who wore a whistle around his neck and taught swimming and Red Cross Life Saving to nurses at Saint Mary's Hospital pool. In his spare time he gave lessons to children and at other times to our mothers. Mother's diary records that Mr. Batz finally cured her of her fear of diving.

One day beside the pool I noticed on Mr. Batz's bench, along with his towel and his notebook, a package with an intriguing picture and label: *Black Horse Chewing Tobacco.* I asked him about it. He said it wasn't for children, which made me want to try it even more. It didn't taste like peppermint, he said. I kept looking at the rearing horse on the package and finally he gave me a little pinch of it which I quickly put in my mouth. In the horrible moment that followed, my mouth went revoltingly slushy. I ran to the dressing room, thinking I might vomit. When I returned to the class I felt chastened, too embarrassed even to look at Mr. Batz.

Cedar Beach

Our pier at Cedar Beach had a ramp attached to a float, with a diving board and swimmer's ladder. It was supported at each corner by sealed, empty fifty-five-gallon oil drums which held the platform high enough off the water so we could swim underneath, out of the sun. At first, it worried our parents when they tried counting heads and came up with a few missing children.

This problem of keeping an eye on us in the water must have reached its peak when some of the boys turned our solidly built wooden rowboat, the *Tortoise*, upside down in the water so we could climb up on its flat bottom and dive off. For the parents, diving wasn't the problem. Worry came when we dove off but didn't come up for air. We would swim under the *Tortoise* and stay in the pale green light a long time holding the gunwhales or the seats, without even treading water, a foot of air over our heads.

Once I was under the boat with Ginny Moersch when David Stark splashed up between us and said, "Helen, your mother thinks you've drowned." He sank out of sight and Ginny and I popped out of the water. Mother, on the float with Aunt Emily, gave a great sigh and slapped her hand to her chest. Then they burst out laughing.

On August seventh, 1932, Mother wrote in her diary:

> Most of us went to Deauville. We get just frazzled when the four families go for dinner *and* supper. Mealtimes as strenuous as counting heads, the big ones in the canoe, medium sizes disappearing under the upside-down Tortoise, and least ones falling off the dock. Ye Gods!

Of the land-based games we played at the cottage, one was Pom Pom Pullaway, or tug-of-war. Another was Annie Annie Over, throwing a ball back and forth over the cottage roof. We skipped flat stones on the lake, and some of the boys brought their slingshots made from a forked tree branch and strips of rubber from an old inner tube. The game we played most was softball. I can still see Uncle John Pemberton, his hair a strident red, organizing softball games. He'd push up his sleeves and grin, throwing his leg up like a real professional as he pretended to throw out a fast one. Baseball was the sport of his youth in sandlots and at the University of North Carolina.

Later, when Uncle John learned that my fiancé was a North Carolinian, he said, "When you get to Chapel Hill, say hello to the natives for me. I have a favorite cousin there you should meet, Frances Grey Patton. She's a writer with a best-selling book out, Good Morning, Miss Dove."

I did meet Uncle John's Cousin Fanny at a North Carolina Writer's Conference weekend in the '60's. By then Good Morning, Miss Dove had been made into a movie.

Uncle John went to med school at the University of Pennsylvania where he heard about "those Mayo boys" in Minnesota. Curious as the young doctors from Canada were, he took the train to Rochester in 1913 and was taken on as an intern at Saint Mary's Hospital. A promotion made him Dr. Charlie Mayo's assistant. Still new at the job, Dr. Pemberton was standing by in cap and mask one day as a goiter patient was wheeled into Dr. Charlie's operating room. The patient's daughter, Anne, a tall, slim new graduate of Wellesley, stood in the doorway, attentive to her mother's tranquil breathing. When she looked up she was suddenly caught by the sight of a tuft of decidedly red hair that had escaped confinement under the cap and mask of Dr. Charlie Mayo's assistant. The assistant met her startled eyes and looked quickly away.

The following day when the red-haired Dr. Pemberton dropped in to check on his patient, Anne Hoagland, the patient's daughter, recognized him immediately and blushed. What made Anne's interest in this young doctor a smoothly developing romance was the fact that her mother, a Minneapolis native, liked him immensely too and didn't mind his Southern accent.

At Cedar Beach, Uncle John Pemberton, our baseball coach, laid out the bases and drummed up a game of softball on level ground that the boys had cleared of scrubby bushes, sumac and goldenrod. First, he selected two big boys as team captains. When teams had been chosen, Uncle John had us line up at bat, cover a base or spread into the outfield. He pitched slow balls to us neophytes, so we often got a hit, and fast ones to the young teens. He also umpired and called *Strike! Foul! Safe!* or *Out!*

Behind the cottage the hills were wild with trees, birds, squirrels, rock cliffs, caves and undoubtedly more snakes than we ever saw. The slope dropped steeply to an arm of the Zumbro River, shallow and sandy-bottomed. The woods were criss-crossed with paths that might have been made by Mr. King's cows but now were just woodsy routes we kids traveled. When I was alone or with a like-minded friend, I pretended to be a horse and raced along those dirt paths at a pounding trot or canter, leaping fallen logs or little gullies. If I saw something strange on the ground, like a discarded Lucky Strike package, I would snort and shy off the path into the leaves. I could imitate a horse's whinny, and often horses in fields answered back. This talent impressed my brothers.

August in Minnesota was usually dry and hot. The level of the lake dropped and often an island appeared straight out from the softball diamond. It was low, flat and oval-shaped. No sooner was that black, muddy river bottom exposed to the sun than all sorts of airborne seeds settled into the ooze and a bright green fuzz of seedlings came to life on the island.

We looked for the return of the island every August. It was as if it had traveled around the rest of the year like a submarine and reappeared at home base in August. Immediately the fathers and older kids hoisted the bulky *Tortoise* off its rack and into the lake. The padlock on the canoe was unlocked and oars, paddles and a dip net were brought from the cottage to take us out to inspect the island. Usually dozens of newly hatched baby turtles, the size of silver dollars, as well as many big ones, would be sunning on the shore. At our approach they all scooted. Tracks of birds were imprinted in the dirt, as well as the wiggly trail of a water snake. Half-buried were the skeletal remains of fish, sometimes tangled with fishing line, hooks and sinkers. It bothered me for fish to die like that. Occasionally we'd find a wine bottle or beer cans among the green shoots.

On one special Sunday in August 1932, we were astonished by a great deal more than the lovely green island. What we saw off our point was caused by a renovation of the power dam. Water was released and our lake dropped so many feet it became a mere stream. The August island with its little trees and grasses was connected to our shoreline by a broad neck of black mud, cracked at its surface by the hot sun. Good, we thought; we can walk to the island. We were out of the cars in a jiffy, running for a closer look. Our parents came too, and reminded us there were chores to do: unload the car, pump water to the tank, collect firewood to boil corn and get the boats down from their racks. We did all that and went back to take stock of the strange new view at the point.

The first boy who rushed out onto that neck of land was Dave Stark. He took a few steps in his tennis shoes and sank to his knees in the slick sediment that had lain for years at the bottom of the lake. Pulling one leg out forced the other more deeply down. His brother Henry went out with a stick for David to grab. Soon both boys were struggling to make it back to firm ground. But the idea of getting to the island had sunk firmly into the minds of the boys. They each seriously took up the challenge of the mud flats. Soon, we girls were in it too.

What we needed was something like snowshoes with rope like a stirrup to pull a foot out of the mud. Everyone went searching for useful foot gear. We found twine in the tool chest and a few boards and roofing shingles under the cottage. An old wooden barrel that floated down to our shore from upstream was commandeered by Henry Stark. He wiggled the rusty iron bands loose and the staves were shared around. Being too long and narrow, they were broken in half and two used for each foot. With a loop of twine to hold the staves to the foot and pull it up when it sank, Henry made a little progress till the two halves fell apart. A shingle worked better. With a shingle tightly under a tennis shoe, one could step onto the dried mud surface and sink only a few inches. Then we'd pull that foot up with a loop of twine and set it cautiously forward while the other foot was hauled up by its loop. I can still envision David Stark with the iron band from the old barrel instead of twine to jerk one foot after the other out of the black, gooey mud. One pair of boys linked arms, inside feet strapped together on a wide slab of plywood, the two legs being pulled up and set down as a single leg while the outer feet, each in a stirrup of twine, sank down knee-deep.

By the time the parents got wind of the activity and came to look, that soggy isthmus was teeming with strange creatures, all of them trailing a unique path in the black mud as they struggled toward the shore of the lush green island. No one who witnessed the events of that afternoon will ever forget them. It is recorded in the memory of many of us, and in black-and-white sixteen-millimeter film, as shot by the Masson duo, Marion and Jim, that on that day, more creative energy was expended, more parental permissiveness was tested and more children got downright muddy than ever before in Cedar Beach memory. All our parents could do was laugh, take our picture in action and marvel at their children's stamina on such a hot day.

My brother Jay was never content with the clumsy *Tortoise* or having to share the canoe. He wanted his own boat. He was in high school when

Cedar Beach

he ordered a kit from *Popular Mechanics* magazine for making a kayak. From the time that kit arrived along with a double-blade paddle, Jay thought of nothing else. He assembled his materials: wood, canvas, glue, screws and paint, and put it together in our basement with a little help from Dad. Bedtime of the last day came and Mother was so proud of Jamie's workmanship she didn't shoo him off to bed. She stayed with him, he tells me, till three in the morning when the paint job was finished. He named the kayak *Penguin* and painted a picture of the erect little bird in black, white and yellow on the sky-blue bow of the boat.

We all admired the beautiful kayak, but Roy Kendall was so impressed he had to build one too. When that was done, the two boys started out on an exploration of the Zumbro River in the spirit of Lewis and Clark taking on the wild Columbia.

Jay doesn't remember if it was Mother, Dad or one of the Kendalls who got up early on a Saturday morning and drove him and Roy to the North Broadway Bridge, the kayaks and paddles in a trailer behind the car. He does remember the leisurely way they plied their little boats north through farmers' pastures and under occasional road bridges. It was an all-day trip up the Zumbro from Rochester to Kendalls' cottage near Oronoco's White Bridge. They stopped once to eat their paper bag lunches. Another time the river was blocked by a barbed wire fence and they had to portage around it. In late afternoon they arrived at Kendalls' cottage, a tired, happy, hungry pair of boys. Mrs. Becky Kendall undoubtedly fed them well.

One well remembered canoe trip was put together by Dr. Kendall and Dr. Robert D. Mussey, a gynecologist. The group consisted of Dr. Kendall and his three sons, Hugh, Roy and Norman, Dr. Mussey and his son Bob, Jay Masson and a guide. Four canoes were rented on the Flambeau River in Wisconsin, a rather spirited stream when the water was high. The boys and their fathers all considered themselves savvy at handling a canoe. In a patch of whitewater, however, the canoe paddled by Dr. Kendall in the stern and Norm in the bow took on a big wave over the gunwhales and turned bottom-up. All their well wrapped bedrolls and backpacks, as well as paddles, jackets and hats, went bobbing down the swirling stream to the quiet water below the rapids. Hugh and Jay both remember how funny it was to everyone but Dr. Kendall, who stood sullenly in water to his waist, a camera safely dry over his head.

The escaping gear was finally retrieved, a bonfire built and tents pitched.

The guide whipped up a good steak dinner with baked beans, canned peaches, bread, cookies and a pot of coffee. By then Dr. Kendall was back in the conversation.

It is well known, as Helen Clapesattle fondly put it, that Dr. Kendall belonged to *"a queer breed of cats,* the research men."[2] He was a perfectionist. He had the patience to privately enjoy the unfolding of a long-range process. What game could require more mental exertion and patient excitement than chess? That was Dr. Nick Kendall's game. In the Kendalls' living room several chess boards were usually set around in different places. Some of his partners were people he'd never met who lived in places like Seattle, Singapore, London or Frog Crossing, Florida. They sent telegrams back and forth to each other, stating their next move on the board.

Some people can't fathom the scientific mind. To them, Dr. Kendall might have seemed a sourpuss, but he wasn't. He was a biochemist who loved his work. Distant goals always beckoned to him, like understanding the part played by the thyroid gland in health and disease. Disharmony among the nations was another engrossing matter to Dr. Kendall. He read three newspapers every day.

My brother Stan and Norm Kendall were exploring the space above the rafters at the Kendalls' Cedar Beach house one day when Stan, not knowing the flimsy nature of masonite, stepped off the rafters onto the masonite ceiling over the porch below. He crashed through, landing in a shower of dust beside the chair where Dr. Kendall sat reading the *New York Times*. A boy falling almost into his lap distracted for a moment Dr. Kendall's attention to the world's news. He looked up. "Norman!" he called. "You and Stanley are going to have to fix this ceiling!"

Bicycles were so much a part of our life on Pill Hill in the 1930's it was just a matter of time before the idea occurred to us of riding bikes to Cedar Beach. This enlarging of our territory was first noted in Mother's diary entry of July 9, 1932:

> Helen, Jay, Virginia and Bob Moersch wanted to go on a bicycle hike, so I told 'em to ride out the Lake City road. In an hour and a half Sylvester and I took the trailer (to bring the bicycles back in) and followed them. They had biked 13½ miles when we picked them up.

Cedar Beach

I don't remember that first bicycle trip, but there are others I could never forget. We were halfway to the Moersch's cottage at Cedar Beach one day when we stopped at a little country church. Ginny Moersch wanted to see if the church had an organ. The doors were locked but Ginny found an open window. Only the cows in the field saw us climb in. There was an organ, a pump organ, and it didn't need a key. Ginny sat on the bench, opened the hymnal and worked the foot pedals up and down, looking calm and respectable as she played "The Old Rugged Cross." The rest of us felt nervous about having broken into this church, but we each took a turn fingering the keyboard and pumping the pedals. Then we left the church as we came, through the window. Finally, our bikes rolled through Oronoco to the dirt road that passed through Mr. King's farm. "Camp Ginibob" was the name of the Moersch's cottage.

Ginny was a regal-looking girl, six feet tall at age fourteen. She said she always felt awkward performing in concert in a long black silk dress, a cello between her legs. Mrs. Moersch would stand straight and masterful, like Hemingway's Pilar giving instructions to soldiers, when she told Ginny, no, she could not skip quartet practice to go ride bikes. Ginny didn't argue. The truth probably is, Ginny was her most serene with the cello in her arms giving out mellow tones at the sweep of the bow. All her life she played with musicians like the Fox Valley Symphony of Neenah, Wisconsin.

Mrs. Agnes Moersch was a tough mom; you had to eat an apple a day, seeds and all. She and Dr. Fred were hardy types, health nuts. Just to prove it, they indulged in a staunch Minnesota tradition continued by diehards long past middle age. They took a swim on the first day of spring when there still was ice on the lake. On one chilly, sunny Saturday in March, a Cedar Beach population of five or six families all witnessed Dr. and Mrs. Moersch in flannel shirts and sweaters set out in a canoe to celebrate the imminent return of spring with some rapid paddling up and down Lake Zumbro. Jean Davis was in the Davis cottage at the time. She didn't see what happened, but she could hardly talk for laughing when she told me about it. She heard a roar from Dr. Moersch and shrieks from Agnes and ran out to see what was going on. Apparently, Agnes lost her paddle, made a lurch to retrieve it, and over went the canoe. There was Agnes in that icy water, clinging to the canoe, and Dr. Moersch in water to his elbows hauling it by the tow line to shore, his floppy hat dripping, his pipe clenched between his teeth.

> **Cedar Beach Grape Pie**
>
> 1 9-inch pie pan and crust
> 4 c. blue grapes (or more), washed and stems off
> ⅔ c. sugar
> 1½ T lemon juice
> 1 T grated orange rind (zest)
> 1 T Quick cooking Tapioca
>
> Pinch skins off "eyeballs." Cut skins with scissors into smaller pieces and put in saucepan with ⅓ c. sugar. Simmer 10 min. and cool.
>
> Squeeze seeds out of "eyeballs"; discard seeds. Put "eyeballs" in small bowl with ⅓ c. sugar, zest, lemon juice, and Tapioca. Let it rest 5 minutes.
>
> Layer eyeballs on pie crust bottom; put skins on top.
>
> Add top crust, seal pastry edges with a wet finger.
>
> Poke holes in top crust in a pattern. Purple juice will make spots in a nice pattern when it bakes.
>
> Bake at 450 degrees for 10 min; reduce heat to 350 degrees and bake for about 20 minutes more.

On another bike trip to Cedar Beach, wild blue grapes were ripe and we picked enough to make a pie at the Davises' cottage. Jean made the crust. Louise Berkman went to their cottage to get some sugar. Ginny pinched the skins off the grapes and Audrey Woltman and I squeezed seeds from the "eyeballs" of the grapes.

Audrey's father, Dr. Henry Woltman, was the neurologist who diagnosed the mysterious and fatal illness he identified as *amyotrophic lateral sclerosis*. It is popularly known as "Lou Gehrig's Disease." Lou Gehrig, the popular baseball player who died in 1939, was Dr. Woltman's patient. Audrey said her father and Lou Gehrig became very close friends. Even after Gehrig's death, Dr. Woltman stayed in touch with his family. On a trip to New York, Aud recalls, he took Mrs. Gehrig out to dinner.

Cedar Beach

Mary Louise (Weezie) Hargesheimer Gibson went along on one of our bicycle trips to Cedar Beach, as did our good dog Barny. Barny followed us; I couldn't make him go home. The fourteen-mile trip wasn't too much for Barny. He had lots of pep left for swimming.

It was corn season. On the way home, there were frequent trucks on the highway loaded with ears of corn, headed for Rochester's Reid Murdock canning factory. With a loud shifting of gears, the trucks groaned slowly up the hills. We found it was easy to grab the side of a corn crib and get a ride to the top. One day we were doing that when suddenly there was a thud, and we heard a yip from Barny. An oncoming car hit him as he ran from behind the truck.

My heart in an uproar, I dropped my bike on the grassy shoulder, all of us did, and ran to Barny, quivering in the road. Weezie got there first. In his shocked state, he bit her, just above the wrist. I was beside myself with concern for Barny. Madly waving my arms, I ran toward a car heading for Rochester. I made it stop. A middle-aged couple in the sedan looked at me in alarm. No! They didn't have room! I couldn't listen. I opened the back door of their car and several of us lifted Barny into the floor. Then we five girls all squeezed together on the seat. Barny was breathing, and he wasn't bleeding. I think he was in a coma. But Weezie was bleeding; somebody's kerchief was wrapped around her wrist and she held it to her chest. The driver I forced into this good deed took us to my house. Dad, fortunately, was home. He came fast in response to my howling. He felt Barney's chest, then lifted him gently out of the car and laid him in the red wagon someone had brought from the garage. Dad thanked the driver of the car for being a Good Samaritan, and then he saw Weezie and the bloody kerchief. He drove her to Saint Mary's Hospital.

That afternoon's experience gave Weezie a lifelong affection for my father, and the feeling was mutual. Years later, Dad would often ask me, "How is Weezie getting along?" I told him about Weezie, a widow at fifty, living in Grass Valley, California, tending a vineyard and making wine with her brother Fred Hargesheimer. Fred was a hero of World War II. He was shot down into a jungle island off the coast of New Guinea, rescued by natives who kept him alive and hidden from the Japanese for nine months. At war's end, in gratitude, he started a foundation, built a school on the island and wrote a book, *The School That Fell from the*

Sky.³ That school has brought many of those native island children into the 21st century.

As for my friend Weezie, she wrote me a letter on January 14, 1997. She recalled that day we rode our bikes to Cedar Beach and caught uphill rides on the corn trucks and how Barny got hit. "Your father," she wrote, "was so kind and gentle, explaining what he was going to do about my arm where Barny bit me, that it didn't need stitches, but a scar would show up. I sat up on the table while he cleaned the cut and put on a bandage. Then he showed me around the big OR. Very impressive."

We lost Barny that day. His last impulse was just a reflex to bite. Weezie still has her scar. She named it Barny, a reminder that we girls did a dangerous thing that day.

◆{ 14 }◆

The Women's Clubs

It is better to think and sometimes think wrong than not to think at all.
Dr. W. J. Mayo, 1935[1]

FLO BARKER, a new bride in Rochester, turned around in panic at the hissing sound that came from the kitchen corner of her one-room apartment on Second Street. Quickly she turned off the bright-red burner and, with hot pads, pulled the large aluminum pot off the burner, dragging with it a gooey overflow of apple jelly syrup. Acrid steam rose up from the blackened coil. Distressed almost to tears, Flo would have cried, but at that moment the doorbell rang and she stiffened. It might be the landlord, who would not like what she had just done to his stove! She opened the door to a well dressed lady in hat and gloves. Flo immediately apologized for the smell of burnt sugar.

The woman laughed and said she knew all about jelly when it boiled over. She was Mrs. Alvarez, the wife of Dr. Walter Alvarez, who would no doubt, she said, be working with Flo's husband sometime during the next three years of his fellowship at the Mayo Clinic. She was making the rounds of the new Fellows' wives, a pet project of the Magazine Club. It was hard, she knew, for young wives to feel settled away from family and old friends, so she and the Magazine Club wanted to speed up the settling-in process by encouraging the new Fellows' wives to come to the next meeting of the Magazine Club. It met every Monday at 3 p.m. at the home of a Mayo staff member. Mrs. Alvarez put a sheet of information and her calling card into Flo's hand.

"In those days," Flo wrote in a letter to a young friend many years later, "engraved calling cards were part of a bride's trousseau."

Flo's husband, Dr. Nelson Barker, after finishing his fellowship, joined the Mayo staff and soon became head of a diagnostic section specializing in peripheral vascular diseases. To the Fellows in his service, including my brother Jay, he was a guiding counselor as they considered their specialties. Two things Jay remembers especially about his first chief were Dr. Barker's unique hobby, recording bird songs, and the courage he displayed as a man going blind. When he retired, he and Flo went full-time into recording Minnesota bird songs. They made records of all the birds in the area using a high-tech microphone that could single out one particular bird at a time.

Flo Barker, after making many jars of apple jelly that didn't boil over, wrote a draft of a book about the history of women's civic organizations in Rochester, beginning in 1894 when the Rochester Women's Club was founded. The club's first activities were cooking classes and a free kindergarten. Another project, which I think was truly inspired, was the "Rest Room" in downtown Rochester. What a boon it was for farmers' wives, who drove in from the country in buggies, to have a place to nurse a baby and change its diaper, to sit down and rest with a bit of privacy.

In 1910 Mrs. Charles H. Mayo, formerly Edith Graham, nurse-anesthetist and secretary to the two Doctors Mayo, was elected president of the Rochester Women's Club. Renamed the Women's Civic League, the group, led by its attractive and sprightly new president, bent its attention to matters of health, sanitation, the teaching of hygiene in schools and, according to the by-laws, "improvement of scenic conditions," which meant Rochester would have an annual Clean-Up Day.

The following year, the Magazine Club came into existence under the leadership of Maud MacCarty, the wife of Dr. William C. MacCarty, a young pathologist known as "Billy." Dr. MacCarty had intended to return to Washington University when he'd finished his graduate training at the Clinic. However, when that time came, his work with fresh tissue diagnosis completely absorbed him. Previously a teacher of botany at Kentucky State University, he found it a joy to be working with delicate living cells instead of tissues pickled in alcohol. He also thrived on the freedom he was given by Dr. Will and Dr. Charlie Mayo to pursue his own research on the structure and function of cells. When he was invited to join the staff, he readily said yes. Ultimately, he was appointed head of the section of Surgical Pathology.

The Magazine Club in the beginning was open only to wives of Mayo Clinic doctors. Later it included the wives of non-doctors associated

The Women's Clubs

with the Clinic: Margaret Harwick, the wife of Harry Harwick, the Clinic's first business manager, and Mary Lobb, whose husband, known as "Bertie," was the Clinic's intrepid legal beagle. Club dues were one dollar. Each member subscribed to a different magazine, from which she eventually presented a program based on articles she had read.

The programs were all planned by the members, for example the one on October 9, 1941: The hostesses, who traditionally served little sandwiches, cakes and tea, were Mrs. Ethyl New and Mrs. Frank Mann. The program consisted of three ten-minute talks: "Lister" by Mrs. F. J. Robinson; "Trends in the Modern Novel" by Mrs. W. F. (Nell) Braasch; and "H. G. Wells" by Mrs. Edith Mayo. Another meeting featured a topic from *National Geographic* by Mrs. Blackford, the wife of surgical pathologist Dr. R. E. Blackford.

The list of Magazine Club members grew steadily. By 1930 there were 250 members. Since few homes could accommodate such a crowd, many of the meetings were held at the homes of the two sisters-in-law, Hattie and Edith Mayo, or perhaps in Daisy Plummer's spacious living room, where its grand piano and supply of folding chairs were always on hand for an audience.

In 1938, Dr. Will and Mrs. Hattie gave their lovely big stone home to the Mayo Foundation and moved to the smaller house they built next door. From then on the Foundation House was regularly the meeting place for social and scientific gatherings including the Magazine Club.

Two specialized groups were spawned by the Magazine Club, a Music Club and a Drama Club. Mrs. Daisy Plummer was hostess to many a musical afternoon at Quarry Hill, the hilltop stone home her husband, Henry, designed and built. At the time, their steep wooded property was almost off the city map. Now its grand tower looks majestically out over U.S. Highway 52 and the populous area that includes Apache Mall. The Rochester Music Club talents included popular high school music teacher Helen Church, Hazel Martin, who gave piano lessons to many of us, and Mrs. John Trost, a frequent soloist at church and civic events. Bob New remembers smaller groups of opera lovers meeting at the New's Ninth Avenue home on Saturday afternoons when the Metropolitan Opera came into their living room via the Magnavox.

Members of the Drama Club distinguished themselves by writing plays and performing them. I have two typed, brittle carbon copies of a play written by my mother. It is a fast-paced comedy in two acts, "Mrs. Oakley's Telephone." It revolves around faulty communication. The four characters are Mrs. Oakley, an inexperienced bride; her friend, Constance, whose fiancé had skipped off to Europe; a romantic Irish maid and a German cook whose sentences in English were strangely constructed. Mrs. Oakley's dinner plans are fraught with complications until the garbled information that passed through the central telephone switchboard turns out to be a fortunate confusion and all ends well.

A popular lead in some of these Drama Club plays was Mrs. George Higgins, the mother of my Rochester High School classmate, Bob Higgins, who later became a World War II bomber pilot and sadly was lost in action.

Carolyn Walters Brown, the youngest child of Dr. and Mrs. Will Mayo's daughter Phoebe, used to attend some of her mother's Magazine Club meetings at the Foundation House. One meeting she said she will never forget was the time my mother came in late.

Cars were parked up and down on both sides of Fourth Street and in the semi-circular brick driveway when Mother, running late, ran across the street and slipped in the front door of the Mayo's house. Carolyn, who might have been nine or ten at the time, saw her stand in indecision in the foyer, listening to the voice from the podium and looking out over the sea of women's hats. The living room was set up with folding chairs, every one of them claimed, as were the comfortable chairs and sofa. At the back of the room was one unoccupied wooden chair tucked under a desk. It was armless, with an intricately carved back like a cuckoo clock. Mother headed for it, tiptoed smoothly around the edge of the arrangement of chairs till, with evident relief, she picked it up quietly, turned it around and sank onto it.

Suddenly, the strident music of a Swiss band swirled into the room, stopping the words of the speaker, causing a quiver in the audience. The sounds came rousingly from Mother's chair! She leapt up, and folding chairs creaked, flowered and beribboned hats wobbled and wagged as heads all turned to her, she with the carved Swiss chair in both hands as if she meant to choke it. Carolyn Walters probably let out the first giggle. (She had seen many a visitor to Granddaddy's house caught off guard by that musical chair.) And then the room exploded with laughter as the tardy member of the club turned with the chair in her arms, its lilting music pouring sweetly forth. She bolted for the kitchen where behind closed doors the melody ran its course.

The Women's Clubs

On April 30, 1938, Mother wrote with abandon about the weather, the flowers and the state of the birds, but her lilting thoughts were like the Swiss musical chair—only a temporary distraction. The next day she was scheduled for surgery.

In those days it wasn't known that iodine in the water supply was a simple defense against the incidence of goiter, a swelling of the thyroid gland. Mother had put off for too long facing the diagnosis that she had a full-fledged goiter. Her surgeon was to be her good friend Pem, Dr. John de Jarnett Pemberton, one of the best thoracic surgeons in the world, but it was a devastating thought that the next day he was going to cut her throat!

She was in the hospital six days, feeling "rotten," till she took on the challenge of writing a rhyming thank-you note to members of the Magazine Club for their gift of a large basket of assorted magazines. After twelve stanzas, naming each magazine, she concluded:

> I can't tell you how deeply I'm grateful
> What more could you kindly friends do?
> I assure you the pleasure you gave me
> Is quite worth a goiter or two.

Mother also belonged to a Sewing Club, a Bridge Club, a Study Club and the College Club, a local affiliate to the American Association of University Women. She was active in the Edison School PTA and the Congregational Church. The pleasure of her spare time was golf. Whenever a free hour or two and weather permitted, she went to the Rochester Country Club and played with one of her golfing friends. They carried their own clubs around nine holes and rushed back home to be there when the children got home from school. Her pleasure in golf had much to do with her love of being outdoors: ". . . When rain had made us green again, the day was too heavenly to be indoors. I love those lofty nine holes with their wide views" (September 25, 1929).

The Sewing Club was a pleasant way to accomplish, in the company of friends, those tedious alterations and mending jobs necessary to keep children in clothes that fit. Also, mothers back then had to make costumes for school events. For an Edison School "Good Health Parade" I once wore a bright yellow butterball costume plumped out with wire that encircled me like hula hoops. Other children were disguised as giant vegetables and fruits, a cardboard milk bottle and a blueberry muffin. One

Pumpkin Chiffon Pie in Gingersnap Crust

Crust:

1½ cups crushed gingersnap crumbs
½ cup butter
1 Tbs granulated sugar
Blend, pat into 9-inch pie plate. Bake 10 min. at 400 degrees.

Filling:

1 cup pureed canned or cooked pumpkin
3 eggs, separated
½ cup granulated sugar
1 cup milk
½ t. salt
½ t. ginger
¼ t. nutmeg
1 t. cinnamon
2 Tbsp. melted butter
1 Tbsp. unflavored gelatin
¼ cup cold water
½ cup brown sugar

Cook pumpkin in double boiler for 10 minutes, stirring occasionally.

Add beaten egg yolks, sugar and milk after they have been mixed together.

Add salt, spices, and melted butter.

Stir and cook till of custard consistency.

Remove from heat and add gelatin which has been softened in cold water.

Stir till dissolved, then chill.

When mixture begins to stiffen, fold in stiffly beaten egg whites to which ½ cup brown sugar has been added.

Pour into gingersnap crust. Chill. Serve with whipped cream and sprinkle with finely shredded pistachios.

The Women's Clubs

October day Mother commented to her diary she had "spent the day making a clown suit for Helen and feel as pleased at the result as Solomon must have been when he looked over the temple he had built."

Those meetings, sitting around someone's living room with a sewing basket or knitting needles and balls of yarn, served, in addition to tea and cookies, nourishment for the spirit. Mother sometimes said, "We had a grand time. We giggled our heads off."

Bob New described his mother and her friends as "a bunch of cut-ups." They were also like the ladies in *New Yorker* cartoons by Helen Hokinson: naive clubwomen, stylishly stout, good-hearted and innocent. Winnie Judd could have been featured in a Hokinson cartoon when she told the Sewing Club an intimate detail of her husband's habits: "After his bath he powders himself all over with my talcum and puff."

I can imagine my mother as the subject for the cartoon about the lady in a sporting goods store saying to the clerk, "I want to surprise my husband with one of those little red caps that lure deer." And another, the lady in a liquor store asking, "Which is the best one for curing a cold?"

Aunt Ethyl New was a superior gardener. She was short, with a round, smiling, sun-tanned and freckled face. When the month of May finally came to Minnesota, Aunt Ethyl and Mother always rounded up a car full of wildflower lovers and took off for the woods with a picnic lunch, a blanket, and an assortment of tools and containers. In those days it was not considered looting to go into the woods in search of fern fronds, trilliums, modest violets and gentians, not to mention common wild daisies and buttercups. Only the showy Lady Slipper, Minnesota's state flower, was not to be molested. To do so would have been a crime against nature, punishable by a stiff fine.

I have a black-and-white photograph given to me by Aunt Ethyl's son Bob of four women in hats, sweaters and dresses sitting on a blanket in a woodsy setting; the clutter of a picnic lunch surrounds them. A coffee pot is supported on a rack over what remains of a fire. The women are Mother's sister, Aunt Lill, visiting from Worcester, Lura Meyerding, Ethyl New and Adlene Broders. Bob New also gave me the following anecdote.

On the way home, my mother driving, there was an urgent call from Adlene in the back seat. She had to "go." So, Marion stepped on the brake and shifted to neutral. Adlene got out, no other cars on that road, and squatted in the shadow of our seven-passenger Buick. In the meantime, my mother, one of the chief "cut-ups" of the Sewing Club, slyly took her foot off the brake. The car, on a slight downgrade, rolled slowly forward, leaving Adlene, as Bob New put it, "helplessly exposed to nature, while the others in the car were helpless with laughter."

The women of the Sewing Club were Pill Hill wives and mothers who had help in their homes and the disposition to entertain visiting doctors, sometimes at a moment's notice. They also had the time and inclination to be creative cooks. Ihla Hartman's pumpkin pie recipe was outstanding.

Conversation was non-stop at the Sewing Club. Clues to the topics are offered in this rhyming summary of one meeting from the pen of Mary Lobb:

> 'Twas the week before Christmas and all through the town
> Was hustle and bustle from preacher to clown.
> The Sewing Club met—BECKY gave us a treat,
> Though down in her heart she wasn't so sweet.
> She was thinking of Hugh, and the section for Nick,
> But it was her turn, so she had it—old brick!
> Now, MABEL was dreaming of Melvin and Ed,
> And ISOBEL's in-laws were filling her head.
> EDNA was trying to settle the "Y"
> And EMILY's children drove her to the sky.
> ANNE, fresh from vacation, had so much to do,
> She hardly could wait till the meeting was through.
> ETHYL had settled affairs far and near
> So knitted in silence on mittens to cheer.
> IHLA was worried—those Latins in Spain!
> She'd send them a card. They might come again.
> And MARION thought, as she pulled out her yarn,
> What school Stanley goes to I don't give a darn.
> WINNIE was home, but she felt like a wreck
> She'd rather be here than nursing her neck.
> And KITTY, remembering, said that she'd heard
> at the meeting last week more than one juicy word.
> Far off in Toronto, GRACE sews all alone,
> And on the Pacific HELEN wants to be home.
> MARY folded her sewing, she thought it was best
> To take up her pen—and you know the rest.

The Women's Clubs

Mother's Bridge Club dates back to the wives of some of the earliest recruits to the Mayo staff. They played Auction Bridge till sometime in the 1930's when an expert came to their meetings and taught them Contract Bridge. From then on Contract was their game. Now and then Mother was asked to fill in at another bridge club. She would squeeze it in, if possible, but she always thought it a crime to play bridge on a lovely day.

A beautiful book by Harriet W. Hodgson, *Rochester, City of the Prairie*, is copiously illustrated with color photographs as well as some black-and-white shots of historic Rochester. One of those black-and-white shots is a picture of a group of seventeen women posing around a long table with a white fringed cloth.[2] The clothes worn by the women are a conglomeration of lace, feathers, flowers, shawls, frilly caps, a fan and at least one bustle. Suddenly several faces popped out at me, including that of my own mother! Over a black skirt she is wearing a waist-hugging, high-necked, lacy white blouse with a cameo pin which I now wear. The event being photographed was an end-of-the-season Study Club costume party. Others I can name in the undated picture are Isabel Helmholz, Anne Pemberton, Nell Braasch, Carrie Balfour, Mrs. Kahler, Dr. Edith Hewitt, Mrs. Bert Eaton and Mrs. Crew, the wife of Rochester's coroner.

The Study Club has a truly venerable history. It was founded in 1892. A member of that early group was Mrs. Augustus Stinchfield, whose husband was a partner in the medical practice of Dr. W. W. Mayo. The Study Club was an offshoot of a group known as the Rochester Chautauqua Assembly, which was itself an issue of the Chautauqua Institution begun in 1874 at Lake Chautauqua, New York. It was then a training school for Methodist Sunday School teachers. It quickly expanded its scope to include The Chautauqua Literary and Scientific Circles which sponsored adult forums, lectures and concerts.

In 1903 there cropped up, in that cultural family of organizations, the Tent Chautauquas. They traveled around the country giving lectures and miscellaneous entertainment to small towns hungry for novelty from the outer world. They staked out their "auditorium" in some farmer's field and, like touring circuses, attracted huge crowds.

The Chautauqua Assembly circulated fliers promoting its traveling programs. One such flier announced "a lecture by Sir Walter Raleigh." That speaker was either uniquely named Sir, like Garrison Keillor's Senator Thorvald, "whose mama just named him that when he was born," or the roving lecturer was a man in swashbuckling costume who went around the country telling the story of the handsome favorite of the virgin Queen Elizabeth. Other cultural offerings on that year's program were a magician, a motion picture company spokesman and a Canadian band "whose drum major was seven feet one-and-a-half inches tall."

In addition to the Study Club, the Rochester Chautauqua Assembly in 1907 influenced the formation of at least three other serious women's groups in Rochester: the Monday Club, the Zumbro Valley Club and the Live and Learn Club. I can well imagine how news of these groups pleased the aging Dr. William Worrall Mayo in the years before his death in 1911. At the age of ninety-one, he was still speaking out his firm opinions, one of them being that the minds of women should be opened to the world beyond their homesteads. Such stimulation would make them better mothers and happier, more interesting companions.

It surprised me to discover among my mother's papers a green booklet from the University of North Carolina in Chapel Hill, *The Conflict of Political Ideas*. It was the Study Club's program guide for 1944 and '45. Mother was the program chairman that year and her handwriting is all over that booklet. She wrote on each week's study topic the names of the hostess and the leader as well as books to supplement the text.

On October 23, 1944, the topic was "The Chinese Individual"; the hostess was Mrs. Slade Schuster, the wife of a Rochester banker, and the leader was Mrs. Donald Balfour. The book to review was *My Country and My People* by Lin Yu Tang. The instructions to the leader would be daunting to any lay scholar:

> List some characteristics of the average American and compare your list with the characteristics of the Chinese.
>
> Discuss the possible effect of the Japanese invasion on the traditional pacifism of the Chinese.
>
> Do you think Lin Yu Tang's description is of the old or New China?
>
> How do you account for the Chinese ability to resist the Japanese in light of the Chinese characteristics?
>
> How close to American conceptions are Chinese ideals?

It was an impressive amount of work these women took upon themselves. They didn't hire professional speakers or book reviewers; they worked up their own programs. In those pre-television, pre-feminism years women all over the country were apparently looking for ways to en-

The Women's Clubs

hance their lives with the sort of post-graduate education offered by this University of North Carolina Library Extension Service.

Every week in 1944, with World War II still dominating the headlines and newsreels, the Study Club continued its assessment of different forms of government. Chapter headings were: "The Communal Man of Soviet Russia," "The Aryan Soldier—Type of Nazi Germany," "The Japanese Warrior," "The Indian Sage and Hinduism."

The green booklet also directed thought to these comparisons:

- Life Devoted to Personality and God—USA
- Life Devoted to the Ethical and Ideal—China
- Life Devoted to "Folk" and Fuehrer—Germany
- Life Devoted to the Emperor—Japan
- Life Devoted to Meditation—India
- Life Devoted to the Welfare of the Masses—Russia

Membership in the Study Club increased over the years until it included daughters of the original group. Margaret Helmholz Burchell, now of St. Paul, joined the Study Club when her husband, Dr. Howard Burchell, a Fellow in Cardiology, was sent to England during the war. She and her baby girl moved in with her parents, Isabel and Dr. Fred Helmholz. It was a happy arrangement for both mother and grandmother. Margie Burchell remembers well the struggle her mother went through preparing a paper to present to the Study Club. With the daughter, the struggle was the same, "like being in college again."

But always, the highlight of every Study Club year was its end-of-the-year party. "Book Titles" was the theme one year. Mrs. Kahler made a dramatic entrance in a slinky, low-cut black dinner dress. Around her neck she wore a long, thin, bright green necktie. Her book title? *How Green Was My Valley*, by Richard Llewellyn.

Another year, the party had a legal theme. A mock trial was presented. Mary Balfour Helmholz, who had married Margie's brother, Fred, was the judge in a black robe and curly white wig. Isabel Helmholz was a clerk and Mrs. Evie Hunt was the lawyer. One felon after another was brought before the judge. Anne Pemberton was accused of sewing sequins on a Christmas angel while someone was delivering a presentation to the Study Club. She was guilty as charged.

Years after Mother died in 1950 of a massive heart attack, when I was back in Rochester for a visit with Dad, I went to Madonna Towers, a retirement and nursing facility where several of my parents' old friends were living. The place had a happy look: potted greenery, country views, smiling nurses and cheerful sounds. A spirited conversation was taking place around a corner on the corridor that would take me to the elevator. I was headed for the room of Mrs. Daisy Plummer.

First, though . . . I knew that voice, high and breathy, like a toy flute; I was thrilled. No one had told me Mother's friend Isabel Helmholz was here. As I walked toward the voices ahead I imagined Isabel's serene, beautiful face, her chin slightly lifted. Suddenly, there she was, her hand on a walker, its basket full of things a woman might carry in a pocketbook and a rag doll with red hair. Her high Katherine Hepburn-like cheekbones hadn't changed. Her white hair was now thin; she was smaller than I remembered. But her smile and her voice were the same as always. At a dinner party years before, a chicken bone lodged in her throat and she was rushed to the hospital. She survived the ordeal, but ever afterwards her voice was light and whispery. She hugged me as I spoke my name, Helen Masson, in case she had forgotten. Of course she remembered me and my mother, the Study Club and her daughter whom we used to call "Rainy." Our conversation there in the hall at Madonna Towers was animated. It was as if there'd been no loss, no change, and her children were all young. When a nurse came to join us I realized that Isabel had no memories; she was an Alzheimer's patient. But she had kept her usual instinct to be interested in people. She was happy going up and down the corridor, calling on friends and neighbors confined to their beds.

I took the elevator up to Mrs. Plummer's floor, saddened and fearful that she too, in her nineties then, would not remember times past. I wasn't prepared for this remarkable lady, Daisy Plummer. She was in bed, the head of it cranked up, pillows around her small, frail body. In front of her was a contrivance that held a bright light, a large magnifying glass and a heavy book. She wore horn-rimmed glasses through which, with the additional magnification, she was reading. I spoke to her, and she looked up.

I was relieved almost to tears when she smiled and said, "Why, Helen, how good to see you. You're up to visit your Dad. Tell me, how is he doing?"

I laughed and said, "I'll tell you what he said when I asked him how he felt. He said, 'Pretty good for an old fella.' He's still living at home with three good nurses. I told him I was coming to see you, and he said, 'Give Daisy my love.'"

I asked about her daughter Gertrude, and she said, "You just missed her; she was here yesterday. She and her husband Bob Thomas have a beautiful place on a lake up north."

I admired the efficient contraption that held the big book in place so she could read in bed. She said she was rereading some of her old favorites, like the book in front of her, essays of Montaigne. "What a blessing it is," she said, "to be able to read."

In addition to awarding scholarship money to a high school senior and sponsoring an International Relations class, the College Club formed a Pen Club for members who wrote short stories and poems. A professional critic read and critiqued their work. A sonnet written by my mother, Marion Masson, was among her papers:

> Midsummer
> I stood upon a lofty, windswept ledge,
> And there below, in shining folds spread wide
> The God of Plenty, for a royal pledge
> Had flung his many-colored cloak aside.
> Dark shaded velvet of a new-ploughed field,
> Pale, washed-blue ribbons of the blossoming flax,
> Gold moire silk, as grain to light wind yields,
> And pine trees weaving in their threads of black,
> Seemed blended in a mantle, richly fair,
> All under-shot with dull, blue-green of oat.
> My grateful heart swelled, seeing it spread there
> In regal splendor—God's most gorgeous coat.
> Such wealth of harvest is His pledge to man,
> Food for the nations from his lavish hand.

Judging from the number of women who came to a Pen Club meeting at our house (sixty-three), it was a stand-up crowd. If they all sat down to listen to a reading, chairs had to be borrowed from across the street at Hattie Mayo's.

On April 25, 1929, the state convention of the American Association of

Pill Hill

University Women met in Rochester. Hundreds of women came in from all over Minnesota. Those who preferred to stay in a hotel did so; others became somebody's houseguest. We put up three. Our guest room had two beds. The third delegate was given my room, and I got to sleep over with a friend.

A tea was scheduled for the second day at our house. A copper tank the size of a window box housed our two baby turtles. It was beginning to smell bad, so Sylvester carried the heavy tank to the backyard and Jay and I cleaned it out with the hose. Speedy and Toots were green-shelled sliders, each the size of a silver dollar, bought at Woolworth's for twenty-five cents each. We fed them angle worms, one at a time. They would each grab hold and have a tug of war.

When the tank was dried off and back on the window bench in the dining room, Jay and I rearranged its landscape, piling clean sand over flat rocks at one end to resemble a rocky hillside that sloped down to the edge of a lake. Sometime after that, Speedy, the more assertive turtle, explored his hill to the top rock, flopped over the edge, and from the window seat dropped to the floor. We didn't see his escape, but discovered he was missing shortly before the AAUW delegates were due to arrive for tea. Frantically, we searched for Speedy till the doorbell rang; women began swarming into the house. My brothers and I retreated, fraught with anxiety, fearing our Speedy was an endangered specimen.

When the crowd had gone we searched everywhere; in the fireplace, under radiators, sofas and the grand piano where my dog Taffy slept on a pillow in the corner. And, of course, we looked on the oriental rug, where our baby turtle could be camouflaged within its pattern and quietly squashed underfoot like a round wheat cracker frosted with green cream cheese and a slice of black olive.

We'll never know where he was when the downstairs and the screened porch overflowed with women, talking and milling around with hors d'oeuvres and punch. But awe fell upon us when Mother turned back the fringe of a rug and there he was, four little feet tucked into his shell, dry and spent, but alive.

On the third and last day of the convention Mother squired her three delegates to their various meetings and finally delivered them to the 4 o'clock train. She wrote in her diary with an exclamation point, "Glad the old convention is over!" Then she and Dad went "out to Balfours' Farm, famous for Aunt Carrie's cheese rarebit suppers."

The Women's Clubs

The listing below will be of special interest to Rochester friends old enough to remember the women mentioned here who frequently enjoyed each other's company playing bridge and doing needlework and repairs and some challenging post-graduate study.

Members of the first Sewing Club were:

Ethyl New	Mary Lobb	Carrie Balfour
Mabel Henderson	Grace Stark	Marion Masson
Emily Haines	Kitty Wood	Becky Kendall
Anne Pemberton	Aila Hartman	Margaret Harwick
Edna Keith	Winnie Judd	
Mary Aldrich	Isabel Helmholz	

Members of Sewing Club #2:

Frances Berkman	Lola Stenner	Mildred Bollman
Lura Meyerding	Alice Anderson	Marion Masson
Nell Crenshaw	Margaret Berkman	
Mary Smith	Faith Randall	

Bridge Club Members:

Carrie Balfour	Gertie Heyerdale	Maud MacCarty
Nell Braasch	Alice Hargesheimer	Corena Plummer
Frances Blakely	Helen Judd	Daisy Plummer
Elsie Crewe	Mabel Henderson	Marion Masson

The membership of the Rochester Study Club, as listed in the University of North Carolina—Chapel Hill study guide for the years 1944 and '45, included this list of Rochester women:

Mrs. D. C. Balfour	Mrs. B. E. Eaton	Mrs. J. C. Masson
Mrs. W. F. Braasch	Mrs. B. L. Eaton	Mrs. W. J. Mayo
Mrs. L. A. Buie	Mrs. J. L. Emmett	Mrs. H. W. Meyerding
Mrs. N. M. Keith	Mrs. H. Z. Giffin	Mrs. J. de J. Pemberton
Mrs. Kilbourne	Mrs. H. F. Helmholz	Mrs. L. M. Randall
Mrs. B. R. Kirklin	Mrs. A. B. Hunt	Mrs. F. W. Schuster
Mrs. E. N. Cook	Mrs. J. H. Kahler	Mrs. Waltman Walters
Mrs. John Crewe	Mrs. J. L. Magaw	Mrs. L. S. Williams

⁕{ 15 }⁕

Prohibition and Social Drinking

> The by-products of human deficiencies, mental, moral and physical,
> are a clog and a burden to the state.
> Dr. Charles H. Mayo, 1917[1]

It was day two of a three-week Western trip in the Buick. After an early start from a hotel in Sioux Falls, South Dakota, we drove about three hundred miles, mile after mile of flat, bleached, crusty land with scattered patches of small yellow flowers, cacti and a few prairie dogs. A sign announced Presho, South Dakota, a cluster of dusty buildings at a crossroads, a gas station, outhouse and cafe. We needed all of it. It was like the sign we saw later in the trip, "Last Chance Saloon." We were on the outskirts of the Bad Lands. No more amenities would be available till we left that desolate and arid land. Dad pulled in at the filling station.

The screened door to the West Cafe let in a few flies and slammed behind us as one by one Mother, Stan, Jay and I visited the wretched little shed out back, then gathered in the miserable little West Cafe. Limp and thirsty, we sat at a table with a slick oilcloth cover. An elderly waitress brought us bottles of cool Orange Crush that made us all smile at her. Dad came in then, having paid for a tank of gas. He was frowning, but he sat down. The place was a mess. A dozen or so men in cowboy boots sat at tables, hunkered over a meal, elbows akimbo on the table tops. We ordered grilled cheese sandwiches, usually a safe bet.

It must have been the astonishment on the faces of my brothers that caused me to turn around in my chair and look at a cowboy at the next table. Mother looked too. Dad had already seen what riveted our attention for a full, speechless minute. The man seemed asleep, his eyes closed, his head relaxed on the table. One arm hung down, his knuckles on the linoleum floor. His cheek and ear were sunk in mashed potatoes and gravy!

Stanley stuttered in a whisper, "Dad, Dad, look! That man, that man ... he—he fell asleep in his food!"

Mother squeezed Dad's arm. "Jimsey, look. That poor man must be sick."

Dad didn't hop up to take the man's pulse. "Don't stare at him," he said. "He's drunk. Let's get out of here."

But our grilled cheese sandwiches had arrived, and as we ate them and drank our Orange Crush our eyes kept returning to the first man we had ever seen in a drunken state.

Back on the road, our giggles erupted again and again as we mimicked the slack face of the drunken cowboy, asleep in his roast beef dinner. We described, over and over, the scene in the West Cafe as we imagined it when he came to; he'd cram his wide-brimmed hat down over his sloppy face, green beans sticking out of his ears and gravy drooling down on his shirt collar.

"It isn't funny," Dad said, but Mother gave a little chirp of a laugh at our performances. Maybe she had never seen a drunken man before either. We recited one of the Burma Shave signs we had seen: "When you're frisky from whiskey, don't drive 'cause its risky." We concluded that whatever the mashed-potato-faced cowboy had been drinking, it didn't make him frisky.

We calmed down, looking out at the awesome landscape of the Bad Lands. Under a dazzling sun, great jagged peaks of knobby clay thrust out of the parched ground at a steep angle. Dad stopped the car to take pictures and let us run around. It was like climbing a hill of stucco, running part-way up a steep, wierdly shaped mound and very carefully coming back down.

We Pill Hill teens didn't know much about whiskey drinking. As young kids we copied the sophistication of the movie cowboys. We'd saunter up to the window in the backyard shack and order a shot of sarsaparilla, which we would toss off with flare. Those movie cowboys, Ken Maynard and Tom Mix, didn't ever get drunk. It was years later when we learned from a movie how a confirmed drinker lost his life. Ray Milland in *The Lost Weekend* showed us the horror of delirium tremens. I still vividly remember the rat of his imagination, as, with little jerks and twitching whiskers, it crawled out of a crack in the ceiling above his bed and squealed!

Social drinking wasn't part of our experience either. Prohibition was in effect from 1920 till 1933, but even after that I don't remember when it became fashionable to serve cocktails before dinner and wine during dinner.

Dr. William Worrall Mayo, the father of Dr. Will and Dr. Charlie, set a tradition of sobriety for the Mayo Clinic staff. In his horse-and-buggy medical practice the old patriarch viewed the weaknesses of many of his patients with a tolerant eye. They came to him time and again, tipsy, muddled, bruised and bloody after fights and accidents caused by excessive consumption of their own home-brewed corn whiskey. He befriended, counseled and patched them up, but no doubt, he rarely cured an alcoholic.

Dr. W. W. Mayo had a double standard; he expected intelligent, educated public figures to be above the corruptibility of the saloon brawler or the weepy housewife. He was no teetotaler, but he believed that those who would lead others should set a sober example. Young Will and Charlie Mayo grew up helping their father care for all his patients, including the habitual drunk. When the workload became too much for the three Mayos and they began to expand the practice, they agreed never to invite a doctor known to be a steady drinker to join their practice, no matter how good a doctor he was when sober.

Dr. Will was the stricter of the two brothers when it came to social drinking. Dr. Charlie, at his country home, Mayowood, offered drinks to his guests and enjoyed a drink or two himself, but Dr. Will, even after prohibition ended, never served drinks in his home.

There's a tale related by Clinic biographer Helen Clapesattle of the time at the annual New Year's Day reception at the Foundation House when Dr. Henry Plummer arrived all aglow with goodwill to the world and whiskey on his breath.[2] Dr. Plummer was not a drinking man, Miss Clapesattle wrote in *The Doctors Mayo*, but on that New Year's Day, he "seemed to have fallen among the Philistines." Possibly, while his wife Daisy was making eggnog for a special occasion, he tested her recipe a few times. However it happened, there he was at the New Year's Day reception for the staff and Board of Governors and their wives, beaming and chatting with extraordinary wit and charm.

It was customary at that event for the staff to form a receiving line to greet their guests. A slowly moving line of at least two hundred persons would be pressing the hand and breathing the air around Dr. Plummer.

Dr. Charlie, knowing how brother Will would frown at their whiskey-enhanced partner if he got wind of the situation, took Henry on as his personal best friend and stuck like glue at his side throughout the festive afternoon. Dr. Will noticed the affectionate banter that went on in the sprightly crowd around his brother and Henry, but he didn't comment. Dr. Plummer was heard to ask, "Charlie, why are you always beside me?" and Dr. Charlie replied, "Oh, because you're so stimulating, Henry."

Another teetotaler of those years was Dr. Gordon Balgarnie New. He was a slim, serious man with a sharp, straight nose, a neat part in his dark hair and a long-stemmed pipe in his mouth. He had the look of a pondering Sherlock Holmes as he sat in a director's chair looking out over the lake at Cedar Beach, sending up puffs of smoke. But the world will remember Dr. New as a renowned surgeon in the new field of plastic surgery, introduced at the Mayo Clinic as a specialty after World War II. He and his friend Dr. Archibald MacIndoe of London refined their skills repairing the severe facial wounds of soldiers and civilians injured during the bombing of London. They did their work in a small English village chosen as a friendly environment where the grotesquely disfigured casualties of war could learn to feel comfortable with the local people, who were used to their presence and accepted them during their prolonged recovery.

Dr. Gordon New came to Rochester in 1912 to attend the marriage of his Toronto Med School classmate, Dr. Donald C. Balfour, to Dr. Will Mayo's daughter Carrie. The trip for young Dr. New became more than a social event. Because of his early training in dentistry he was asked to stay on as an intern at Saint Mary's Hospital, where he proved himself adept at facial surgery. Another good reason he was happy to be invited to join the Mayo group practice was his pleasure in the company of Dr. Charlie's anesthesiologist, the perky Ethyl Margaret Bailey, a fellow Canadian. He later succeeded in persuading her to marry him.

Bob New, the youngest child of Ethyl and Gordon New, remembers a day in his childhood when he learned that alcoholic beverages can "explode." He was playing in the Meyerding's basement with the Meyerding's daughter Anne Louise and some other children when one of Dr. Meyerding's prized bottles of homemade beer worked up a head of steam and popped its cork. It reeled into the bottle beside it. Like a row of dominoes, those agitated bottles shot off their corks and crashed, scaring the wits out of the children. Little Bob New ran all the way home. Hardly able to get the words out, he told his mother there were explosions going off at the Meyerding's house. I can imagine Aunt Ethyl calling Lura Meyerding to ask if something was wrong over there and could she help? Lura was embarrassed. "Oh dear, no. It's just Henry's beer. He didn't get the tops on tight."

Bob New also remembers with a laugh when he first realized his father could not be induced to take liquor in either sickness or health. Their neighbors across the street, Uncle Mel and Aunt Mabel Henderson, were invited for dinner one night when Bob's father was coming down with the flu. He felt miserable. He had a headache and a fever and his eyes were bloodshot, but he didn't complain.

When the Hendersons arrived, Uncle Mel looked at his friend, felt his forehead and agreed with Ethyl, Gordon did look bad; he might have the flu. "Give him a jigger of brandy and get him to bed," Uncle Mel advised. "I'll be over in the morning, and we'll go from there."

Bob told me his father said no to the brandy. "Uncle Mel laughed and said to Mother, 'Okay, Ethyl, let the son of a bitch die.'"

Bob, being a little boy unaccustomed to cussing, glanced at his mother and Aunt Mabel. Since they and Uncle Mel Henderson were all snickering, he burst out laughing too, knowing that whatever it meant it was cussing.

The family next door to the News on Ninth Avenue was the Crenshaws, John and his wife Nell and their three children, Jack, Meg and Bill. Dr. Crenshaw was known at the Mayo Clinic as a likeable fellow and a skilled urologist. He was more famous in the neighborhood as a master of arresting language. The Crenshaw children, as well as the children of the Lobbs, the Broders and the News, among others, had been cautioned by their mothers not to repeat what they heard in the Crenshaw's backyard when dogs, weeds, lawnmowers, automobiles or children frustrated Dr. Crenshaw.

Dr. Crenshaw had interned at Saint Mary's when the future Ethyl Bailey New was a student in anesthesiology. He caught her attention one winter day as she was cautiously crossing the icy, unpaved street in front of Saint Mary's Hospital. She was bundled up in the long skirts of the day, her nurse's cape with hood, overshoes and wool mittens.

"Hey, Billy!" the brazen and handsome John Crenshaw yelled at her, "Look out, you'll break your goddamn neck."

For a little while John kept Ethyl Bailey's attention. He took her ice skating, to movies and to the Sunday open house at Daisy and Henry Plummer's. Then Gordon New came to town for the wedding of Don Balfour and Carrie Mayo, and he began paying close attention to Ethyl Bailey, a fellow Canadian. At the same time, John Crenshaw caught the eye of another attractive girl in Dr. Charlie's class of nurses studying anesthesiology. She was Nell from Little Rock, Arkansas. I don't know if Dr. Crenshaw swore out loud to catch Nell's attention, but he eventually got her to marry him. The Crenshaws built a house beside the News on Ninth Avenue south of Tenth Street. As neighbors then, John continued to hail Ethyl as "Billy."

My grandfather Knowles was well known to be a bigoted man, as firmly set against liquor drinking as he was biased against Catholicism. Because of him, Mother didn't drink. Wine made her wobbly, she said. At our house Mother's silver service was on the sideboard; Mother and her friends were tea drinkers. Dad, though, came from a household where there was always a decanter or two of something alcoholic on the sideboard.

One rainy day in a prohibition year, my friend Virginia Moersch and I, looking for something indoors to do, decided to investigate a certain blind window in our dining room. Its glass panes had been replaced by mirrors. Our house had become too small for us. It was enlarged every year or so, up, down and sideways, since 1921 when Dad bought it. A sleeping porch and crib room were added upstairs; downstairs a screened porch extended into the back yard; off the china pantry, more cupboards, an extra sink and a breakfast alcove were added. It was that breakfast nook that backed up to the window in the dining room and caused the panes to be replaced with mirrors. Ginny and I wondered what was behind those mirrors.

We moved the tea cart out of the way, loosened the brass latch, and pushed up the window to a shaft of empty space, dark as midnight and full of cool damp air that drifted up as if from a cave. I ran to the basement workshop and got a flashlight. I can still remember Ginny's whinny of laughter when the beam of light hit the bottom of that deep dark pit, revealing a dozen or more sealed bottles.

"Booze!" Ginny cried gleefully.

> Wild Cherry Bounce
>
> 2 quarts wild cherries
> 1½ quarts Brandy or Scotch
> ⅔ cup sugar
>
> To measure, pack the cherries in two quart jars.
>
> In a large bowl strew sugar over each layer of cherries. Pound the cherries hard with a wooden mallet to bruise them and allow juice to escape.
>
> When the sugar and cherries are well mixed, fill the jars and pour as much Scotch or Brandy as can find room for itself between fruit and sugar. It will be gradually soaked into the fruit.
>
> Return to each jar till contents are saturated and the liquor stands on top.
>
> Screw on covers and do not trouble yourself to think of the Bounce again for four months.
>
> Turn the contents into a bowl, pound and crush the cherries with a potato masher and strain and squeeze, a cup at a time, through a cloth (to get the pits out).
>
> The liquor will improve with age and keep for years.

"No, it's not!" I said, embarrassed and defensive. My parents didn't drink booze, and hers sometimes did.

"What else?" she said. "It's homemade stuff."

At the dinner table that night I told what Ginny and I had seen in the black hole behind the mirrored window panes. My brothers were out of their chairs in a flash, eager to have a look, but Mother made them sit down. "What's in those bottles, Dad?" I asked.

His answer was prompt. "Cherry Bounce," he said with a grin. In his "palmy days" he and some friends had made it. That was in Dunnville when he lived in the little white house in the shade of the big oak tree. The cherries were a gift to him from a patient. He was saving the Cherry Bounce, he said, for a special occasion. That occasion was June 2, 1945, my wedding reception.

In none of my cookbooks could I find a reference to Cherry Bounce. A woman at the Charlotte Public Library, however, found a recipe in the book *Beverages*, edited by Time-Life Books.[3]

Pill Hill

According to Berton Roueché in his book *The Neutral Spirit* "the casual use of alcohol was first mentioned in cuneiform writing on clay tablets fifty-thousand years ago. Since then distilled aqua vitae (water of life) was thought to be the mistress of all medicines. But its use for pleasure became highly controversial. Christians felt the barbs of jokes aimed at them, such as "To drink is a Christian diversion unknown to the Turk or the Persian," from William Congreve's sophisticated comedy, *The Way of the World*.[5] A chorus for reform followed the publication of the poem "Gin" by the Reverend James Townley of London.

In the United States, the Puritanism that came in with the Pilgrims gradually relaxed in a free-spirited approval of beverage alcohol. Then the moral current shifted in an equally vigorous reaction against the flamboyant style of the 1920's. Whether or not the government should have a yea or nay over the right of people to drink alcoholic beverages has been a hot topic in this country for more than a hundred years. Before the Civil War, thirteen states had passed prohibition laws. Then, except for the state of Maine, all repealed them. The liquor business boomed. Then again, public reaction tipped toward the "drys."

Adding strength to the Prohibition Party in 1874 was the advent of the Women's Christian Temperance Union (WCTU). Its most powerful voice was that of Carry Amelia Moore Nation. She was arrested many times for disturbing the peace, but many conscientious people marched in her parades, admiring her as a woman of courage and Christian character.

Mrs. Nation's first husband was a drunkard. She divorced him and found another with sober habits. In 1890 she began in earnest a crusade against the scourge of beverage alcohol. Ten years later she deserted her second husband, but she liked his name and kept it; combined with her own name it had a prophetic ring—Carry A. Nation.

Carry Nation was a frightening sight to those men who slid past her at the threshold of their favorite watering hole. Six feet tall in her black button shoes, she would burst into a saloon, wearing a bulky black worsted dress, a leather sack belted around her hefty waist, a tight bonnet framing her fervent round face and a small sharp ax glinting in one fist, a Bible held aloft in the other. She wrecked many a saloon, hacked their smooth bars and bar stools, broke mirrors, jugs, bottles and barrels of beer. Cartoons of Carry Nation in riot mode appeared in newspapers from coast to coast. To her credit she never killed anyone, as did the notorious Lizzie Borden of Falmouth, Massachusetts, who, with her ax "... gave her mother forty whacks, and when that gory deed was done, she gave her father forty-one."

An anecdote from the days of Carrie Nation is remembered still in Rochester: a rumor was buzzed around that the dreaded crusader was headed for Rochester. An Oronoco lady who came to shop in Rochester was accustomed to taking a shortcut to Broadway by going through a vacant building on First Avenue and coming out on Broadway. Recent construction had eliminated her usual door, so she went in a different one. No doubt with a confused frown on her face, she found herself in a well patronized, smoke-filled saloon that had suddenly gone silent. Every man, seated or standing, gaped at her, awe on his face and slightly hunched, as if poised for a quick getaway. Flustered though she was, the lady was no quitter. She kept on walking and went out the swinging door to Broadway, leaving in her wake a stunned silence as the men at the bar shivered with fear that this lady was the hatchet-bearing Carrie Nation.

It was not just women who pressed for national prohibition. The Anti-Saloon League, founded by Wayne Wheeler, a lawyer, had a following of prominent and influential men at all levels of society. The League agitated for an amendment to the Constitution prohibiting the sale of alcoholic beverages. Arguments flared hotly and quickly on the issue of government intervention in the debate. With our entry into World War I, under the food-control bill, Congress voted for a proposal disallowing the manufacture, sale and use of beverage alcohol. The drys won; saloons were shut down. The eighteenth amendment to the Constitution took effect on January 16, 1920. All social drinking, from the mildest of beers and wines to the stoutest of whiskey made in England, Scotland and Bourbon County, Kentucky, became illegal. The drys won because the French wine makers, German brewers and the distillers of hard liquor in every country could never get together and agree on a strategy. However, twelve years later, under President Roosevelt, Democrats and Republicans in Congress united to put the question before the people, and the eighteenth amendment was repealed.

In 1917, while the national debate was raging, Dr. Charlie Mayo was ushered in as president of the American Medical Association. In his presidential address he spoke of two subjects at the top of everyone's mind: the war in Europe and the issue of alcohol. On the latter subject Dr.

Pill Hill

Charlie amused his audience with a witty account of the medical use of tea and alcohol in the annals of Oriental and European literature: "Virulent bacteria in polluted water were unwittingly killed by boiling the tea water in the Oriental cultures," he said. "In Europe, the same end was achieved by diluting the drinking water with a pure distillate made from a fermented mash of various grains or fruits. In the Southern states, this mixture was referred to as 'bourbon and branch water.'"

Dr. Charlie pointed out to his audience of doctors that since they now had an abundance of pure water in this great country, "there was no longer a necessity to fortify our drinks with alcohol. The policeman and the doctor," he said, "know better than anyone else the disturbing correlation between intemperate liquor drinking and life's main miseries: poverty, sickness, immorality and crime. Medicine has reached a period when alcohol is rarely employed as a drug, being replaced by better remedies." He concluded, with a wink to the audience, "The only place for alcohol now is in the arts and sciences. The medical profession, therefore, would welcome national prohibition." Always warm and full of fun, Dr. Charlie had those doctors on their feet, cheering.[7]

Mayo Clinic policy has always been to accept, as members of the staff, only those men or women who had "the right stuff." Weighed into the decision, in addition to professional judgment, was public behavior. If a fellowship student was known to be a regular drinker, that person had no chance of being asked to join the staff, regardless of who his or her parents were or how skillful a doctor.

A nephew of my father and Uncle Morrie Masson came to the Clinic as a post-graduate fellowship student. He was charming, kind, intelligent and a highly qualified doctor. But being well known as a party boy, when he finished his fellowship, he was not invited to join the Clinic staff. Drinking would go with him throughout his life. He found his place to practice medicine in the little Canadian town of Nipigon on the edge of Lake Superior. "They loved him," my cousin Allan said, "drunk or sober." He lived there till he died of alcoholism at age 58.

One icy cold December night in the early 1940's, according to Dr. O. C. Clagett, a group of Clinic Fellowship men organized a party at the Valencia, a popular night club on the edge of Rochester. The place was a magnet for young people, its atmosphere murky with cigarette smoke, the music live, lights low. Small, slowly revolving mirrors hung from the ceiling above the dance floor, reflecting candles on tables. Mixed drinks were served or soft drinks with ice, popcorn, pretzels and peanuts. "Brown-bagging" was permitted, the bottles stashed under the tables as if prohibition were still in effect. On this winter's night at the Valencia, the Fellow's party, it was said, became "a bit boisterous." Dr. Will was informed of "a wild party." He let it be known to the officers of the Fellows Association that there was not to be a repetition of such parties. Future dances were to be held at the Masonic Hall above the Weber & Judd Drug Store, where drinking on the premises was prohibited.[8]

It was long ago when my brothers and I saw the drunken cowboy in the West Cafe in Presho, South Dakota. As he lay with his face in his dinner, it seemed terribly funny. Even Mother laughed when she said, "Wasn't that awful!"

I remember the similar shock I felt when I saw the mother of two of my peers in the card room at the Rochester Country Club behaving very strangely. Other people in that room were playing cards at square tables. It was the Clinic's annual Fourth of July celebration. Parents and children all mingled outdoors in the late afternoon. There were pony rides, a parade with flags, games, hot dogs, lemonade and ice cream. When darkness fell over the fairway, fireworks bloomed from a distant hilltop. I was coming back from the Ladies' Locker Room when I glanced into that card players' room and saw a tipsy woman in a slim yellow sleeveless dress, a long loop of pearls and high heels. She circled a table of four men playing bridge, a glass in her hand. As she passed behind each chair, she fluffed up the man's hair. When she came to a bald-headed man, she walked her fingers around on his scalp. He ignored her till she put her glass on the table, kissed the top of his head and wrapped her arms around his neck, laughing. He put down his cards and untangled himself from her as onlookers watched, mildly bemused. I went to watch the fireworks.

A revered figure of the Greek Orthodox Church in the late fourth century was Saint John Chrysostom. In one of his homilies he commented on foolish cures for drunkenness:

> Many cry over the deplorable excesses of mead, saying,
> Would there were no wine, Oh folly! Oh madness!
> But, is it wine that causes this abuse? No. If wine
> causes drunkards, it would be as reasonable to say,
> Would there were no night that causes thieves
> to steal, and Would there were no women
> because of adultery."[9]

In our country and everywhere, prohibition by government mandate was found ineffective at curing the addicted alcoholic. Carry Nation and her true believers had no lasting effect on them either. In 1935, an organization began in New York City led by three men—an alcoholic New York stock broker, an alcoholic physician from Ohio, and an alcoholic Peabody of Boston. With great hope they started Alcoholics Anonymous. Sixty-nine years later it still seems to be working for many of those who want to be cured.

⊰{ 16 }⊱

In Times of War

> When knowledge is translated into proper action
> we speak of it as wisdom.
> Dr. William J. Mayo, 1920[1]

LONG before there was a Mayo Clinic in Rochester, each state was entrusted with a duty to offer soldiers and doctors to the country when a war had to be fought. Such a war was the war between the northern and the southern states, America's terrible Civil War. Word reached President Lincoln that a certain "little doctor" named William Worrall Mayo, an immigrant from England, was a brave friend and protector of his neighbors during a Sioux uprising. Therefore, in preparation for the impending danger of civil war, President Lincoln dispatched a summons to Dr. Mayo of Le Sueur, Minnesota, to report for duty at military headquarters in Rochester, Minnesota. His job would be to verify the good health of southeastern Minnesota's troops.

When the Civil War ended, a new baby boy, Charles Horace, romped in the Mayo household, making four children for Louise Abigail Wright Mayo to raise. So, Dr. W. W. Mayo, who had moved many times in his life, settled into Rochester as his permanent home.

What Dr. W. W. Mayo taught his two boys, William and Charles, went far beyond how to care for the sick. He instilled in them, and doubtless also his daughters, Gertrude and Phoebe, a broad interest in helping people. He wanted to sharpen the wits of the area's hard-working farmers, expose them to books, upgrade their lives. He felt gratitude for the freedom of his adopted country and would willingly help win its battles whenever the need arose.

Pill Hill

The old doctor didn't live to see another war. But at his death in 1911 at ninety-one years of age, the dark clouds of an approaching war in Europe dominated the news. The Mayo sons, Will, a graduate of the University of Michigan, and Charlie, a graduate of Chicago Medical College, were then partners in their father's practice, which had expanded to include more doctors and more personnel. That was a time of lingering distrust by some members of the profession who couldn't believe in the honesty of the Mayos' unusual business arrangement, now known as group medical practice. By 1914 the group had treated thirty thousand patients. To clarify their honorable intentions, the Mayos put into binding legal language what they had for years been offering, free post-graduate education for medical students and a certificate from the University of Minnesota in Minneapolis. The Mayo Foundation for Medical Education and Research formalized that relationship between the Mayo Clinic and the University of Minnesota. It further defined how money earned by the practice beyond expenses and salaries would be spent. The completion of the first Mayo building in 1914, on the site of the old Dr. Mayo's homestead, marked a new phase in the history of the first group practice to appear anywhere in the world.

On June 28, 1914, the world was alarmed by the news that the popular Archduke Francis Ferdinand, heir to the throne of Austria-Hungary, and his wife Sophie were assassinated, shot by a deranged student who was thought to be in league with the government of Serbia, Bosnia's neighbor. Those pistol shots in Sarajevo marked the start of World War I. Germany immediately declared war on Russia, which had mobilized an army on the borders between Austria and Germany and soon nearly all the civilized world was involved. The United States' early help to the Allied side was limited to the shipping of supplies.

On October 15, 1914, four months after the murder of the Archduke and his wife, my parents were married at the Knowles home in Worcester, Massachusetts. There was no talk of war then, no indication that hostilities were rampant anywhere in the world—except, unfortunately, in the breast of my grandfather, Frank Poole Knowles, who could hardly bear to look at the handsome young doctor from Canada, "a foreigner," who had stolen his precious daughter and would take her to a little one-horse prairie town in far-off Minnesota. He had, however, exacted a promise from the bridegroom that Marion could come home to visit whenever she chose.

My father was first referred to as a "foreigner" on the society page of the Worcester paper when Mother's engagement was announced. Soon after the wedding, when Jim Masson accepted the Mayos' invitation to join the Mayo Clinic staff, he changed his nationality to "American citizen."

A yellowed newspaper account of the Knowles-Masson wedding in the *Worcester Daily Telegraph* details in flowery prose the blossoms, the greenery, the gowns of the bridesmaids, and the lovely bride in "white charmeuse, draped and veiled in rose point lace." On the back of that clipping is a grim reminder that men were being killed and wounded in Europe. An Associated Press report follows boldface warnings that private loans to belligerent countries "are in the same class as munitions of war and other contraband."

The summer after Jim and Marion Masson moved into a small frame house at 212 S. Grove Street (later renamed Second Avenue Southwest), Marion was pregnant. In those prudish times women didn't go out in public in the awkward later months of pregnancy. In order to ride the train, with eight hours to spend in Chicago, while she was still slim, she made her promised first return visit home to Worcester in June. She saved her almost-daily letters from Jim, letters that told of his work as assistant to Dr. E. Starr Judd.

When Dr. Judd was out of town for two weeks, Jim was restless. The work was easier with no new cases, but he preferred being busy, especially with his Marion half a continent away. He made rounds of Dr. Judd's cases and others at the Kahler. Back home he had time to write letters to Marion, sit in the big chair reading the *National Geographic* and feel lonesome. An interesting sidetrip he wrote about was a call to Dodge Center to see a boy and girl injured in a runaway buggy accident. He spent the night in the village and returned on the train the next morning. One day, after finishing his rounds, he went out to the traps to shoot clay pigeons with "Pem" (Dr. John Pemberton). After dinner they listened to the Victrola and smoked cigars. Another day, he wrote, they "... took a spin in the car up the big hill back of the State Hospital on

Pill Hill

high, the best pulling the Reo has done yet. We took Garby along and I made him run about two miles on the way back. He is developing into a regular tramp. I met him down on Broadway yesterday playing with a couple of 'yellar' dogs."

Jim wrote often of being invited out to dinner by friends, especially the Balfours, News and Hendersons. Once a week the staff met after dinner at someone's house where the past week's work was discussed and problems aired. Someone reported on important articles read in one of the medical journals. Jim's letters also told about babies born. Corina and Will Plummer had a boy; the E. V. Smiths, a little girl. He mentioned how tall Marion's "hop vines" had grown; how he missed her while listening to music at the new band shell in the park; how Garby missed her, the flowers missed her. The good news in one letter was that Pem was promoted to resident at Saint Mary's Hospital. Always he sympathized with her early symptom of pregnancy, nausea, and gave everyday advice: drink plenty of water and get plenty of rest. He never complained that six weeks was too long for her to be gone, but every day she was gone, he wrote, meant one day closer to her return. What he grumbled about was "the pesky blackbird babies" in the nest outside their window. "They set up a hunger cry about half an hour before daylight, and I am almost tempted to get my gun and put an end to them."

His letters always returned to the subject of the war in Europe:

> July Fourth . . . heard a very good sermon, and of course it was a patriotic one. I must say Mr. Woodbird was quite careful not to offend any of us "foreigners." I heard, though, that Mr. Vogelsonger is pro-German. If that is so, he had better be very careful not to make any pro-German statements from the pulpit.
>
> News from home is that Morris will soon be leaving Canada for England. Stanley's battalion has arrived in France. . . . He is apt to go to the firing line any day. From now on, dear, you won't blame me if I am even a little more anxious than ever to see the paper and to read the Roll of Honor, because each day I do not see his name will lift a great weight from my heart. Poor little Mother. I just know how she will scan the paper and already I picture her giving a great sigh of relief as each day passes and we are assured that he is safe by his name not appearing. Just think, there are millions of mothers in Europe doing that very thing every day and already there are 55,000 Canadian mothers with children

In Times of War

or husbands in France and another 1,000,000 preparing to say goodbye to soldiers who expect to cross the Atlantic this year.

On July 12th, full of jubilation, he wrote:

Everything has started with a bound today. Judd back and full of pep which meant a busy morning and, what do you think? This afternoon I was listed as the surgeon for the Colonial and have six cases. I had just about finished the Kahler when they got word to me . . . .

Rumblings of trouble ahead seemed remote to the new bride and her friends in Rochester. Their husbands went early to work in the hospitals and Clinic and came home late. Patients came to the Mayo Clinic at an ever-quickening pace. Publicity given to the proposed alliance with the University of Minnesota and the Mayos' ardent critics had energized journalists all over the country.

A short time before Great Britain was drawn into the war, Dr. Charlie Mayo and his wife Edith were in London for a somber meeting of the Clinical Congress of Surgeons of North America. Dr. Charlie was elected its president. Talk of war had slipped into every conversation. But as the couple was returning home, sound asleep on the *S.S. Mauritania*, the ship's engine suddenly roared into reverse. The whole ship lurched in the quiet sea, jogging the passengers awake in their beds. The *Mauritania* swung to a new tangent at high speed. Edith, thoroughly alarmed, wanted to join the excited passengers who rushed into the corridor outside their staterooms, but Dr. Charlie, in his calm and reasonable manner, coaxed her back to bed; the captain was in charge; the sailors were doing their job and there was nothing the passengers could do but get in the way. Edith went back to bed, but not to sleep. In the morning the ship landed at Halifax, Nova Scotia, not New York. The *Mauritania* was draped with canvas tarpaulins. Blankets covered the portholes. Information spread quickly among the passengers that a wireless message from a British cruiser had warned of a German raider sighted in the area.

When Canada entered the war, there was great personal concern among the Canadians at the Mayo Clinic. The News, Hendersons, Balfours and Massons all had relatives and friends gearing up to defend Mother England. My father's brother Stanley put on the uniform of the Royal Canadian Artillery. His youngest sibling, Duncan Morrison Masson, our Uncle

Pill Hill

Morrie, winner of Canada's highest top student honor, the Prince of Wales scholarship (top grades in all subjects), was in his first year in medicine at the University of Toronto when he followed his brother Stanley into the RCA. Their beautiful sister Louise, in nurse's training in New York, found the red tape involved with trying to join a unit of Canadian nurses so cumbersome, she took a ship to London using her own savings and joined the Queen Alexandria Nursing Corps. For the duration of the war, Aunt Lou cared for wounded soldiers in France and Belgium.

"I loved those boys," she said, ". . . so patient, uncomplaining, so seriously hurt, but grateful for every little thing I did." She had tears in her eyes as she lit a cigarette. "I learned to smoke in those hospitals," she said. "The stench was everywhere."

As a child I used to watch the ash on the end of Aunt Lou's cigarette as she knitted baby things for nieces and nephews. She always seemed to catch it in an ashtray before it fell on the little pink or blue sweater she was knitting. She had a deep smoker's laugh and a memory bank of marvelous nursery rhymes.

At first, the wartime letters from Jim's brothers, Stanley and Morris, were full of fun, like letters from boys at summer camp. They were making new friends and seeing old schoolmates.

From Otterpool Camp in Shorncliffe, England, came a letter from Uncle Morrie written on guard duty, September 9, 1915:

> . . . We have been here three weeks today and have begun to feel at home. We are in old leaky tents but expect to move to barracks. . . . In a week we'll . . . get back the $10 deposit taken from our first pay to pay for the uniform etc. and will be classed as full-fledged soldiers. We have all our equipment now and will be able to go right ahead with our training. The 16 eighteen-pounders of the brigade, each with its two ammunition waggons [sic] all in a line, make a very formidable showing. We have right up-to-date guns marked 1915 and with several new improvements, chief of which is an 18 inch higher shield which affords much greater protection for the gunners.
>
> We got our horses last Sunday, 720 for the brigade. They're a very fair bunch and pretty well broken in. I was one of the bunch detailed to go for the horses. We got an early dinner, and started off for the station at

noon. A good 8 mile walk, and as it was a beautiful day we all enjoyed the tramp. The country scenery here is beautiful—everything is a lovely green and the roads, though very narrow for the most part, are all well paved and bordered by high hedges or stone walls. No road is straight for any distance and some of them are very hilly and have some dangerous curves. I never saw such a place for automobiles and reckless driving. A uniform is a license for speeding, it seems. Motorcycles are more than plentiful, army service transports are passing every few minutes. There are no railways here and the traffic is carried by large motor buses. It's a wonder there are not more accidents as they come down hills and around bad curves at full speed and, considering the narrowness of the roads, it is certainly very reckless driving.

We found the horses watering at the station and after an hour or so our battery got their bunch. It was a long walk back leading two horses and we were all fairly tired when we got back to camp at 6 p.m.

The letter from Uncle Morrie was interrupted when someone brought news that his brother Stanley, on active duty in France, had had an attack of appendicitis and was at Shorncliffe Military Hospital for surgery. When finally Uncle Morrie was able to visit his brother, Stanley was recovering from the operation and expecting to rejoin his unit in France. Aunt Lou received a letter from Stanley describing the distant roar of the heavy artillery on the continent that he could hear from his hospital bed.

Again on guard duty, Uncle Morrie wrote about their first zeppelin raid, a black-out, water shortage, and a swim in the channel:

About 9:30 we were startled by a loud explosion. The flash lit up that part of the sky. "Lights Out" was sounded all over camp and we experienced our first Zepplin Raid. About 40 bombs must have been dropped, some of them not more than a mile away. It lasted about half an hour. It was a very dark night and nothing could be seen. They missed their target by quite a bit though. A few bombs if dropped in the horse lines would cause a stampede that might cause a lot of damage. All headlights on motors and all the lights in the villages around were ordered extinguished by the military police. The towns here are very dark at night anyway. No street lamps are lit except a few at busy corners, and there they are so shielded by heavy blue glass as to give very little light.

Pill Hill

... We had a swimming parade Friday down to the sea, or rather Channel. The tide was in and quite a roll on. It felt mighty cold at first, but I never felt it better after one got in. Had a great swim and felt a lot better for the wash. We're awfully short of water. Have to walk the horses about a mile to drink three times a day, and for the last week we have had no water in the taps at all, but have to bring all the water for washing and cooking in the water waggon.

Give my love to Marion.
your affectionate brother, Morris

A letter from Uncle Stanley gives a young man's first impressions of war as an exciting display of pyrotechnics. He then describes the sights and sounds of an "almost every day" fight in the air and the digging of trenches topped with frozen bags of sand:

... rockets, certainly do look fine as fire-works. There are often half a dozen in the air at once.... Some big 12 inch naval guns around a mile behind us heave their big shells every now and then. The flash from the gun lights up the whole sky, and the roar shakes our old barn. The shell goes whizzing over us and hits a target ten miles or so away.

... The [sand]bags were so rotten they had to be handled with care. They were all practically one mass, and it was cold work pawing in the wet earth picking them out, for there was a heavy frost. You could imagine how busy we were ... time was everything. The job had to be completed before daylight. It was quite misty, though bright moonlight. We were mud from head to foot. We roofed the dugout with the galvanized corrugated iron from the old one (built by the Germans) and piled sandbags several layers deep on top. There was quite a lot of activity in the trenches, rifles and machine guns and the trench mortars which make a great roar and flash. Several bullets whizzed past us within a few feet, but they were only spent ones and not directed at us. We got through about 3 a.m. and it was 4 a.m. when we crawled into our blanket back at our billet.

This week I expect we will be digging gun pits. That will be some job too. I expect to go up to the guns next week. That is a lot better than here, for one gets sick of slopping about the horses and wading in mud.

An almost everyday sight is a fight in the air. Every fine day the aeroplanes are up and German ones come across reconnoitering to find gun positions or horse lines etc. as targets for their guns. Our anti-aircraft

In Times of War

guns are mounted on large motor trucks and follow them up, blazing away at them all the time. Their shrapnel bursts all around the aeroplane and leaves a bright round ball of white smoke. They make a very difficult target and are seldom brought down, but half the purpose is accomplished if he is kept up high and scared off. We saw one brought down yesterday.

Today there was quite a raid. A number of hostile craft came over and our men went up after them. There were seventeen of them in the air, and the sky around the Germans was dotted with bursting shells. When they came in close quarters they went at it with their machine guns. It was some exciting battle. None of them were brought down, however. It is rather risky watching such a fight as the shrapnel is bound to fall somewhere. It whistles through the air quite a piece, and one must take cover. Some of it lit quite close to us.

Another letter from Uncle Morrie, somewhere in Belgium, was dated May 31, 1916: "... This peace talk seems absurd when one considers the only terms that would be at all acceptable to the allies. Fritz is far from being smashed at present, even if the potential strength of the allies exceeds his."

Uncle Morrie once asked Dad to send him "... one roll of bandage, a little adhesive, a little cotton, and some suitable antiseptic." Then he asked for "a catapult." When the slingshot, as we call them in the U.S., arrived he wrote that he had had "quite a bit of fun" shooting with the catapult, using shrapnel pellets as ammunition. He didn't mention the target of this sport. Perhaps it was out of consideration for the gentle folks at home like my mother, who wouldn't have known about the scourge of rats who bit the boys asleep in trenches during World War I. Uncle Morrie then wrote with compassion of a tragedy in our family. Mother's first baby, a perfect little boy, died at birth. It always gave me a lonesome feeling when I tried to imagine that brother who would have been four years older than I.

By 1917 the United States under President Wilson declared war on the Second Reich of the German Empire, and American soldiers were sent to fight in the frozen or muddy rat-infested trenches of that devastating war's front lines. But the good news in Dad's letters to Morris, Stanley and Louise was that his Marion was again pregnant. Letters of hope came back. Aunt Lou wrote:

Marion dear, I shall so anxiously look for your news in January, and I shall get something French for the little stranger if she is a girl. If, however, he is a boy, I'll get something English.

Uncle Stanley, in his letter of congratulations on the birth of my brother, James Knowles Masson, added what he considered his own good news:

> I am no longer a driver but a gunner at the waggon lines for anti-aircraft work. I have no more horses to groom or feed, only the bright blue sky to peer into, and when a Fritz appears, shower him with bullets with the hope of bringing him down. It is a wonderful job and I am envied by many. I cannot tell all I would like, and hope the day is not far distant when I can.

That eagerly awaited day in the future for Stanley was not to be. His name appeared in the paper shortly after the Armistice was signed. The Roll of Honor listed the soldiers killed by the enemy, who hadn't yet heard that the war to end wars was over.

Somewhere in that wasted corridor between us and them, a scrawny German Shepherd puppy, frightened out of its wits, cowered in a shell hole. An American soldier found it, fed it, and brought it home at the war's end. He named it Rin Tin Tin. There wasn't a movie starring Rin Tin Tin that I, as a child, didn't see.

Back in 1914 when World War I was in its first year, the Mayo Clinic's people were rejoicing over the completion of the new 1914 Building and the end of the squabble that had followed the news of an alliance between the Mayo Clinic and the University of Minnesota. Many perceptive people, though, were apprehensive about the long-range security of the world. News of Germany's prodigious war machine came over the air waves with every radio broadcast from England. What forced the United States to declare war on Germany, April 6, 1917, was the ominous presence of German submarines that lay deep in the ocean off our Atlantic shores.

For several years there had been shuffling at the White House to come up with a plan to bolster medical preparedness. Finally, President Wilson, the Red Cross and the surgeon general, in 1916, established The General Medical Board under the Council for Medical Defense. The Mayo Clinic was asked to sponsor one of fifty base-hospitals with up to five hundred beds and responsibility for supplies and staff.

In Times of War

This was a ticklish proposition for the two Doctors Mayo. To avoid possible criticism that the Mayos were seeking publicity, Dr. Will, in his diplomatic way, suggested, and it was agreed to, that the University of Minnesota would be a more proper sponsor for a base-hospital. The Clinic would be available to help. That help began with a check for $15,000 to the University for supplies and a promise of personnel. As it turned out, one-third of the Clinic's employees, including doctors on its permanent staff, were ushered into the army.

Minnesota's base-hospital #26 was mobilized December 13, 1917. After two weeks in makeshift housing on the University of Minnesota campus, the group was sent to army barracks in Atlanta, Georgia. There, they received intensive briefings on army protocol and battlefield medicine.

They had an impressive sendoff. Aboard the British ship *Adriatic* they headed for England with an escort of submarine chasers, destroyers, a cruiser, five hydroplanes, a dirigible and a balloon towed by a destroyer. All this festive display seems excessive for a ship wanting to sneak across the Atlantic the day after German subs had sunk fifteen vessels in American waters. When dawn broke the next morning, the only chaperone in sight was the cruiser, *S.S. Leviathan*. The others had turned back.

Safely across and at anchor, base-hospital #26 heard the bad news. They had lost their nurses! Their nurses were stolen, detached from hospital unit #26 and sent elsewhere for service. In army parlance, the nurses were "requisitioned," as were socks, Scotch whiskey, garlic cloves, batteries and crankshafts, by a soldier, a chef or a general who wanted them too avidly to put the request on paper.

Another surprise for the Minnesota unit was their first view of their destination in France. Allery, Saone-et-Loire was in total chaos. Construction was underway for much more than Unit #26. Fifty-three buildings and barracks for ten base-hospital groups were being built, plus a convalescent camp for five thousand ambulatory patients. The baffling scene that confronted our Minnesota group is described by Helen Clapesattle in her book, *The Doctors Mayo*:

> The Minnesota Unit was the first of the ten on the scene, and all its members pitched in to help finish the plumbing and wiring and dig the sewers. The wounded were coming in from the front long before supplies arrived from Minneapolis, so the staff contrived a hundred and one

ingenious makeshifts—tubs and sinks and laboratory receptacles out of biscuit tins; bathing slabs out of lumber and roofing materials; sterilizers out of empty barrels; and refrigerators from gunny sacking stretched over frames and kept wet by dripping water. The doctors scoured the surrounding villages for whatever drugs, dressings, and suture materials they could find, to serve until their own supplies arrived a month or so later. As the great summer offensive of 1918 continued, Base Hospital No. 26 received hundreds of wounded a day, and when its sister units arrived it became solely a surgical hospital, while the other units took over other specialties such as contagious, venereal, and nervous diseases. By the time the unit was ordered home, it had treated seven thousand two hundred men.[2]

Many people asked to see the famous Mayo brothers at the front and were disgruntled to be told they weren't there. The Mayos were kept at home by the Surgeon General, Dr. William C. Gorgas, the man who is credited with conquering malaria and yellow fever in Panama.

Dr. Gorgas appointed a rotating board of ten outstanding doctors to enlist civilian doctors to serve the military at home and abroad. Too many differing opinions, personal egos and bureaucrats prevented much of anything from being accomplished. A board member would serve his two-week turn, then a new man would arrive on the scene. It took him his whole rotation to find out what was going on. To sort out that tangle, the Surgeon General asked Dr. Charlie Mayo, who was famous for smoothing ruffled feathers, to do the job for three weeks. He would be relieved by his brother Will, then Dr. Charlie would return to the post. That system worked till close to the end of the war when one and then the other of the brothers became too ill to travel. Dr. Charlie came down with pneumonia and Dr. Will developed an infirmity even he couldn't identify for sure.

Their job was to ensure the high standard of character and professional ability of the forty thousand or so civilian doctors taken into the service. Later, Dr. Henry Plummer was brought in for a special purpose: to pass judgment on the scores of devices, inventions and new methods proposed by would-be inventors. Also wanting to be given rank in the medical corps were men with no credentials from a medical school but claiming an apprenticeship as chiropractors, osteopaths and chiropodists. Dr. Will and Dr. Charlie didn't discourage their zeal because they could be of service in the rehabilitation of disabled soldiers. But the Mayos couldn't advise the Surgeon General to give officer's rank to unlicensed medical personnel.

Back in Rochester, the Mayo Clinic was under stress to stay afloat. At all levels its people had put on the uniform and left for active duty. At the same time, patients continued to need treatment. Many of the supplies the doctors had become dependent on were unavailable due to shipping restrictions and wartime priorities. A certain methylene blue dye made in Germany, for instance, was greatly needed by pathologists for staining tissue samples. But necessity, that good mother, came to the aid of the Mayo pathologists. Dr. Benjamin E. Terry, an independent researcher, learned of the need for the dye. He moved his ongoing work to the back burner and set himself to the task of finding a formula that would reproduce the much-needed blue dye. In six days he came up with a dye every bit as reliable as the one produced by the German firm.

At this time, an epidemic of influenza was sweeping the country. When it arrived in Rochester it almost overwhelmed the resources of the Clinic. Almost everyone took a turn being down with "the bug"—doctors, desk girls, elevator boys, the General Service men and women, nuns at Saint Mary's and the nurses; they all worked until they too became victims of "la grippe." Volunteers from the city, including Dr. Will's younger daughter Phoebe, came in to relieve the shortage of personnel.

For several years Dr. Will and Dr. Charlie had admired the work of a promising young bacteriologist in Chicago, Dr. Edward C. Rosenow. When asked if he'd like to join the Clinic, he politely declined; he was happy where he was.

However, in 1915, Dr. Will wrote again to Dr. Rosenow. He described the purpose of the newly instituted Foundation for Medical Education and Research and added the following wistful sentence, his heart on his sleeve: "We have always had it in our minds that someday you might join us, on your own terms, to do what you wanted to do in your own way."[3]

What scientist could turn down such an offer? Dr. Rosenow moved his lab to Rochester. He had been there a year when influenza began its epidemic surge. He gave it his full attention.

Finding one species of streptococcus predominant in the sputum samples he examined from Rochester patients, Dr. Rosenow made a serum of it. To test it, he offered to administer it free to Rochester citizens whose progress he could keep track of. The results were so positive that the story got into the papers that Dr. Rosenow had invented a vaccine for flu. Scientists don't want their work to be publicized until testing is complete. But before Dr. Rosenow could demand a retraction from the newspaper editor, a writer from the *Journal of the American Medical Association* (JAMA) had zipped into Rochester and was at Dr. Rosenow's door. All Dr. Rosenow could say was that his experimental serum seemed to help a lot of Rochester residents avoid the flu.

But "seeming" to a scientist is not the same as having proof. The day after the news of his testing was published in JAMA, the Clinic received four hundred telegrams from all over the country asking for the serum. Of course Dr. Rosenow couldn't answer the demand, but his "recipe" was free for the asking to any qualified bacteriologist.

Another burden for the overworked Clinic personnel during the first World War was the Clinic's commitment to numerous training programs for the Army Medical Corps. Classes were held for noncommissioned officers and privates who would serve in the ambulance corps. Civilian doctors had to be updated in new techniques in surgery. Many of the staff surgeons, including my father, were mustered into training positions which required their attending a course at Camp Crane in Allentown, Pennsylvania. They were given the rank of Major and assigned to a special Surgical School at Saint Mary's Hospital for members of the Armed Forces. The program was under the direction of Dr. E. Starr Judd with Dr. James C. Masson as co-director.

In the fall of 1918, Dr. Will returned from his last rotation in Washington, D.C., a sick man. He went directly to the office of the Clinic's business manager, Harry Harwick, and sat down with a sigh. They needed to talk, he said.

Dr. Will had first heard of Harry Harwick ten years before, in 1908. He was riding horseback with his friend and frequent riding companion, Burt W. Eaton, a Rochester attorney and officer of the First National Bank. After a brisk canter on a dirt road, Dr. Will asked Mr. Eaton how things were going at the bank. Mr. Eaton bragged a bit about the bank's training program for future managers. They had some fine young men learning the business. He mentioned especially one crackerjack lad from a local family, a tall, handsome, dark-haired young fellow, quick to learn and trustworthy. His name was Harry Harwick. Dr. Will's ears perked up.

In Times of War

When his horse was back in the paddock at Dr. Charlie's farm, he located his brother somewhere on the property and asked him if he knew a bank teller named Harry Harwick. Soon after that conversation between the brothers, they asked Harry Harwick to join them. Mr. Harwick was glad to be asked. He accepted the job as assistant to the Clinic's overworked business officer, William Graham, the brother of Charlie Mayo's wife Edith. Harry Harwick became more than an assistant. He soon met the boss's daughter Margaret and that was the start of another Mayo Clinic romance that ended in marriage.

Burt Eaton might have been miffed at the Mayos for co-opting the bank's prize pupil, but it didn't end a lifelong friendship or interrupt those evening horseback rides with Dr. Will.

Ten years later on that fall afternoon near the end of World War I when Dr. Will returned from his last war-time duty in Washington, he walked into Harry Harwick's office in the 1914 Building and sat wearily in a chair. His face was a dark, sickly yellow.

In his matter-of-fact way Dr. Will told his young administrator that he had either a case of jaundice that would cure itself, or he had cancer of the liver and not long to live. If it was the latter, there were things he wanted seen to, "and you're the man to do some of them," he said.

For almost two months a new routine was instituted. At nine every morning Dr. Will's driver, Louis West, would pull up at the curb in front of the Clinic. Mr. Harwick would get in the back beside Dr. Will. Sometimes Mrs. Hattie Mayo came along and sat with Louis. They would head for the country, stop for lunch someplace, then continue their drive into the afternoon. Dr. Will did all the talking; his young associate listened. It was an invaluable education for young Harry, like a bonding of father and son. To get his daily work done in those two months, Harry Harwick arose at four in the morning, grabbed some breakfast without disturbing his wife, his young son Bill or the baby Margaret (my friend Mary Ann had not yet been born), and drove to the Clinic. He finished yesterday's work before his rendezvous with Dr. Will.

What filled Dr. Will's mind was concern for his brother. He and Charlie had been devoted partners since childhood. No decision was ever made without the other. Any differences of opinion just hung around till something tipped the balance and the two could agree. In that uncertain time, there was no advanced technology to pinpoint the source of Dr.

Will's illness. If he were to die, he wanted to know there was someone who understood the business end of keeping the Clinic on its intended track.

When Mr. Harwick had first come to work at the Clinic in 1908, the practice was a loose partnership of the Doctors Mayo, Stinchfield, Plummer, Graham, Judd and Balfour. Now, with the Clinic still growing and a new generation of doctors in training, there needed to be safeguards in place, some form of trusteeship, an ongoing Board of Governors, hedges against a loosening of medical standards, a defined policy for fees and payments. Another weighty problem was what to do with all the extra money wealthy patients were giving to the Clinic with no strings attached but to help the sick who couldn't afford to pay. It awed Harry Harwick, only thirty-one at the time, that he had been chosen by Dr. Will as the one to help Dr. Charlie with decisions that would lead the Clinic into the future.

It was jaundice Dr. Will had, and he recovered, leaving Harry Harwick relieved, and a much wiser administrator.

On a morning shortly after the Armistice was signed, Dr. Will sent cables of greetings to some of his old friends, including doctors and suppliers in Germany and Austria. Later that same day, he opened his door to a grim-faced secret service man who demanded in a stern monotone, "Dr. Mayo, why have you been communicating with the enemy?"

Dr. Will, in that post-war time, had committed an act of political incorrectness that would trail for years in the unexamined feelings of the general population. Such nonsense irritated Dr. Will. Facts were facts. They should not be denied by irrelevant emotions. He gave the questioner an icy stare. "*I thought the war was over!*" he said.[4]

❧{ 17 }❧

The Great Depression

> Adversity, if faced up to and beaten, is not a bad thing.
> Harry J. Harwick[1]

IN his memoir of forty-four years as the financial custodian of the Mayo Clinic, Harry Harwick writes that a great good sometimes follows the bad.[2] And so it happened after the Great War. Our side was victorious, our people came home, and good cheer was evident everywhere. It seemed that "the country was on a rising tide of prosperity." But it didn't last. In the autumn of 1929 the stock market took an abrupt downturn. On Thursday, October 24, 1929, headlines such as these—STOCK MARKET PLUMMETS, 19 MILLION SHARES SOLD, PANIC ON WALL STREET—shocked our parents as they sipped their morning coffee. Day after day newspapers showed pictures of seething crowds and mounted policemen in front of the stock exchange in New York.

The grim story of the Great Depression has been recorded in detail in television documentaries, newspapers and books. It deeply entangled the presidencies of Herbert Hoover and Franklin Delano Roosevelt. The loss of millions of dollars in "paper" money was a disaster that caused men to leap from the windows of tall buildings. Companies that closed their doors when their stock became worthless had to dismiss employees or lock their doors forever. Men without jobs often left home in search of work. Some became hobos, riding the rails on freight trains to places where pastures might be greener. Some became migrant farm workers in areas where short-term work was available. Others, depressed and confused, roamed city neighborhoods asking for work or food.

My first confrontation with joblessness was a hungry man at our kitchen door. I was blithely rushing through the kitchen to the back door when I almost fell on him. He was sitting on the brick steps with a plate of food on his lap. Our eyes met as I fumbled to back out of his way. My embarrassment was enormous, but I'm sure his was even more so, caught as he was by a ten-year-old girl in this humiliating predicament, a man who had probably had a job until suddenly the job was gone, he had spent his last cent, and there he was, a beggar at a kitchen door on Pill Hill.

The Salvation Army in Rochester served thousands of meals to hungry men during the Depression. What those men really wanted was a job that would let them know they were worth something to the family they belonged to. My mother was concerned for these often very young men needing work. Her heart-warming short story of such a young man, "Freddie" (printed at the end of this chapter), could have been inspired by one of those pathetic young men who came to our door hoping for a job, not just a plate of food.

Some of my friends' parents who didn't have a regular yard man like our Sylvester Robinson found work for these jobless men. Jean Davis Warman said her father, Dr. A. C. Davis, usually gave them jobs raking leaves or, if he had gasoline rations to spare on a Sunday, they might drive to the Davis's cottage at Cedar Beach to repair a leaky boat, refinish furniture or dig up bushes and young trees in the woods and replant them near the cottage.

Rochester, I always thought, was a clean little city with tidy yards on all sides of town and no miserable-looking shacks beside railroad tracks. But that was an uninformed view of conditions. The State Bank Building, which had closed its doors as a bank, was a center for the collection of used clothing for needy families. Mother's diary of November 18, 1933, confirms there were 1,100 Rochester families in need, and tons of clothing she helped sort for distribution.

My neighborhood friends and I knew very little about the country's woes. We were sheltered from the facts of ordinary life. At our house my father and mother sometimes talked privately in the library behind closed doors and we children knew something bad was happening in the adult world, but it was never fully explained to us why the banks were going broke. We knew nothing about the stock market.

Harry Harwick said the early 1930's were the most difficult years he ever lived through. For the first time in his life, he said, he "knew what it was to go to bed but not to sleep."[3] The number of patients coming to

The Great Depression

the Clinic for treatment was greatly reduced. In 1932 registration of patients dropped to fewer than fifty thousand, nearly a forty percent drop over a three-year period. Many patients, too seriously ill to put off treatment, came but were unable to pay.

After no more borrowing from banks was possible and no new ways were found to reduce the Clinic's operating costs and pay salaries, Mr. Harwick went before the Mayos and the Board of Governors with a bitter recommendation. No one need be let go, he said, but all salaries had to be drastically cut. Dr. Will, as early as 1930, had proposed such an across-the-board cut of staff salaries. There was disagreement at the time, some suggesting that fees be raised and pressure used to collect accounts. Dr. Will answered that opinion on August 31, 1931:

> Since, in this time of hardship the common man is trying by frugal living to establish a new basis of living The Clinic must . . . follow him in his retrenchment and scale down its charges. We must meet him halfway, and not by more severe methods of collection add to his already great distress. We must adjust the accounts to his ability to pay, and give him such time as is necessary. . . . We must send out, not collectors, but adjusters. We must not sacrifice the ideals of the Clinic because of temporary inconvenience to ourselves.[4]

The need for "retrenchment" was accepted by most of the staff with grim goodwill, but some did leave the Clinic to practice medicine in more profitable climates. Mr. Harwick believed the Depression was the most unifying influence in all the Clinic's history. In adversity, the members of all staffs pulled closer together.

Robert C. Roesler, as chairman of the Mayo Department of Administration (1976–1982), came upon unforgettable records of patients treated during the Great Depression. A man from Wisconsin, for instance, in need of a serious operation, told the business office that he could indeed pay for the surgery; he had mortgaged his farm to do so. He paid his bill when released from the hospital. Back home he received a letter from Dr. Will containing his uncashed check and another check from Dr. Will with his hopes that it would help with the extra expenses his serious illness had caused his family.

Many patients who said they couldn't pay a bill but would do so when they were able, did, sometimes in small installments. One big surprise was the patient so obviously without funds that no second bill was ever sent to him. Forty years went by, and he surfaced again as a patient. This time he didn't wait for a bill. He gave the Mayo Foundation five million dollars for construction of the Baldwin Building for Community Medicine, a diagnostic and treatment center for Rochester area residents.

Mother, in her diary of June 6, 1932, wrote, "Jim gets his third cut in salary this month." A year later she wrote that FDR had ordered "bank holidays"—all banks would stay closed through Thursday. "President Roosevelt has vested himself with wartime authority for this financial crisis. At Study Club there was no apparent excitement. People seem to realize this moratorium is necessary."

This was not the first financial crisis to hit Rochester. In the old Dr. Mayo's time there were several slumps in the market. In 1893 the *Rochester Post* ran stories of a severe drop in the New York Stock Exchange. One Rochester bank shut its doors and there was grave concern that the First National Bank might be the next to fold. Panicky farmers came to town in their wagons and carts to withdraw their savings. The bank complied, handing over large sums of cash. Quickly, a meeting of the town's business leaders was organized. They came up with a list of twenty-one citizens who signed a statement of support for the bank. Among those men willing to go out on thin ice for the sake of the community was the partnership of Dr. William Worrall Mayo and Dr. Augustus Stinchfield. They promised $5,000 as security money from their medical practice. That list, a "Who's Who" of Rochester businessmen, pledged $400,000 to sustain the First National Bank through its crisis. It appeared on the front page of both Rochester papers, the *Post* and the *Record and Union*. Their faith in the community quickly ended the run on the banks.

The economic Depression of 1929 that hung over the whole country was deeply set by 1932. With staff incomes at the Clinic cut by one third, family spending was severely trimmed. People didn't buy new cars or take vacations far from home, if at all. We children weren't aware of the subtle changes in our lifestyle. Mother didn't buy expensive meats anyway. We grew our own vegetables and we made do with the clothes we had. To send a child to college would have required sacrifice. Margie Helmholz Burchell said her father, Dr. H. F. Helmholz, "let his life insurance go so the boys could go to college"; Margie's mother, Isabel Helmholz, got a job with the Works Progress Administration.

The WPA was one of President Roosevelt's job-creating programs of

The Great Depression

the National Recovery Act (NRA). One of its projects in Rochester was the construction of Silver Lake Park. Since jobs for men out of work were easier to find in warm weather when crops were planted, harvested and canned at the Reid Murdock canning factory, Silver Lake Park in northeast Rochester was created in the fall and winter months when the problem of joblessness was the most severe.

Children of the Depression had their ways of making a little spending money. Robert C. Roesler began his working career in 1930 at the age of twelve caddying for golfers. The going rate for eighteen holes was a ten-cent tip. A few golfers, like Harry Harwick, were extra good tippers; they gave the caddy a quarter. Mr. Harwick might have noticed that Bob was an extra good caddy. He kept his eye on him when he got his first Clinic job in the department of General Service. Bob learned the Clinic's business from the ground up, serving for thirty-seven years in many key positions, including secretary of the Board of Mayo Governors and vice-chairman of the Board of Trustees of the Mayo Foundation.

Surely, the lot of the Mayo Fellows was the toughest of all who worked for the Clinic. Their three-year fellowship, a "free" post-graduate education under the auspices of the University of Minnesota, paid a meager stipend for long hours of work.

In his autobiography, Dr. O. T. (Jim) Clagett writes that when he was a Fellow in the 1930's there were thirty Fellows, some with wives, living on $70 a month. When the Clagett's old car overheated and the block cracked, they sold it for junk for $125 and went without a car for the next four years.[5]

Dr. Jim Clagett's introduction to surgical service was with Dr. John Pemberton, whose first assistant was Dr. John Waugh. Each day was an exciting adventure, he wrote. He lived at Saint Mary's Hospital most of the time, occasionally getting home to his wife Alicia for a few hours or overnight. Early every morning he visited all Dr. Pemberton's patients to take care of any orders or treatments necessary. He changed dressings as required, administered any intravenous or subcutaneous fluids indicated and checked for any complications or problems.

Shortly after breakfast, he, Dr. Waugh and Dr. Pemberton made rounds of all the patients. They also looked in on patients wanting Dr. Pemberton's surgical opinion of their problem. On alternate days a list of surgical operations was performed, beginning as soon as morning rounds had been completed. On the non-surgical days Dr. Pemberton consulted on surgical problems at the Clinic. When patients were referred to Dr. Pemberton's service it was Dr. Clagett's responsibility to review and condense the patient's history, see that the patient was listed for surgery and order the appropriate preoperative preparations and medications. On operating days he acted as second assistant in the operating room.[6]

That was a typical week for surgical Fellows. When a little free time was available, they often went to the Clinic library to read up on the various conditions with which they were dealing, which at this time for Dr. Clagett were thyroid and colon surgery.

Somehow, the well known privations of living on a Fellow's salary during the Depression didn't diminish the zeal of the young men and women applying for the chance to live that poor, arduous apprenticeship. The schedule Dr. Clagett had to keep might have finished off many a marriage, but he and his wife Alicia remember those years as some of the best of their lives. Where else could a doctor find such challenge among such congenial fellow learners and splendid teachers? The senior staff, including the Mayos, worked as hard as the new Fellows on the team. "They made us feel important to the success of the Clinic," Dr. Clagett wrote. "They gave us time off for study and money for the wives to go along on study trips. In spite of our poverty, we were happy. We lived in a wonderful, enthusiastic environment.... I was excited about all the things I was seeing and learning and the opportunities that were opening up for me."[7]

Some of the Fellows, though, did leave the Clinic before finishing their three-year course. Some left because the work was too long and hard and the winters too cold. Others returned to families back home who were hard-pressed by the Depression, and a secure salary from him was the primary need.

As I mentioned before, as a child I was not hurt by the hardships imposed on my generation by the Depression. It is evident, though, in the following story, "Freddie," written by my mother, how deeply *she* understood the anguish in many American families.

The Great Depression

Freddie

It was five o'clock on a cheerless November afternoon, and Mrs. Wilbur sat at the kitchen table wearily paring potatoes. Her feet were sore and her back ached. Since early morning she had been working hard, directing the men where to put each piece of furniture, and trying to get the pictures and curtains hung before Myron arrived. Annie had just gone upstairs to make the beds while Mrs. Wilbur started dinner.

Moving day or not, Myron must find dinner ready when he came home—meat, potatoes, a vegetable, a substantial dessert. Myron was like that. He was a little man, not very clever in business. With men he felt a smothering inferiority complex, which perhaps accounted for the joy he took in lording it over his wife and son.

Mrs. Wilbur was thinking of Myron now as she painstakingly cut the thinnest possible parings from the potatoes, and her thoughts were tinged with bitterness. Myron was always so sure he was right. She had usually given in meekly to his decisions, but why couldn't Myron see that it was different with a lad of seventeen?

It was now almost three years since that awful night when Freddie had come home full of enthusiasm with his plan to leave school and accept a job in a garage. She could still hear the boy's eager young voice—"Gee, Dad, it's a swell chance. Bill says I know more about a car now than half the trained mechanics. I'll be owning a garage before you know it."

Freddie's mother lived over painfully the scene that followed. Myron, tired from a hard day at the office, had lost himself completely. He had said scathing things which none of them would ever forget—about working his fingers to the bone to give his son a fine education, about the pigheadedness of youth, about rank ingratitude. He had dealt the boy's fine confidence in his own ability blow after blow.

The final scene was indelibly etched on Mrs. Wilbur's memory: Myron, red-faced and dogged in his refusal even to discuss Frederick's plans; the lad, white to the lips, his head thrown back like a thoroughbred colt that resents a heavy hand on the bridle rein. "All right, Dad. I'll go. I can take care of myself." Flinging his schoolbooks on the table, Freddie had gone without a backward look. That was three years ago. He had stepped out into the shifting, seething world and disappeared, like a pebble thrown carelessly into the ocean.

Mr. Wilbur had been horrified at the results of his unreasoning tirade, but it was too late. He had left no stone unturned in his effort to find the lad, but all to no avail. Freddie was gone. Business worries began to pile up for Mr. Wilbur. The Depression had started, and he was on the toboggan. This was the third time they had moved in three years—and each time a step down—from the comfortable old house on Essex street with its wide yard and two-car garage, to this little six-room cottage.

As soon as they were settled Annie would leave. There was no need of a maid in such a doll's house. Mrs. Wilbur was going through her usual period of restlessness and anxiety that followed every moving. She was never comfortable till their new address was in the city directory and the telephone book.

A sharp ring of the doorbell startled her back to the present. "Annie," she called, "Answer that, please. My hands are wet." The front door opened, then shut smartly with an impatient exclamation from Annie, who appeared immediately in the kitchen. "I hain't got them bells straightened out yet. Guess it must of been the back door," she said as she squeezed between Mrs. Wilbur and the sink on her way to the entry.

A low murmur of voices ensued, and in a moment Annie stepped back into the kitchen. "It's a tramp, Mis' Wilbur," she said. "Wants to know if we got any work he could do."

Mrs. Wilbur put back a lock of gray hair with the hand that held the paring knife. "Oh, dear, Annie," she said. "He's the third one since we came in this morning. Give him some bread and butter and a glass of milk. There's no work for him."

When Annie returned to the outside door and delivered her message rather tartly, the man's voice rose on a protesting note. Mrs. Wilbur caught her breath in a painful gasp, and the knife clattered into the pan. She put the back of a shaking hand to her forehead. It was damp, and she could feel little shuddering chills creeping over her flesh.

Annie called back over her shoulder, "He says if you ain't got no work he don't want no food."

"Annie!" the word was sharp, compelling. "Tell him to come here."

Steps sounded presently from the entryway, and still Mrs. Wilbur sat rigid, her back to the door. Very slowly, in agonizing terror lest she be wrong, she turned to the man standing now just behind her.

Then with a sighing little moan of "Freddie!" she slipped limply from her chair as the tramp sprang forward and caught her.

❧{ 18 }❧

A Century of Progress

The keynote of progress in the twentieth century is system and organization,
in other words, "team work."
Dr. C. H. Mayo, 1938[1]

EVEN before the Great Depression settled over the United States like dense fog and, to a lighter extent, over the European continent, planning began for a World's Fair in Chicago in 1933 and 1934. It would be known as the Century of Progress International Exposition. It would mark Chicago's 100th anniversary. Forty years earlier, in 1893, Chicago hosted the World's Columbian Exposition, in celebration of the 400th anniversary of the discovery of America by Columbus. The marvels exhibited then included the linotype printing machine, Pullman cars and the Ferris wheel. That fair used more electricity than was then used by the whole city of Chicago.

The purpose of the 1933 Exposition, in addition to providing the wild fun of a fair, was to introduce to the non-scientific public the remarkable scientific achievements of the past one hundred years and to showcase the cultures of participating nations, including our former enemies in the first World War. It showed visitors the marvels of science: strange robots, efficient new telephones, digital radios, automobiles, airplanes and fabrics. New power sources were demonstrated. Science fiction of the 1920's was virtual reality in 1933. The Exposition was intended to entertain and coax the nation out of its severe depression. It was not only a financial success, it enabled many Chicago businessmen and women to stave off bankruptcy.

Also in Chicago, undeterred by the prevailing economic downturn, construction was underway for a new museum, the Museum of Science and Industry. That museum was to become one of the world's truly important museums. Located at 57th Street and Lake Shore Drive in the Jackson Park area, it was described by the American Association for the Advancement of Science as "Chicago's top draw." But it was the World's Fair that drew the huge crowds to Chicago in 1933 and '34.

The fair organizers extended an invitation to the Mayo Foundation to contribute exhibits that would demonstrate a half-century of progress in medicine and surgery. The Foundation gladly accepted the challenge. Dr. Arthur H. Bulbulian, formerly with the Natural History Museum at the University of Minnesota, was put in charge of the Mayo exhibits. He assembled photographs, lantern slides, charts, motion pictures and his own wax models that told the story of the progress of medicine in the previous fifty years. When the World's Fair was over, most of those exhibits became the nucleus for the Clinic's Museum of Hygiene and Medicine.

Dr. Bulbulian's colored wax models of an appendectomy-in-progress were so popular that when the Exposition ended, Major Lenox R. Lohr asked if Chicago's new Museum of Science and Industry might keep it a while on loan. After an extended stay in Chicago it was sent back to Rochester. But they missed it in Chicago and after a polite interval, asked for it back. Dr. Bulbulian, like so many of his peers, was a stickler for accuracy. The techniques involved in snipping off the veriform appendix had changed since the doctor/sculptor first made his models. He would send some new models to Chicago.

The new exhibit was bigger and better. At twelve feet long, it was too long to be loaded on the standard side-opening freight car. After some disconcerted huffing and puffing and shuffling of cars onto other tracks, a freight car with a rear opening was found to accommodate the popular attraction.

The veriform (worm-like) appendix, which projects from the cecum end of the large intestine, has no function in humans; it is a useless remnant which evolution failed to discontinue. Helen Clapesattle, Mayo historian, speculates that the surprising popularity of this particular exhibit is due to the fact that a fourth of the adult population, after a painful flareup of that superfluous little outcropping of flesh, have lost their appendixes to a surgeon's knife.[2]

Another popular exhibit in the Mayo section of the Century of Progress Exposition was the stately Transparent Man. "T.M." was six feet tall,

A Century of Progress

moulded from a transparent material called cellon. He stood on a slowly rotating pedestal, his arms raised as if in supplication. His internal organs were fully visible, especially when individually illuminated as a demonstrator described the function of each organ. Transparent Man was constructed at the Deutsches Hygiene Museum in Dresden, Germany. It was purchased by Dr. Will, who admired it greatly, was loaned to the Chicago Fair and then returned to Rochester.

The Mayo exhibit in Chicago told the story of one hundred years of progress in our understanding of the human body and the treatments found to cure many of its diseases. Detailed information was given in layman's language on the function of the digestive tract, the thyroid gland and the sympathetic nervous system. The "speaker" for the explication of the digestive tract was a mechanical marvel himself; a robot in shirt, coat and bow tie who "told" the crowd what happens to food when we eat it. Dr. Bulbulian's wax models and the accompanying text made clear the important steps in operations on the stomach, colon and gall bladder.

Another featured Mayo exhibit was a large, modern x-ray laboratory. Beside it, in contrast, was a small room similar to the one in which the first x-ray studies of the stomach were carried out in 1896. Two large transparencies showed an operation performed fifty years before in a physician's home and the same operation undertaken in a contemporary operating room.

One day in 1932 as the Mayo exhibit for the fair was being planned, my mother returned from a trip east to see her parents. In Mother's suitcase was a beautiful blue silk dress with lacy trim from the 1880's that my grandmother, a diabetic under the care of Boston's famed Dr. Frank Leahy, used to wear before she gained too much weight. Being a budding pre-teen, I tried it on, a perfect fit. Dad came home, and I was still wearing the dress. Dad was apparently in on the Exposition plans, because a day or so later Dr. Bulbulian called me on the phone. He asked if I would kindly do him a favor. Would I, wearing my grandmother's dress, pose for pictures of the way the patient of yesteryear was examined by her doctor? The pictures, he said, were needed for the Mayo exhibit at the World's Fair. The old-fashioned doctor he had in mind, Dr. Rollin T. Adams of Mantorville, Minnesota, would be the doctor in the pictures, wearing his own frock coat, stiff collar, tie, a trim white beard and a gold watch chain across his vest.

Pill Hill

On a trip with my family to the Century of Progress Exposition, I saw myself in a series of photographs with Dr. Adams. The "office" where we were photographed was a drab little room with heavy velvet drapery, a rolltop desk, a bed, a Victorian chair and Dr. Adams' bulky black bag containing the cutting and probing tools of his trade, some unsterile bandages, iodine and a bottle of brandy. The Hall of Science brochure explained, ". . . on one side is the old doctor looking at his patient's tongue, pressing various areas of her abdomen, listening with his ear to her heartbeat."[3] In contrast were photos of the tools routinely in use by doctors examining patients in 1933: a thermometer, an otoscope, a microscope, an ophthalmoscope, an x-ray machine and others.

Another Mayo Clinic exhibit especially intrigued the Fair's older visitors. It was a large electrical tremometer, a hands-on device that enabled visitors to measure the temperature of their hands and test the steadiness of their nerves.

Of special interest to educators were maps, charts and motion pictures that tracked the places in the world where the incidence of goiter was high. The prevalence of that disease of the thyroid gland was closely related to localities where a lack of iodine was in the drinking water. Pictures were shown of dwarfed and feeble-minded cretins in Switzerland where the incidence of goiter was high. Dr. Henry Plummer's simple recommendation that iodine be given to goiter patients before attempting surgery reduced greatly the mortality of that operation and changed the way goiter patients everywhere were treated.

"Legitimate" doctors have always insisted on the free exchange of their good ideas; they published their news and views. Dr. Will once complained that quacks "educate" the public with their vividly colored posters of medicines containing mystery ingredients. Early in the practice of Dr. W. W. Mayo and his two sons, it used to rankle them that across the street from their offices was a charlatan who advertised patent medicines. The components of his bottled "cure-alls" were closely guarded secrets. To the three Doctors Mayo it was criminal to so deceive the public. They solved the problem of having him for a neighbor by buying him out, making room for a legitimate druggist in Rochester.

An important phase of patient care at the Clinic was teaching the patient to manage his or her own care at home. The elder Dr. Mayo wrote detailed instructions to his arthritic patients on the use of jelly-jar paraffin for heat treatments and how to make other cheap and simple substitutes for expensive equipment. In later years, lessons from technicians in the Mayo Clinic Diet Kitchen taught patients how to prepare the foods their doctor recommended.

Dr. Will and Dr. Charlie considered the Chicago Museum of Science and Industry an effective forum for communicating accurate and worthwhile scientific information to the general public. The museum's medical exhibits, they felt, reinforced a favorable image of the medical profession and its standards. The Mayo Foundation's relationship with the Chicago museum didn't end with its gift of the now-famous appendectomy models. Subsequently, the Foundation sent them five more anatomic models, clarifying for the layman the "architecture of the human body." By a cut-away method, these models revealed, under the skin and muscle layers, the deep-lying organs in the body. Later, exhibits on the five senses were added to the museum's collection.

Arthur Koestler said that scientists are "peeping toms at the keyhole of eternity." A true scientist, he meant, never gives up the effort to learn more today than he knew yesterday. When investigation of an illness being confronted at the Mayo Clinic seemed stalled, Dr. Will in frustration used to refer to the sneaky perpetrator of the disease as "a parasite of diagnostic obscurity."

Because a doctor, stuck with such a problem of diagnosis, can't devote all his time to one patient, the Mayo Foundation, with "eyes at the keyhole of eternity," initiated a new service for special clinical investigation. In that category were laboratories in bacteriology, biophysics and biochemistry, as well as the already established laboratory for experimental medicine located a mile or two southwest of town on Dr. Charlie's country property, the place we used to call "the dog farm." All sections of clinical work, when they got mired down with a baffling case, could call for help from these four investigative teams.

For many diseases there was no known cause or treatment. Meniere's disease, a neurological disease of the inner ear, was one of those. It was named for the Frenchman who, in 1861, first described its symptoms of dizziness and nausea. Many headaches were also of unknown origin. Investigators at the Clinic had learned to distinguish among the many types of headache and found one that they successfully treated with histamine. One day, a patient was presented to their department with a history of that kind of headache as well as a bad case of Meniere's disease. The patient was treated for the headache, and, to everyone's astonishment, it also vanquished the Meniere's disease.

Rarely do these tireless researchers have the pleasure of meeting the excited and grateful patient whose life is suddenly made whole again through their efforts. But one spectacular exception was the experience in the early 1920's of Dr. Charles Sheard. Dr. Sheard, formerly a physicist at Ohio State University, gave a lecture to Mayo ophthalmologists on applied optics. Following his presentation he was invited to come to the Clinic to set up a division of physics and biophysical research to devise the apparatus and techniques deemed necessary by doctors in the different specialties. When Dr. Sanford's hematology laboratory, for instance, needed help accomplishing three hundred or so hemoglobin tests a day, Dr. Sheard contrived a device, the Sanford-Sheard photolometer, that made light work of many different kinds of chemical tests without the human propensity for occasional error.

Dr. Sheard's inventions benefitted many thousands of patients, but he agreed with the poet John Ciardi, who said that giving a poem to the world was like dropping a rose petal into the Grand Canyon: the researcher rarely receives a word of gratitude from a patient. One day Dr. Sheard was made an exceptionally happy man by what he was able to do for a patient of Dr. Gordon New. Dr. New had removed the man's cancerous larynx, leaving him alive, but miserable; he was unable to make a sound. Dr. Sheard was called in for consultation. Could he devise a "voice box?"

What Dr. Sheard came up with in his laboratory was a first for a problem of this kind. Dr. Sheard said, "You can't explain electric potentials to the man on the street, but he doesn't have any trouble understanding a little tube and box that make him able to talk. There is a real thrill in seeing a man who is without hope, discouraged, unable to speak, turn into a whole human being again by a simple contraption that lets him speak as well as we can, from Alaska, Arizona, or anywhere, as clear as a bell."[4]

The tone of the patient's new voice was somewhat monotonous, but restored communication was a great gift. After the success of that first artificial voice box, Dr. Charles Sheard created more than three hundred custom-built larynxes for cancer patients, heavy smokers all, who had lost the ability to talk.

A Century of Progress

The question almost every oncologist, with every patient, sooner or later has to face is, "How long can I live, doctor?" Dr. Albert Compton Broders, a surgical pathologist, set his sights on finding an answer. From a study of thousands of cancer cells collected from cancer patients during surgery at the Mayo Clinic, Dr. Broders noticed several differing configurations of cells under the microscope that he correlated with the number of months or years the patient lived following surgery. He graded the different patterns of cells from one to four, Grade Four being the most aggressive. A longer life expectancy could be predicted if the patient had Grade One–type cancer cells. This grading system is still being used today all over the world. It allows the doctor to more intelligently treat the patient and predict the course of the malignancy.

The practice of medicine in the twentieth century introduced countless ways for people to stay healthy, avoid accidents, prepare food and keep house. But none of it has slowed the hectic pace at which we live. Speed caught the attention of my generation. "Going like sixty" meant you were really traveling. The cars we grew up with had running boards. Their engines often backfired. They chugged unwillingly up an ordinary hill and sometimes stopped dead in the middle of puddles because their underbellies got wet. But every year cars were built to go faster and perform better in new styles and shapes intended to please us, the public. One of our Canadian cousins came to visit us in a marvelous novelty, a Nash car with a rumble seat and a saucy brass horn with a rubber bulb.

Of special importance to this century's progress was the astonishing advent of the airplane. The first airplane to actually get up off the ground was the well known fragile craft flown in December of 1903 by Orville Wright at Kitty Hawk, North Carolina. It traveled a mere 120 feet at 6.8 miles per hour. From then on the airplane was big news. In my childhood, daring young pilots came barn-storming into Rochester, invited by the board of the Olmsted County Fair Grounds. In their little single-engine planes, they did loops and wobbled their wings to amuse us. They landed and leaped down to our sod runway like heroes. As early as 1911 a journalist for the Olmsted County *Democrat* waxed effusive over these daredevil airmen, ". . . manipulating their wonderful Curtis Machine in the depth of the ethereal blue, trifling with treacherous currents of air in a nonchalant manner, sailing aloft in company of feathered brethren, gliding giddily downward, cutting capers."

At one time on that grassy strip, a drama unfolded. An urgent message to the Mayo Clinic announced that a patient was at that moment being flown in from the Dakotas needing immediate medical attention, probably the result of an accident. What I know of the impelling circumstances was told to me by a friend who was there, Isobel Lobb Jones. The small rescue plane would be approaching Rochester's airport in minutes and an ambulance had to be there to take the patient to Saint Mary's Hospital for emergency treatment. That would have been a routine request in the daytime, but the emergency happened at night. Rochester's little airport had no field lights.

The situation was relayed to Mr. A. J. "Bertie" Lobb, the Clinic's lawyer, and he flew into unprecedented action. His daughter, my friend Isabel, remembers vividly how frantic and exciting it was. Her father called several people and told them to call all their friends and tell them to drive immediately to the airport. Isabel went along with her father and joined a parade of cars and an ambulance gathering on each side of the runway, their headlights blazing as they faced each other across the grassy corridor where the private plane would land.

Although the plane with its patient never arrived, the event was the start of Mr. Lobb's attention to the Clinic's need for an adequate landing strip and lighting for planes arriving in all seasons and at night.

The Mayo Clinic "think tank" had for some years been considering Rochester's need for a better airport. In 1928 a decision was made that the Mayo Properties Association would subsidize the construction of a new airport, one fully up-to-date with comfortable passenger facilities. Its paved runways would be lighted at night and able to accommodate large planes offering regular passenger service to Chicago and Minneapolis. That modern airport was in use and turned over to the city of Rochester before time was found to christen it. Finally, in 1952, after it had been extensively used commercially and during World War II as a refueling stop for military planes en route to Alaska, it was formally christened Lobb Field. Rochester's mayor presented a bronze plaque, eloquently inscribed to Mr. A. J. Lobb, "whose unlimited vision and confidence in Rochester... was largely responsible for providing adequate air transport to Rochester."

Immediately after Lobb Field was constructed and regular passenger service began, private planes often brought patients to the Clinic. Mother's diary is full of references to airplanes coming and going from the new Lobb Field. On January 10, 1929, she wrote, "... the tri-motor monoplane (?) came down after 150 hours of continuous flying. First really successful test of refueling a plane while flying. Isn't it wonderful!"

Sometimes a plane would come for my father, and he would be whisked off to Chicago to see a patient. Once, "Speed" Holman piloted a plane that brought a visitor or patient to Rochester to see Dad. His nickname, "Speed," came from some feat in the air he was famous for, but it wasn't that for which we children remember him. He had lunch with us while the man he chauffeured in his Ford Tri-Motor plane was having lunch somewhere else with Dad.

We sat around the dining room table, I in my usual place beside Dad's chair, Mother at the other end and Mr. Holman beside her. His brown hair was slicked back, his tan, handsome face grinned around at me and my brothers as if trying to put us speechless children at ease. We were on our best behavior. In the presence of our august guest we didn't slouch on an elbow, reach past a brother for the grape jam, or talk with our mouths full. In fact, we hardly talked, being so agog having lunch with an airplane pilot. What we all wanted to ask and didn't dare to was, would he take us up for a ride? He and Mother were having a lively chat about airplanes and we listened, almost too excited to eat our chicken pot pie.

Mother glanced at the plate of muffins in front of me and said, "Mr. Holman, would you like another blueberry muffin?"

"Thank you, ma'am, I believe I would," he said.

Quick as a slingshot he reached his long arm over Stanley's glass of milk, past Mother's arrangement of yellow chrysanthemums and the dish of celery and olives, toward the plate of muffins. Astonished, I saw the fork in his hand stab a muffin and swoop back to his plate. Miraculously, we kids didn't all burst forth with wild giggles. Wide-eyed, we looked at each other and at Mother, who winked, and we held it in.

"Speed" Holman buttered his muffin. Mother asked him a question like where did he get his nickname, and he never knew that his boardinghouse reach with a fork was what suddenly put us children at ease. We were all over him with questions, but he said with regret he wasn't allowed to take us up in the plane.

Pill Hill

Our first flight, and Mother's first too, came on October 21, 1930. Dad's boyhood friend, Stuart Pritchard, flew into Rochester in his own Stinson plane. He took us all for rides after school and spent the night. The next day Mother wrote, "Quite a thrill to take our guest to the airport after breakfast and watch him fly off to Chicago. He expects to be in Battle Creek for lunch. Whew!!"

A totally unexpected problem developed for some of the Clinic's patients flying out of Rochester in the late 1960's. Mayo Clinic surgeons began replacing diseased hip bones with a prosthetic joint. These patients, able to walk again thanks to their polyethylene hip socket with its two-inch ball and seven-inch stem made of highly polished metal, were forcibly detained by airport security police. They made it out of Rochester, so accustomed to patient problems, with a simple explanation from the Clinic, but at O'Hare in Chicago they were sure to be held and searched down to the skin, suspected of carrying a concealed weapon that had set off alarm bells at their gate. That was the beginning of the time when "skyjacking" was in vogue for criminals wanting to flee to Cuba. It is noted in the July 1973 issue of the *Mayo Alumnus* magazine that patients with artificial hip bones now leave Rochester with a personalized and illustrated card which describes the total hip implant for the benefit of vigilant airport security guards.[5]

On October 23, 1933, Carrie Balfour called Mother and suggested an adventure for some of their friends while the men were off in the duck blinds. Not much would be known of their exuberant trip to the Century of Progress Exposition were it not for Mother's diary record and a rhyming thank-you note she wrote to Carrie on their return.

Nels Twedt, the Balfour's man of many talents, agreed to chaperone six women in the car plus a seventh who joined them in Chicago. An ordinary man might have been daunted, trailing around with seven talkative women on a spree without their husbands, but Nels Twedt enjoyed it. He was a cheerful, slight-built man from Norway who talked slowly and confidentially in a droll and sensible way that made him popular with children and adults alike. Once during the tense days when Hitler's name was in every conversation, he told young Bob New his own personal grief. He was "a man without a country." His native Norway had been overrun by the Nazis.

A Century of Progress

The adventurous group on that trip to Chicago included Kitty Wood, Anne Pemberton, Marion Masson and the Root sisters, Jess and Mabel. Mabel was Harry Harwick's Girl Friday in the Clinic's business office. Anne Pemberton's friend, Esther Stillhammer, a Wall Street investment banker, flew to Chicago from New York to join them. It was Indian Summer weather the day they left for Chicago, Mother wrote, ". . . the sky a clear blue, a nip in the air, the leaves so beautiful they take your breath away. Had a picnic lunch and got to the Plaisance Apt. at 5 p.m. to find Esther and tea waiting." They were revived by dinner at Le Petit Gourmet, then went to a play, "Her Majesty the Widow."

The next day was a full day at the fair, everyone on her own till they met for lunch. Notable in my mother's diary were The Swiss Village, The Black Forest Village, the Pabst Casino and fashion show, the Ford Building, the skyride tower and, everywhere, lagoons of blue water and flowers. When they met at 5 o'clock they were "too tired to be sensible," but another wonderful meal at Le Petit Gourmet put them in high spirits, and they went to a musical comedy, "Take a Chance."

The next morning began with "a hilarious breakfast in our apartment." As the seven women and Nels left their hotel, they were "suddenly struck with wonder. The uniformed doorman and people on the sidewalk were gazing fixedly upward. An aluminum behemoth hovered just over the tops of tall buildings like a big oval balloon afloat in the blue sky. The Graf Zeppelin circled majestically over Chicago. It was to leave Akron, Ohio, October 28, and would be in Berlin, Germany, two days later. That seems incredible," Mother wrote.

The Graf Zeppelin, a lighter-than-air vehicle, was German-made, 800 feet long, and traveled at 70 miles per hour. It had luxury accommodations for fifty people and their luggage. Earlier models were used in air raids against Great Britain during World War I. But the strategy was discontinued. The big balloons were easily shot down.

Mother went two other times to the Century of Progress International Exposition, once with the whole family and once with her two sisters-in-law, Aunt Lou from Toronto and Aunt Laura, Uncle Morrie's wife. But as she wrote in a rhyming thank-you note to Carrie, the three-day spree with six good friends without children or husbands was the most unforgettable excursion.

Dr. Charlie's daughter Louise is quoted in Harriet Hodgson's book, *Rochester, City of the Prairie*, as saying that the secret of the Clinic's usefulness was that the doctors aimed at improving the future; they didn't look back.⁶ Years before, it was her grandmother, Louise Abigail Mayo, the Little Doctor's wife, who first made that observation and added, "Looking backward is not a good thing for one's soul."

⋅≼ 19 ≽⋅

World War II and the Korean War

> We are more than ever firmly convinced that war
> is what Sherman called it . . . Hell.
> Dr. Charles H. Mayo, 1917[1]

THE International Exposition in Chicago closed its gates in the fall of 1934, its participants glad to have been a part of its multicultural success. But reports from around the world gave ominous signals that people in many countries were in grave danger. Newspaper headlines such as these were alarming:

HEINRICH HIMMLER BEGINS STATE BREEDING PROGRAM
TO PRODUCE PERFECT ARYANS

NUREMBURG LAWS PASSED WITH DEATH PENALTY FOR
INTERMARRIAGE

ADOLPH HITLER DENOUNCES VERSAILLES TREATY

One snowy December 25th, when Aunt Laura and Uncle Morrie Masson were at our house for the Christmas turkey dinner, Uncle Morrie somberly read aloud a letter both he and my father had received from Dr. Walter H. Judd, a former surgical assistant to my father. We underinformed young people sat around our decorated Christmas tree enthralled, hearing the passion and authority in the voice of the writer. Dr. Judd wanted all his friends and peers at the Mayo Clinic to understand why he was giving up the practice of medicine to run for a seat in the Minnesota House of Representatives. His message, based on what he learned as a medical missionary in North China, was later widely distributed in a pamphlet, "The Basic Themes for Survival" by Rep. Walter

H. Judd. It was published by the Reserve Officers Association from an address he gave in 1959 at the nation's first National Strategy Seminar for Reserve Officers.

Dr. Judd, a graduate of the University of Nebraska Medical College, had two tours of duty as a medical missionary in China, the first from 1925 to 1931. Often, while in Shaowu, China, Dr. Judd had no choice but to blunder into an operation he knew nothing about. He needed more training. He applied for a fellowship in surgery at the Mayo Clinic. As he said to Dr. Louis Wilson, then director of admissions, who thought Dr. Judd was a little old to begin a fellowship, "Sir, I am more useful to you now, because now I know what I don't know."

In May 1934, six months before the end of his fellowship, Walter Judd received a cable from the American Board of Missions. The director of the 160-bed Congregational Hospital in Fenchow, North China, had just died of a heart attack. Yes, Dr. Judd responded, he would be willing, even eager, to get back to the Chinese people he had grown fond of, and it was also fine with his wife Miriam, formerly a missionary in India. In North China they and their new baby girl would be safe from malaria, the disease Dr. Judd had repeatedly contracted in his previous assignment.

He didn't know it then but the danger in the North would be potentially more fatal than malaria.

As a doctor, Walter Judd met all classes of Chinese people. Some of his patients told alarming stories of communist soldiers entering their villages to steal and rape. But other patients who came to him were those same zealous communists, eager to explain to him, the American doctor who spoke their language, the strategy of their leader that would bring even the American capitalists under the red banner. It appalled Walter Judd how these true believers justified the planned starvation of whole areas and categories of people who would stand in the way of the Marxist goal of world conquest. Judd also learned from his communist patients the intent of the Japanese expansion into Manchuria, to link up with the Chinese fellow-communist, Mao Tse-Tung. Mao would fight on the side of the Japanese to overthrow their number-one enemy, the Chinese nationalists under Generalissimo Chiang Kai-shek.

Dr. Judd worked uneasily at the Fenchow Hospital until the risk of losing his life in a Chinese prison became intense. Wave after wave of Japanese troops surrounded Fenchow. With the ingenuity of a James

World War II and the Korean War

Bond, Judd planned his family's return to the United States. He had hardly gotten Miriam and the two children on a plane to freedom when his own ticket to escape miraculously dropped into his lap.

A Korean interpreter came to him one day with a message from the commanding general of the Japanese Yamahoka division headquartered in Fenchow. He wanted to speak with Dr. Judd, privately and at night. With some fear, Judd agreed. The following night the Japanese general walked into Judd's office accompanied only by the Korean. The general revealed he had contracted a venereal disease from a Chinese woman and would like to be examined and treated. Obviously he couldn't go to his military doctor.

Judd agreed to treat the Japanese general. To have refused would have been risky. He told the general he must abstain from alcohol and sexual relations for two weeks and come to the doctor's office every night to have his urethra irrigated, the only treatment available then. Lee Edwards, author of Dr. Judd's biography, *Missionary for Freedom*, described the unfamiliar surge of power and satisfaction Dr. Judd felt, having this "exalted Japanese General, under the son of Heaven, emperor of Japan" in the palm of his hand. In shame the general crept in after dark like a frightened deserter, then took down his pants before an American doctor who subjected his genitalia to the humiliation of the irrigation procedure.[2]

When the ordeal was over, the patient cured, Judd received what he asked for—supplies for his hospital and the necessary papers for a flight home. For the general, it was the safe way to be rid of the man who knew his damaging secret.

Dr. Judd left his hospital in the hands of a Chinese doctor and a Mayo-trained head nurse, Emma Noreen, from Minnesota. On the train from Peking he was the only living passenger in a railway car stacked high with the boxed ashes of dead Japanese.

Back home, Dr. Judd set up a medical practice in Minneapolis, but it did not keep him from speaking out about the predicament of the Chinese people and their ancient culture. As a speaker, Walter Judd was a spellbinder. He was elected in 1942 to a seat in the House of Representatives from Minnesota's fifth district, where he served for twenty years.

The letter Uncle Morrie read to us that Christmas day in 1938 was my introduction to the honorable passions of patriotism. Dr. Judd was leaving the practice of medicine because time was precious. He must be an alarm bell for America, tell what was happening to the Chinese people, why that war was being fought, and what was ahead for us. "The United States is all that stands between the communists and Marxist domination of the world," he said in his letters to the Mayo staff and in his address to the Reserve Officers Association.[3] His message was radical. The enemy was without mercy; preparation for war was the only way to peace.

The economic hardship that followed World War I was the main reason Europe was quick to react on September 1, 1939, when the German army marched into Poland. Two days later Britain and France declared war on Nazi Germany. It caught Hitler off balance, accustomed as he was to the appeasement-prone leaders of those two countries.

As the war in Europe escalated, my generation of carefree Americans was gradually awakened to the collapsing world of the people we had met in Chicago at the Century of Progress Exposition. We listened to the earnest voice of Edward R. Murrow on the radio and read accounts of plundering Nazi troops entering Poland, Finland, Denmark, Norway, Holland, Belgium and France. Late in May of 1940 the blitzkrieg forced the Allies to retreat to the French port of Dunkirk. Surrounded by the German army on land and German ships in the English Channel, the Allied troops were saved by one of the greatest spontaneous military rescues in history. One thousand British and French vessels of all types, from destroyers and mine sweepers to private yachts and rowboats, took part in the evacuation of nearly 350,000 Allied soldiers across the English Channel to the English coast, losing very few lives in the process.

By then the enemy had become a despised target, a tyrant with a small, black moustache, raising a clenched fist. The U.S. draft began that summer. Many young men volunteered. On a battleship in the shipyard at Newport News, Virginia, a smiling, muscular "Rosie the Riveter" became a poster girl, inviting women to join the workforce. Women rallied to the call at hundreds of industries shifting from peacetime to wartime schedules. My future mother-in-law, Kathleen Jones Copeland, of Newport News, became personnel director for the women who worked in the shipyard. At Consolidated Aircraft's plant in Fort Worth, Texas, it was learned that women's fingers were often more nimble than men's in assembling airplane parts. To do their part for patriotism, many celebrities made public service announcements, such as the glamorous film star Veronica Lake, who demonstrated the danger of long hair being tangled in a drill press.

Japan's control of Manchuria was almost a chokehold when President

World War II and the Korean War

Roosevelt ordered a ban on our shipping to Japan. Japan had been our polite trading partner. We bought large quantities of their beautiful silk; we sold them junk, scrap iron, gasoline, cotton, rubber and aircraft equipment. Our embargo on shipping to Japan was like poking a hole in a wasp's nest.

For most of us unworldly students, the Japanese were an enigmatic people. Their language was strange, childlike; their manners humble; their art, a delicate reflection of nature, serene and uncluttered.

When I was in junior high school, a Japanese friend of my grandfather in the textile business brought his wife to the Mayo Clinic for surgery. We saw quite a lot of Gumpei Kawada. Once, when he came for dinner, I asked him what his children did for fun. He said, smiling, "I show you."

With a sheet of paper and a pair of scissors he made a flower. Then he spoke to my mother in a whisper. She laughed and cleared everything off the glass-topped coffee table. From the kitchen she brought a canister of sugar. We watched, rapt, as Mr. Kawada poured sugar on the coffee table. From his pocket he brought out some little tools with sharp and blunt points and a feather. On his knees by the coffee table he created a simple scene; a bird in the sky, a bridge arching over a river, a clump of reeds, a little boat, a distant mountain peak. We were enchanted. Gumpei Kawada embodied our concept of the Japanese people.

Then came that terrible Sunday, December 7, 1941. While our soldiers, sailors and pilots slept, 360 Japanese attack planes rose from the decks of aircraft carriers and headed for the Hawaiian port of Pearl Harbor where much of our Pacific fleet lay at anchor. At nearby Hickman Field, trim rows of army aircraft were parked. That infamous bombardment by dawn's early light sank or badly damaged 18 battleships and other naval vessels, destroyed 200 aircraft, and killed or badly wounded 3,000 American military personnel. That day will never be forgotten by those of us old enough to comprehend so merciless an attack. It was "a day that will live in infamy," said President Roosevelt.

The attack on Pearl Harbor transformed the limited war into a global one. The United States declared war on Japan, Germany and Italy. Dr. Herbert A. Bruce of Toronto, my father's mentor and friend, described our country's predicament as like Canada's at the start of World War I, forewarned, but unready.[4] With speed and efficient organization Japanese forces subdued most of the islands of the South Pacific, the Philippines, the Dutch East Indies and the northern half of New Guinea. It is a tribute to the fighting will of our Pacific fleet and airmen that they, after the devastation of Pearl Harbor, were able to win back island after island, culminating in the battles of the Coral Sea and Midway. An advantage we gained was the cracking of the Japanese communications code in April of 1942, allowing us to anticipate their movements. The Japanese, in retreat, became desperate; they would sink our carriers or face humiliation.

Then Ota, an idealistic young Japanese soldier, humbled himself before a superior officer and suggested a way to win. Quickly, a fleet of terrible new weapons was assembled. We called them suicide bombers. Their Japanese name, Kamikazi, meant "Divine Wind." Many thousands of young Japanese fliers died, strapped into a cheaply built small plane carrying a deadly missile. Their objective was to guide the plane through a hail of antiaircraft bullets to the hull of an American vessel. Their reward was reunion in paradise with their Kamikazi comrades. A shrine was built in Japan to encourage and honor these volunteers. Every day the boys, some as young as fourteen, with as little as thirty hours of flight time, prayed at the shrine, tears on their cheeks, as they waited for the hour when their number would be called.

Dr. Will and Dr. Charlie Mayo didn't live to know the enormous cost of our unpreparedness in this second World War, but Dr. Charlie's son, Dr. Charles William ("Chuck") Mayo, carried the Mayo name into World War II. Dr. Chuck served as unit director and executive officer of the original Mayo Army Hospital formed in 1940. As one of several surgeons at the Mayo Station Hospital in the jungles of New Guinea, Dr. Chuck cared for the victims of the Japanese offensive in the South Pacific. Like his father and his Uncle Will in World War I, he surprised the career officers by forgetting to change the ensignia on his uniform when he was promoted from major to colonel. What mattered to Dr. Chuck as he made the daily rounds of the wards of the Station Hospital was not his rank but the mood among his patients. When spirits needed lifting, he would sit on the edge of a soldier's bed, and they would talk over options open to the veteran, like education under the G.I. Bill. Dr. Chuck had a way of leaving a depressed patient with a brighter view of the future.

Since much of World War II involved flying at high altitudes, several technical problems had to be solved before a pilot could fly into thin air without passing out. A Mayo Clinic physiologist, Dr. Edward J. Baldes, developed the human centrifuge to test the effect of gravitational forces on pilots. In the process, other important information was learned about the cardiovascular system under stress. Dr. Baldes studied the problem of helicopter pilots and the physiology of paratroopers, whose heartbeat may exceed two hundred beats per minute in anticipation of the jump and the chute opening.

A team of three Mayo doctors collaborating with Canadian and British researchers and industrial experts combined their skills and came up with a system that would provide oxygen to a high-flying pilot. They devised an oronasal/nasaloxygen device, more simply called the B-L-B Mask. It was named for the three Mayo physicians who invented it, Dr. Walter M. Boothby, a pioneer metabolic researcher; Dr. W. R. (Randy) Lovelace, head of a Mayo section of general surgery who had soloed in the 1920's under a Naval Reserve program; and Dr. Arthur H. Bulbulian, the sculptor for museum exhibits and master of maxillofacial reconstruction. Dr. Bulbulian's contributions to aviation medicine included the development of oxygen masks and pressure suits, the original models for NASA's "space suits."

Dr. Randy Lovelace served on the Clinic staff only two years, one year before and one after the war. After his fellowship in surgery he took a leave of absence to attend the Army School of Aviation Medicine and was called to active duty in the Air Force as a flight surgeon. As chief of the Aeromedical Laboratory at Wright-Patterson Field, he made the initial test of the B-L-B Mask. Although he had never before made a parachute jump, on June 24, 1943, with himself as guinea pig, he jumped from a plane at an altitude of 40,200 feet, demonstrating the efficiency of his oxygen equipment. That record stood for years and earned Dr. Lovelace a Distinguished Flying Cross. While flying over Europe in a B-17 bomber, equipped with the B-L-B Mask, Colonel Lovelace and his crew were attacked by German fighters, but high flying made it possible for them to make it back to base. The air evacuation of many wounded GIs was accomplished because of Dr. Lovelace's contributions to air safety.

Soon after the war ended, heartbreaking tragedy hit Dr. and Mrs. Lovelace. Their two young sons came down with the epidemic disease poliomyelitis, which struck Rochester in 1946. Both boys died. The devastated parents returned to their home in Albuquerque. Randy Lovelace was known as "space medicine's family doctor." But in 1966, just a year after he was named Director of Space Medicine in the Manned Space Flight Division of NASA, he and his wife in their small private plane crashed shortly after takeoff on a snowy Colorado mountain.

Young American high school graduates who went off to serve their country in the early 1940's came back, when they came back, mature men. One such guileless boy was my brother Stanley, named for our Uncle Stanley Masson who was killed in World War I on a battlefield in France.

My brother Stanley, whom Rochester friends still call "Mud," had just finished his sophomore year at Carleton College when a letter from the U.S. Department of the Army arrived in the mail. Stan was ordered to report for duty on June 18, 1942, to the Commanding Officer of the 531st Amphibian Engineer Shore Regiment at Camp Edwards, Massachusetts. I can't do it, Stan thought. Our brother Jay was going to be married on the 20th of June and Stan was to be his best man. So he wrote to the general a nice personal letter about his commitment to his brother, a medical student. He asked for an alternate date, and said he would gladly report then for induction into the army.

A no-nonsense telegram arrived for Second Lt. S. F. Masson (he had earned that designation in ROTC at Ft. Snelling): "You will report as ordered."

Stan left for Camp Edwards on June 16. Mother's diary records her trepidation and pride:

> Stan and I packed Jim's old army trunk now marked 2nd Lt S. F. Masson. He's only 20. How can I let him go? My heart is a hard lump, but I did manage to send dear old Stan off without weeping on the 8:30 in a fine drizzle of rain. He looks so stalwart and young in his uniform.

A few letters came from him, and then a month of silence, till Mother could hardly bear the waiting. Where was "the dear lad"? Then on the second of August at 11:10 p.m. the phone rang—Stan at Camp Edwards. He was leaving the next day; he didn't know where to.

Stan, it seemed to us, was just a kid, like so many of the boys signing up to go out and shoot the enemy. He had shot pigeons with a BB gun and handled a rifle on the Crack Squad at Shattuck Military Academy; those things were just games. But there was one terrifying event in Stan's life he didn't tell at the dinner table. He was seventeen, in a summer job at the Reid Murdock canning factory. He was a pea grader, paid 45 cents an hour for ten hours a day. He spent his savings on a good camera.

The peas arrived at the canning factory in truckloads from the farms around Rochester, having been run through a threshing machine which separated the vines and pods from the peas. Stan's job was to send a container of peas from each truck through a grader. The peas rolled down an incline in the rotating steel cylinder with exit holes from small to large. The peas would fall through the holes into the appropriate basket below. The weight of these baskets was the basis used for putting a value on the truckload of peas. The farmer was paid more for small peas.

One day the bottom of Stan's T-shirt was grabbed by the revolving mechanism. The shirt was wound around and around, tighter and tighter, and the cutoff button was out of Stan's reach; it was too late to peel the shirt off over his head. Trembling, his hands braced against the wooden frame of the grader, he fought the unstoppable pull of the machine. When he heard the first rip of the cloth across his back, he knew he had won. A lesser fighter would have become an industrial accident statistic.

What we also didn't know about Stan, that day he called from Camp Edwards, was that he had qualified for the most rugged of infantry units, the Rangers. The Rangers, like today's Special Forces and yesterday's Office of Strategic Services (OSS), were given especially tough training in advanced combat, demolition techniques and intelligence gathering for missions behind enemy lines. Two weeks later a card in Stan's handwriting mailed in New York City said he had reached his destination safely. Mother was frantic to know where he was. A phone call to the Postmaster General, made by an influential patient of Dad's, found that Lt. S. F. Masson was in London. The next day a cable came; Stan was in Scotland.

After all the worry and uncertainty came a moment of calm. Scotland was safe. Then the worries began again. All across America, and in fact all around the globe, the same cycle of worry and relief afflicted the hearts and minds of those who loved the boys "over there."

Wives on Pill Hill saw very little of their husbands during the war. The men who had joined the Medical Reserves went when they were called. Others signed up for the training. The staff and Fellows remaining at the Clinic worked long hours. Every section of the Clinic was short-handed. My father, who was known to be a speedy operator, sometimes kept his assistants busy from dawn until after dark to complete twelve to fifteen major surgical cases in one day. Nurses being in short supply, relatives often helped care for hospitalized patients. Blood supplies were low since many of the Clinic's professional donors had left Rochester in uniform. When Mrs. Nora Giere, who often catered Pill Hill receptions and dinner parties, was hospitalized with severe anemia, Mother and others of Nora's friends and customers gave blood on her behalf.

Dr. Howard Burchell in 1942 was a Clinic Fellow in surgery when he was called for duty in London. His wife Margaret, with their new baby, moved in with her parents, Dr. and Mrs. Fred Helmholz. Isobel Helmholz worked for the Red Cross in the morning and took care of her granddaughter at night, freeing Margie to be a Red Cross nurse's aid in the evening. A letter from Margie told of her work with the Red Cross:

> When the Second World War broke out, thousands volunteered to work with the Red Cross—knitting, rolling bandages, and doing Home Service, which was a link between the service man and his home. In Rochester we often had requests from the military to verify the illness of a serviceman's relative who was a patient at the Mayo Clinic. The serviceman either wanted information or was requesting leave to see the sick relative.

Mrs. Gordon New (Aunt Ethyl) was a very young Red Cross nurse during the first World War. With the onset of World War II she was immediately recruited to teach classes in home nursing throughout Olmsted County. She was given a "B" sticker for her car, which gave her the privilege of buying gasoline to drive nursing students to and from her home.

In the early days of the war the civilian population had their radios on all day as a constant updating of Hitler's sweep of bloody victories filled the airwaves. Patriotism was high. Few people grumbled over shortages; food and raw materials were needed in industries filling orders for the armed services. Households were issued coupons by the Ration Board for meat, sugar and butter. Oleomargarin, a soybean substitute for butter, came to us pure white with a little gelatin capsule containing a concentrated yellow oil which we vigorously stirred into the lardy-looking oleo. On toast, the yellow color seemed to give it a better taste.

Gasoline rationing kept us at home unless we could convince the Ration Board of real need. In 1943, the year after my graduation from Wheaton College, Norton, Massachusetts, I applied to the Ration Board for extra gas coupons to drive to my new job at the National Institutes of Health. Washington, D.C., was bustling with soldiers and sailors during the war. Places to live were almost impossible to find. For a short while I stayed in an apartment with my Rochester friend Isobel Lobb and her roommates, all of them officers in the Navy unit called WAVES, (Women Accepted for Volunteer Emergency Service). They helped me find another group of WAVES renting a house in Bethesda, Maryland, which was closer to my work, and I moved in with them. Again I went to the Ration Board and they gave me gas coupons to drive to work one day a week, as part of a carpool. A year later the Board supplied me with coupons to get me and my 1937 Chevy back to Rochester for my marriage to Herbert Jones Copeland, a fighter pilot home from New Guinea.

On July 1, 1943, in Rochester, Dr. and Mrs. William A. Plummer, Corena and Bill, received a letter from their son John, a junior officer in the Coast Guard, saying he had, by stunning coincidence, run into "Mud Masson on a ship in the Mediterranean." Corina Plummer, of course, called my mother with the sketchy bit of news.

Stan remembers the encounter with John Plummer in every detail. Stan was a platoon commander in the Amphibian Engineers of the First Ranger Battalion at the port of Oran on the coast of North Africa. His platoon was assigned to an LCT (landing craft tank), the *Joseph T. Dickman*. It was one of many ships, each carrying fifty men or a tank that would deliver the Amphibian Engineers and all their supplies across the sea to Sicily. Their mission was to clear the beach of mines and clutter and ready it for the arrival of the Allies' main assault force. When Stan's platoon had all climbed aboard the *Joseph T. Dickman*, and Stan had seen the men to their assigned space, he went to find the stateroom assigned to him. The door was ajar. He kicked it in. In one hand he carried a submachine gun, in the other, a backpack. His webbing bristled with a pistol, bayonet, several hand grenades, a wire cutter and magazines of ammunition. "I must have looked dirty and unpleasant," Stan said mildly as he described the scene to me. Across the room, leaning against the wall, was a red-headed "boat driver" who eyed Stan suspiciously. For some time they stared at each other. Then Stan dropped his backpack and said, "Gee whiz! It's John Plummer!" He was looking at a friend from the Pill Hill neighborhood, the older brother of his high school sweetheart, "Peg" Plummer. It was a grand reunion.

After two days and one night on the LCT the small flotilla of ships reached Sicily. The men of the 531st Amphibious Engineers began clearing the beach of mines and tangled barbed wire. That night Stan settled into a dry ditch for whatever rest was possible. Tracer bullets from machine gun fire flew back and forth as the U.S. Beach Defense held back the German/Italian army. By dawn German soldiers were all over the beach and the Rangers engaged them in close combat as the clearing of the beach continued.

On the second day of the battle, Stan was hit by a blast of machine gun fire and artillery shrapnel. The last thing he remembers before he passed out was wrapping his right upper arm with his belt as a tourniquet to stop the profuse bleeding and, with his bayonet, tightening it. Combat medics carried him on a litter to the battalion aid station, where a sorting process, triage, was constantly going on. The wounded as they were brought in were evacuated in order of urgency. Those who might live if tended immediately were evacuated first; those with a lesser injury, like a broken leg, waited; and those who were dead or dying were removed last. My brother was laid in the row of unmoving men, each covered over by a blanket.

When Stan's friend Mitch came looking for him, Mitch, stricken with grief, began folding back the blankets from the faces of the dead, then covering them up again, one, then another and another and another. Suddenly, the bright sun flashed on Stan's face. He winced; his whole face froze in a squint.

Mitch yelled as he leaped to his feet, "Hey! This man's not dead!"

Stan, with the rest of the wounded, was put aboard an LST headed for a navy hospital ship. He doesn't remember the thunder of the German dive bomber that attacked the LST—a direct hit. The ship trembled, but stayed afloat long enough for the crew and the wounded to be transferred to another ship. Then it sank. Stan vaguely remembers the transfer, swinging on a stretcher in a net suspended from a mechanical hoist.

Back home in Rochester, Mother went about her job at the Ration Board, often typing letters at home in the evening. She and other Rochester women knitted socks, mittens, hats and scarves at home. At the Red Cross building the women worked toward a quota for September of 570 wool dresses. "Cut out 60 flannel nighties," she wrote in her diary. On July 10th, 1943, she wrote this news of the war:

> Allied forces invaded Sicily today! At last the invasion of Hitler's Europe has started, and I can't help being glad Stan is in Syria, even if it is only postponing his part in this horrible thing.

Postponed for her was the knowledge that Stan *wasn't* in Syria, but in that action on the beaches of Sicily. Three weeks later a letter, dictated by Stan to a Red Cross nurse, reached Rochester. He had been hurt, an injury to his writing hand. Very slight, he said, but they were keeping him in a hospital. The next day another letter, a few lines picked out on a typewriter. A month went by. Then a special delivery letter arrived from someone at the Twenty-First General Hospital in North Africa. Stan was to be sent home for recuperation and a thirty-day furlough as soon as possible. "He has a compound fracture of the right elbow and a leg injury, not serious." Mother was giddy with mixed pain and relief. She accepted another job. She became a "lieutenant" in a third War Bond drive. The radio continued to pour out the voice of Edward R. Murrow. To lift the spirits of listeners, a popular pair was brought back to the airwaves, Edgar Bergen and his little wooden sidekick, Charlie McCarthy. Franklin D. Roosevelt, in his third term as president, continued his weekly fireside chats. He assured us that soon this dastardly war would be over, and we would be on the winning side.

On September 22, 1943, a naval ship brought Stan to Halloran Hospital on Staten Island. My parents, by plane, train, subway, ferry and "six miles in Captain Baker's car," got to Stan's bedside and learned the truth about his "slight" injuries: a smashed elbow, bullet through one lung, several dozen shrapnel wounds, and two arteriovenus fistulae, at first thought to be aneurysms (a swelling in a blood vessel). Twice, a bullet had pierced between a vein and an artery, nicking each and causing arterial blood to be shunted into the vein, a weakening and potentially fatal condition. Stan had lost sixty-five pounds. "But his spirits were fine and courage high," Mother wrote in her diary.

The next day he was moved by ambulance, sirens screaming through New York City to Penn Station. On a stretcher he was shoved through the window of a train into a compartment beside that of Mother and Dad. "He was in terrible pain on that jerky train from his chest wound," she wrote. I don't know how Mother stood the strain when Dad too became seriously ill with a cough, chills and fever. The day after Stan was wheeled into Ashford General Hospital in White Sulphur Springs, West

Virginia, (the former Greenbriar Hotel), Stan's doctor, Col. Daniel Elkin, put Dad in the hospital with pneumonia.

Mother's days were spent shuttling between Dad and Stan, the Hart Hotel, the Greenbriar Casino and

> ". . . now and then, a game of shuffleboard with an ambulatory patient in a maroon bathrobe. The oaks and maples are gorgeous and I enjoy my walk to the Casino at sunset. Today I was escorted by a man who can carry a 640-pound bull.

Dad was hospitalized fifteen days, not allowed to visit Stan except once in a wheelchair wearing a mask. Extreme caution was being taken because Stan was a guinea pig for a new drug, penicillin, being tested in a few army hospitals. Penicillin is credited with saving his life. This germ-killer was discovered in 1928 by Dr. Alexander Fleming in London. He noticed that beads of liquid on a mold cultured in his laboratory killed bacteria. Purified and tested, penicillin ushered in the age of antibiotics.

On October 13, Mother and Dad were flown home in a private plane owned by Mr. Al Lodwick, whose wife, Dot, was a former patient of Dad's. They left Stan, knowing he was in good hands. Dr. Dan Elkin, Dad said, was perhaps the best aneurysm surgeon in the world. Stan was recovering well from a three-hour operation on the arteriovenus fistula on his leg. His multiple wounds and several skin grafts were healing.

On October 29, Dad was feeling well again. He and Mother were in Chicago staying at the Palmer House. Dad was to deliver a paper, "Endometriosis and Its Serious Complications," to a meeting of the Interstate Postgraduate Medical Association of North America. At 4:30 p.m. Mother had returned to their room from a day of Christmas shopping.

> . . . Jim was reading his paper (to the postgraduate students) when Dr. Elkin phoned from White Sulphur Springs. Stan's arm has to be amputated. I dreaded so to tell Jim. It is a terrible blow and we both feel dazed. No accommodations out of Chicago so we came home tonight.

The following day they took the night train back to Chicago and the next train to White Sulphur Springs.

"I'm worried about Jim," Mother wrote. "He feels it so keenly. Stan's plans for the future had always been to be a surgeon like his father. Thank God Helen is with him. She got there Tuesday."

At that time I was working as a lab and research assistant at Brown

University. In the same week that Stan's arm was amputated, two other crucial events in my life happened: my fiancé, Herb Copeland, left Grenier Air Force Base in Manchester, N.H., for parts unknown, and my boss, Dr. Ivan Taylor, died suddenly of a heart attack. I quit my job at Brown and drove down to be with Stan, settled into a room at the Hart Hotel where my parents had stayed before, and met their train when it arrived in the early morning. After breakfast we went to the hospital. Mother wrote,

> ... Stan had a smile, and Jim and I held back our tears. It nearly killed us both to look at the poor arm with four pound tractions attached to it. Stan is simply wonderful. So brave and strong. Oh! this boy has what it takes, just as his father has.

On a bleak Sunday morning during that time in White Sulphur Springs Mother went to an Episcopal Church nearby. Stan had had many painful days, the stump of his right arm in traction. Dad's fatigue was also a constant worry, and the everyday presence of the severely wounded young soldiers at the hospital reminded her of the savagery of the war. "Church is hard for me now," she wrote. "I am a rebellious Christian, still trying to hold fast." It was that thought that must have powered the poem I found among her papers:

Hold Fast

> We must remember that the sky is blue
> Though hoards of Messerschmitts obscure the sun.
> We must remember that the grass is green
> Though red-streaked where the refugees have run.
> We must remember sun, and moon, and stars
> Pursue their courses *calmly* year on year,
> And not forget that faith in *right*—rock-firm—
> Must triumph always over hate and fear.

Across the nation, families became accustomed to shortages and rationing. Victory Gardens were in. On Pill Hill, the Haineses and Helmholzes

Pill Hill

tilled and seeded a lot that had lain weedy and unclaimed between their two houses. They brought in a bumper harvest of vegetables. They were like tenant farmers, except that the owner, whoever he was, didn't show up to claim a share of the produce.

The Masson backyard had always produced vegetables, tended mostly by Sylvester, but during the war my father had his own plot for his specialty, tomatoes. His patch was the fertile soil behind the Old Garage which had been a pen for chickens, goats, pheasants and, for one month, a horse. Dr. John Pemberton, whom I knew as Uncle John, grew tomatoes too. He proffered a challenge to Dad that he could, in his good ordinary Minnesota soil, produce a tomato larger and heavier than any my father could grow in his famous chicken-poop soil. Dad took him up on it. The loser would buy the winner a box of good cigars.

Yellow flowers bloomed on Dad's tomato plants and he plotted a strategy. He selected the strongest of his twelve healthy plants growing in full sun by the path that cut through the lilac hedge by Dr. Dripps' garage. He pinched off half the flowers on that one plant, thereby directing more strength to the remaining buds. When the green tomatoes were mostly the size of ping-pong balls, he eliminated the slow growers. Finally, he had one lustrous, red-orange globe, staked and supported by ribbons of cloth.

Uncle John, too, had a pampered and perfect specimen. The due date came, and the Pemberton tomato was brought to our house. It filled the palm of Uncle John's hand. Dad stroked his chin and shook his head sadly, "You win by default," he said. That very day his giant tomato, as big as a melon, he said, disappeared—plucked, undoubtedly, by some mischievous kid taking a shortcut down our driveway to the Edison school playground.

Anticipating the housing shortage that would hit Rochester when the war ended, the Mayo Clinic's Board of Governors voted to build close to three hundred small homes and apartments. One new addition, the Homestead, reserved for Clinic Fellows, was located on part of the farmland bought by old Dr. W. W. Mayo. Another group of homes, in northeast Rochester, was the Carroll addition. The Graham addition, reserved for Fellows with families, was a cluster of Quonset huts known as "the Prefabs." It was located across the highway from the Olmsted County Fairgrounds and Rochester's landmark water tower, shaped and painted

World War II and the Korean War

like a giant ear of corn. Maintaining a V-Garden was a way of life at the Prefabs long after the war was over.

All hostilities should have stopped when Japan surrendered in 1945, but they didn't. Political discord between North and South Korea continued to smolder. The United Nations tried to settle things by backing a joint occupation of that nation. The United States would act as protector of the weaker southern half of the island and North Korea would be occupied by Russia. UN-sponsored elections resulted in an agricultural Republic of South Korea and a Communist North Korea whose elected premier, Kim Il Sung, had fought with the Soviet army in World War II. Diplomatic efforts to keep the peace failed. The war that began was as bloody as any other war, though it was often referred to as the Korean conflict. Again, men from the Mayo Clinic were called to serve.

My brother Jay, a Naval Reserve Officer, had completed nine months of his fellowship in plastic surgery when he was ordered to report to Camp Pendleton in California. From there he was whisked across the Pacific and assigned to Marine Medical Company "C" located near the 38th Parallel in South Korea. It was March 1952; the war was in a furious last-ditch stage, four months before a truce was signed by the United Nations and the North Korean Communist Commander.

The Marine field hospital, where Jay's group treated the daily flow of war casualties, was made up of tents set in "nice rolling hills somewhat like southern Minnesota." They were well supplied with good medical equipment and six operating tables on a dirt floor. "Suddenly one day," Jay wrote, "we got a surprise. We had a scrounger in the unit, a sergeant who could get us most anything we needed from the army. This time he stole a truckload of cement, and we had a new floor."

Often, their hospital had to be moved. Three times in one year they were ordered to pack up for another location, for reasons known only to the strategists. Patients who needed specialized treatment were flown to a U.S. Naval Hospital in Japan.

Shortly after the truce, the doctors were restless with no new patients coming in. The Marine Medical Company asked permission, which was immediately granted, to help out with the civilian patients at Seoul Medical School. Jay wrote,

Thereafter, every Wednesday about four of us medical officers with the First Marine Division, went to Seoul, about 35 miles south. We saw and operated on some patients in the hospital. It was good for us, as we had time on our hands once the war activities stopped. But it was only one day a week.

Then, I got lucky. There was no one in Korea doing plastic surgery at that time, and when the word got out, quite a few Korean civilians sought me out and showed up in my regular sick call. Through interpreters I could talk with them, and arranged to treat them at our Marine Field Hospital. They were mostly patients with burn injuries and congenital problems like cleft lips, birth marks, and hand and face deformities. We were given a tent for them to stay in a few days after surgery or until the stitches could be removed. Infants and children and some adults were allowed to have their families stay with them. They cooked their own meals, and the family members made good nurses. It was surprising how good the little ones were. In spite of the rather primitive conditions there was very little infection.

One day a six-year-old boy appeared on my sick call list. I found out from the interpreter he came by himself, hitchhiking from several hundred miles away to find me and ask to have his cleft lip repaired. The next day I repaired his lip deformity and he disappeared for about eight days. Then he returned in my sick call lineup. He pointed to his lip and asked to get the stitches out. He apparently had stayed with a Korean family in a nearby village. After the stitches were out he left with a "thank you," and I assume he hitchhiked back to his home village. All of the kids we saw were old for their age and knew how to manage very well for themselves. This boy was only six!

The whole experience was very gratifying, being able to offer something I was trained to do, something these people, in that time, couldn't get there.

In all wars there are unsung heroes. One such man, whose stated desire was to be a litter bearer in the Korean War, was considered by members of his platoon too weird to be real. Private Austin's story, reported first in the Sun Coast group of newspapers, Port Charlotte, Florida, by his former platoon leader Fred Farris, was later reprinted in Farris's book of columns, *Times Recalled*:

World War II and the Korean War

> That night we pulled off a good one.... We ambushed a full company of Chinese and wiped them out....
>
> Two nights later we were hit pretty badly by the Chinese. Sgt. Nitschke took the survivors and all the wounded, except Private Sutherland, back to our lines. Private Austin and I remained with Sutherland who had been hit by a mortar shell fragment which literally scalped him. His scalp was peeled and lying on one side of his head. The chance for infection was higher than normal because we would have to carry him back across several miles of terraqueous terrain where the rice paddies had been fertilized with human feces.
>
> Private Austin had a sewing kit in his first-aid kit. Threading a needle on either end of some thread we sewed Private Sutherland's scalp back on figuring that was the best way to avoid infection. Several days later we got a message from the area M*A*S*H* recommending that whoever sewed Private Sutherland's scalp back on should be given a decoration.

In the unwinding after the battle, with some black market whiskey, Private Austin opened up his secret to me. He, Private Austin, was really Doctor Austin, a psychiatrist who wanted to experience combat first-hand so he could, with understanding, treat veterans after the war.[6]

Eventually, following those war and Depression years, the great shuffling of the population stabilized. Northerners met Southerners. City people learned to harvest vegetables and can them. Career plans changed. Veterans enrolled in colleges on the G.I. Bill. As the bombing of Pearl Harbor had been a bugle call that woke us up to what loomed on the horizon, rousing an army of patriots, now in peacetime, President Hoover warned that it was a foolish notion that the economic engine in this nation was out of steam. Ahead, he said, there will be a chicken in every pot and a car in every garage.

In this century hundreds of innovations such as penicillin, rapid transport of the wounded to field hospitals and the fully-equipped "Hospital in a Box," which unfolds like an umbrella on any terrain, have made quick emergency treatment of wounded soldiers possible. Civilian medicine, too, has learned something useful from the wars of the twentieth century. For the first time, doctors worked as teams with doctors of different specialties. This Group Practice idea was first found successful as long ago as 1892 when the Mayo team of three, Dr. W. W. Mayo and his sons, Dr. Will and Dr. Charlie, began inviting other physicians to join them in Rochester. An English surgeon, commenting on the phenomenon of the Mayo Group Practice, told Helen Clapesattle, the Mayo historian, that "the most amazing thing about the Mayo Clinic was the fact that five hundred members of the most highly individualized profession in the world could be induced to live and work together in a small town on the edge of nowhere, and like it!"[7]

❧{ 20 }❧

On the Social Side

> When you start to educate the people you should begin with the
> women because they will fight for the health of their children.
> Charles H. Mayo, 1928[1]

WE who grew up on Pill Hill in the 1920's and '30's agree that our childhoods were unique. Like all children, we tested our limits, but there was no escaping the magnetism of the concepts held by the Mayo Clinic's elder statesmen. Trust in the scientific method was an ineffable lure, like an established religion, which we absorbed into our lives. The sublime Plummer Building was itself a beacon in downtown Rochester. Young men and women came to it as students from med schools and as nurses, technicians and high school graduates wanting to work at the Clinic. They often married each other and automatically energized a social environment good for raising families.

My friend, Jean Davis, told me her father said there were some people who thought the Clinic doctors had even begun to look alike. Dr. Davis, with five other Clinic men in the 1930's, took the train to Chicago to attend a medical meeting. They were met by two Chicago doctors. It was a cold winter day, and the six men stepping down to the platform were dressed in bulky coats with fur collars and Russian-style fur hats. One of the Chicago greeters was heard to say to the other, "My God, they've got them in uniform now."

Before the Mayo practice became a group of many specialties, a reunion could gather all its doctors and their spouses at Dr. Will's or Dr. Charlie's house for a sit-down dinner. But, in 1946, the group of former staff and Fellows that came back for the reunion was so huge the Clinic began its week-long celebration with one big party at the Mayo Civic Auditorium with a well known band for dancing and left the rest of the socializing to the hosts and hostesses of Pill Hill. In a letter, Mother wrote:

> ... after the arrival of Dr. and Mrs. Eric Larson, our houseguests, on their heels came about 500 docs and spouses [staying with friends around town or in hotels]. ... We spent the week hopping from one tea to another with oodles of cocktail parties and a few dinners. Dad gave a luncheon here for 10 of his former first assistants.
>
> The week was pretty hard on Dad [who had retired the year before at the mandatory age 65]. He had no service at St. Mary's and it made him feel badly to be out of the operating room completely. Everyone was so nice to him, but the nice things they said nearly floored him a couple of times.

A P.S. to that letter mentioned another rousing occasion, the retirement of Uncle Don Balfour: "At the banquet they gave him, the applause was so long that when he got up to speak, he began, 'You needn't sound so glad to get rid of me,' and they clapped more than ever."

Dr. Donald Church Balfour's career at the Mayo Clinic took off in 1912 when he became head of a section of general surgery, doing everything from tonsillectomies and varicose veins to diseases of the spleen and the gastrointestinal tract. In addition to his reputation as a surgeon of great skill, Dr. Balfour is remembered as a man of exceptional warmth. He was just naturally adored by all who knew him. He was as much at ease with heads of state as with children. He was "a stopper-of-people-in-corridors," as one young associate said. He was a lifter of spirits.

However, a tense encounter between young Doctor Balfour and Dr. Will Mayo turned up in a Mayo Alumni Association collection of memories.[2] With a patient undergoing surgery in Dr. Will's operating room and a gallery of visiting doctors watching and listening, a fly landed at the foot of the table. Dr. Will stood motionless, glaring at the intruder. One of Saint Mary's nurses handed a fly swatter to Donald Balfour, a newcomer in Dr. Will's service. The young man took a swing at the fly. Somehow his grip was loose and the swatter fell into the sterile field. Dr. Will stepped back while the drapes, gowns, and gloves were changed in total silence. The young assistant perhaps expected a fierce look from Dr. Will that would mean "You are fired!" But, as we know, he was not fired. He later married the boss's daughter, Carrie.

For twenty years Dr. Donald Church Balfour earned international acclaim in his specialty, surgery of the upper gastrointestinal system. Visitors from everywhere crowded his galleries to watch him work and hear his lucid and folksy discourse on the surgery he was performing. Then his health let him down; he contracted tuberculosis, for which in 1933 there was no cure. One might expect a surgeon with a brilliant reputation to be dismayed, depressed even, at having to leave his chosen field. Not Dr. Balfour. He went smoothly into another career that allowed him the rest he needed and the satisfaction of giving his time and support to promising young doctors. He became Director of the Mayo Foundation Graduate School. Every young man and woman who came through the three-year course came to look upon him as a surrogate father. They often asked his advice, and he gave them his full attention.

I remember many occasions when Uncle Don, as I came to address him, gave *me* his full attention. One Saturday afternoon in the summer of 1939, the Balfours had a mother/daughter party at their farm. I was home from my freshman year in college, working a summer job in Dr. Sanford's hematology/serology lab. I loved the Balfours' farm, a place we often lived in when the Balfours were out of town for a week or two. The barn was painted red and white, the house built of native stone cut from the hillside. Its picture window faced a stream that meandered through the pasture.

For that tea party in the country I didn't have a little straw hat of the sort women in those days wore to garden parties. "A little flowered thing would be perfect," I said to Mother and she, as a joke, offered a bunch of daisies she had brought in from the yard, white with yellow centers.

"Good idea," I said, and soon I had a beret of daisies pinned over a coil of my upswept hair.

"Nobody would ever guess it's not a hat," Mother laughed.

Cars were parked on the gravel driveway from the barn to the house and around the circle. Uncle Don met us at the front door. Mother joined the crowd inside, but I stayed with Uncle Don, who had me by the arm, looking with interest at my headgear.

"I like your hat," he said.

Then he asked how my college work was going. What English courses was I taking? I remember telling him about little, bald Mr. Boas, who turned me on to Shakespeare. Was I enjoying Biology? Did I get in to Boston on the weekends? Was I still riding horseback? Now and then he glanced at the daisies. Finally, he gave me his wonderful smile and a nudge. "Yes, that's some hat. And she's some girl who wears it even though it has little black bugs crawling all over it."

The doctors at the Clinic made a practice of being active in many of the hundreds of medical and surgical associations in the United States. Those meetings served as social mixers and ongoing education for doctors wanting to keep up on new information in their fields. One of the many lifetime friends Dr. Will and Dr. Charlie made in the early 1920's through these social/educational meetings was Dr. Albert J. Ochsner of Chicago. Dr. Ochsner's hospitality included invitations to the Mayo brothers and their wives to visit him and his wife at their ranch home in Mexico. A visit to the Ochsners led Dr. Will and Mrs. Hattie to a meeting with Mexico's President Obregon.[3]

On a later trip to visit Mexican hospitals, Dr. Will was accompanied by Dr. Plummer and Dr. Balfour. Dr. Will made a courtesy phone call to President Obregon, who promptly invited the three Rochester doctors to a bullfight the following afternoon. Dr. Will accepted the invitation, though bullfighting was not his idea of sport.

The first daring young man to come before the overflowing grandstand crowd bowed to his fans and then to President Obregon and his party. With a flourish, he dedicated his bull to President Obregon's guest, Dr. William J. Mayo of the U.S.A. The crowd cheered, and the matador unfurled his red satin cape. He saluted the curious, snorting bull and stepped neatly aside when the big head lowered and attacked the fluttering cape. When the bull was finally slain, the crowd cheered wildly. The second toreador to enter the arena was Luis Freg, young and handsome, idolized by all of Mexico City. The applause was thunderous. He dedicated his bull to President Obregon, bringing on another burst of cheers. Like a ballet dancer Luis Freg sought to dazzle his president and the crowd. His daring was excessive. The bull caught him on a wicked horn and tossed him. The fans groaned. The three doctors from Minnesota were horrified. The young man had just been carried from the field when the news swept back to the crowd that Luis Freg was dying. President Obregon asked Dr. Will to see if there was anything he could do.

The small first-aid station behind the wall where the matador was taken was full of weeping friends and relatives of the injured man. Doctors attempting unsuccessfully to stop the hemorrhage in the groin area by external pressure gladly stepped aside for President Obregon and the three doctors. Dr. Will called for gloves, a gown, and scissors, but settled for soap and water, an apron and a knife. By simply cutting the skin above the bleeding femoral artery he was able to take hold of the vessel and tie it. The speed and ease with which he stopped the bleeding and thereby saved the life of the popular young matador made a profound impression on everyone. The story was all over Mexico and the United States the next day. It no doubt accounted for an influx of new patients to the Clinic from south of the border.

The Mayos were also inadvertently in the news when journalists wrote about famous personalities going to the Clinic or when Dr. Will or Dr. Charlie Mayo were summoned to some important bedside. One of the Mayos was called to see President Taft and, at another time, the wife of President Harding. Franklin Lane, Secretary of the Interior under President Wilson, was sent to Rochester by his New York physician. Helen Clapesattle quoted Lane, the jester of the Wilson administration, as saying he had to find out if it was true that his stomach and his gall bladder were becoming too intimate. "Rochester," Lane said, "was the Reno where such divorces were granted."[4]

During his stay in Rochester, Franklin Lane wrote many letters comparing the Mayos and their Clinic with Henry Ford, Louis Pasteur, Thomas Edison and Charlie Schwab, the shipbuilding magnate. He added, "Fine reputation, eh, what? for two young chaps who never went to Harvard."[5]

Many Hollywood celebrities came to Rochester and made long-lasting friendships. The handsome cowboy actor, Randolph Scott, a native of Charlotte, North Carolina, was a frequent checkup patient and guest of Dr. H. R. Butt. He made his biggest splash in Rochester when he accompanied Dr. Butt and Mr. G. Slade Schuster, a Mayo financial advisor, to a father-daughter party at Rochester High School. He danced with several of the daughters and later told a journalist, "They put up with the old man."

The band leader Benny Goodman came to Rochester by charter plane in 1940, but he didn't have much of a party while in town, though he was a dinner guest at the home of Dr. and Mrs. W. L. Benedict. He came to the clinic for treatment of a "slipped disk" and stayed for surgery and recuperation at Saint Mary's hospital. Comedian Jack Benny entertained the country on Jack Paar's television show, describing his checkup at the

Mayo Clinic and his meeting with Dr. Chuck Mayo during World War II in New Guinea.

Cowboy comedian/philosopher Will Rogers, in his newspaper column "Will Says," wrote this bit of foolishness on April 25, 1934:

> Dr. Mayo and his accomplices held spring practice on the body of Knute Rockne, the Notre Dame coach. They extracted some of his poison and gave it to rabbits . . . . the rabbits went into a huddle and came out with an Easter egg. Mayo then took a larger dose of this poison from Knute's infected leg and gave it to 11 baby guinea pigs. They immediately defeated the rabbits 58–0.[6]

Some well-known people attempted to avoid publicity by registering under assumed names. But some, like Ernest Hemingway, who used a Spanish pseudonym, couldn't fool the public, and the news made the rounds.

On a sultry summer day in 1934 President Franklin Delano Roosevelt came to Rochester for the dedication of a new park to be named Soldiers Field. Dr. Charlie's son, Dr. C. W. "Chuck" Mayo, in his autobiography, *Mayo, The Story of My Family and My Career*, states that the Clinic had always honored veterans, never charging a fee for treatment. Chuck Mayo was one of six children growing up at Mayowood at the time of the dedication of Soldier's Field. "This pioneer respect," Dr. Chuck wrote, "eventually flowered into our present network of veterans' hospitals."[7]

On the day before the dedication Dr. William D. Haggard, a formal and distinguished man then president of the American Medical Association, was a houseguest at Mayowood. He had agreed to prepare some remarks for President Roosevelt to speak at the ceremony the following day. He took the task seriously and stayed up late to do it.

Houseguests at Mayowood in those years were sometimes the victims of pranks perpetrated by the mischievous children of Dr. Charlie and Edith Mayo. This time it was the ebullient Esther and Alice who, with giggles, stuffed a large, lifelike doll and a few suggestive pillows under the covers in Dr. Haggard's bed. It was three o'clock when the tired gentleman returned to the guest room, his speech-writing duty done. He turned on the light. One can only imagine the shock the dignified Dr. Haggard must have felt to see a woman in his bed, her blond curls loose on the pillow. He stood in utter silence for a minute or so, then turned off the light and went back downstairs. He slept on the lounge. In the morning he complained to a mystified Dr. Charlie that his hospitality was "excessive."[8]

Rochester welcomed President Roosevelt with a parade that muggy summer day. The route was lined with flags and cheering crowds. FDR rode in an open car with Dr. Will and Dr. Charlie, followed by a motorcade with other dignitaries including the governors of four midwestern states and two Mayo grandchildren, "Muff" Mayo, the daughter of Dr. Chuck and Alice Mayo, and Waltman Walters, the son of Dr. Waltman and Phoebe Mayo Walters.

Rochester parades sometimes included the high school marching band, Girl and Boy Scout troops, a flashy red fire engine, a green John Deere tractor and perhaps the old duo Rogers and Rasmussen on their fifty-year-old tandem bicycle. Rochester's early history was remembered with ox carts, covered wagons and the "First Stage Coach West of Worthington," drawn over Broadway's brick surface by a pair of sturdy white horses.

What I remember of the parade for President Roosevelt was my role in it as part of a troop of young girls riding horses rented from Hap Cartwright's Stable at the fairgrounds. Sixteen-year-old Jack Pemberton had a more significant role to perform. He was part of an Eagle Scout Honor Guard escorting the president to the platform where he made his speech. The two Mayo grandchildren unveiled the American Legion plaque, which was presented to the mayor of Rochester.

Jack remembers how surprised he was by the lack of security around the president. "I could have reached out and touched him," he said.

In those days few people were aware of the extent of President Roosevelt's handicap from polio. It was not considered morally correct for journalists to publish a picture of a prominent citizen in a weakened position, certainly not the president of the United States in a wheelchair. With a cane in one hand, he was helped from his wheelchair, the leg braces locked. Standing firmly at the podium, in his strong public voice enhanced by a loudspeaker, he delivered the speech written by Dr. Haggard the night before. He paid tribute to America's veterans. On behalf of the American Legion, he presented citations to Dr. Will and Dr. Charlie. The event was broadcast nationwide over two radio networks. His words and Dr. Will's acceptance speech were heard live by 125,000 people, six times more than the total population of Rochester in 1934.

Four years later, FDR came again to Rochester. Mrs. Eleanor Roosevelt was already in Rochester with her son James, who was scheduled for abdominal surgery. His surgeon was to be Jack Pemberton's father, Dr. John de Jarnett Pemberton. Customarily, Jack told me, his father met with relatives of the patient before an operation to answer any last-moment questions or concerns. On the day of the surgery, Jack said his father came home saying he'd had a most unusual session with President Roosevelt. Surrounded by his entourage, FDR in his wheelchair was rolled into the conference room all smiles. He didn't mention his son Jimmy or Jimmy's operation. The meeting turned out to be not an occasion for the doctor to give comfort to an anxious father and mother, but for the team of surgeons to hear a "grandstanding" speech for FDR's reelection to office.

The operation was a success and the president returned to Washington in his private railway car. Mrs. Roosevelt stayed while Jimmy, minus his peptic ulcer, recuperated. Jimmy enjoyed his time in Rochester. He met and fell in love with a Saint Mary's nurse whom he later married. Mrs. Roosevelt was entertained royally at teas, luncheons, rides in the country and dinners at Mayowood and at the Balfour's farm. When Jimmy was released from the hospital, mother and son went to the Ringling Brothers circus with Dr. Will and Mrs. Hattie Mayo. In her newspaper column, "My Day," a down-to-earth Eleanor Roosevelt related her pleasure at being in Rochester. And as for the circus, it made her day. She enjoyed seeing an elephant lie down "for her beauty treatment." That elephant loved having her back swept clean by a man with a broom.[9]

Twenty-three years later, Mrs. Roosevelt came again to Rochester. She addressed a United Nations Day program. Her hostess was Mrs. Howard K. Gray, then president of the Rochester Chapter of the American Association for the United Nations. Mrs. Roosevelt was a special guest at a concert presented by the Rochester Symphonic Orchestra conducted by our venerable Harold Cooke at the Mayo Civic Auditorium.

Danny Kaye, comedian and star of stage and film who had previously had some medical training, came to Rochester with a request to have Dr. Chuck Mayo remove his appendix. Dr. Chuck recalls in his autobiography that just before the surgery Kaye was lying on a gurney, a little sedated; he reached out and touched his surgeon's gown, then quickly pulled back his hand.

"I'm sorry," he apologized. "I'm scared. I forgot you were sterile." Then he murmured, as the anesthesia began to take effect, "What am I saying? He's got six kids."[10]

Dr. Chuck's hospitality, when he and his wife Alice were raising children at Mayowood, was as generous as that of his parents. A Hungarian movie director, Gabriel Pascal, a guest at dinner one time, said in his passionate Hungarian accent, "I love Mayowood. I will stay!" So he did. He lived with his young wife Valerie in the gardener's cottage for three months. He was often encountered in the woods, like a satyr, "striding along in the briefest of briefs, displaying, as Helen Clapesattle put it, "a considerable amount of hairy pelt."[11]

Medical meetings were often great fun for the wives as well as for the Mayo doctors. The Minnesota State Medical Society met one year in Minneapolis in the 1930's during a week of Grand Opera. The Massons drove up with the News. While Dad and Uncle Gordon attended meetings, Mother and Aunt Ethyl went to *La Boheme*, *Faust* and *Thais*. The third night, Mother wrote, "We got into our evening clothes and the men accompanied us to a vivacious *Carmen*." Sometimes the women went to Minneapolis to shop. At other times they attended open meetings. Mother loved hearing Dad make a speech and listening to other women say flattering things about him.

On October 22–24, 1931, when the Interurban Surgical Society met in Rochester, Mother wrote, "Jim was busy as a wet hen with his Interurbans, Dr. Gallie and Dr. Scriminger, our house guests. Jim's luncheon went off very snappily—34 men. They were fed and gone by 2 p.m."

That many people for lunch at our house must have meant ten in the dining room and six card tables in the sun room, living room, and library. We had help in the kitchen, of course, but Mother must have been "busy as a wet hen" too.

Sometimes dramatic things happened on the road to Minneapolis that were laughed about for a long time afterward. In January 1933, three Clinic men and two wives set off for St. Paul—the Massons; Dr. G. W. Stephenson, Dad's first assistant, and his wife; and Dr. Al Snell. "Icy roads," Mother wrote in her diary; ". . . on the cut-off, we skidded in a rut and in no time, were piled on top of each other, the car on its side in the ditch. No one even scratched and only a broken running board. Two men in a Chevrolet turned over almost on top of us. The men pushed our Buick on its feet again, and off we went."

On October 12, 1933, Mother went with the Bannicks, the Browns and Frances Berkman to hear the beautiful Lily Pons, a coloratura soprano who for twenty-five years sang leading roles at the Metropolitan Opera House in New York City. On another visit to Minneapolis, Mother, Anne Pemberton, Ethyl New and her daughter Marion went to see Katharine Cornell in *The Barrets of Wimpole Street*.

Rochester, with its population of barely twenty thousand, had its share of talent too. In addition to our home-grown musicians who gave concerts at Mayo Park, the Community Concert Series brought exceptional artists to Saint Mary's Auditorium, an annex to the School of Nursing. Mother used to take us children to those concerts when we were old enough to stay awake after 9 o'clock. I certainly stayed awake for the Vienna Boys' Choir! I was thrilled by the glorious sound of the boys' treble voices. I paid special attention to the handsome face of one tall boy in the back row on whom I had a romantic crush. After the concerts, there was always a rite among us children—to acquire a famous signature. We pre-teens and high school kids lined up backstage with our programs for our moment of glory when a famous person or a handsome boy signed our program, and we said, shyly, "Thank you." The boy soprano I had fallen for, whose name I have forgotten, signed his name and smiled at me, but I'm sure he kept no swooning memory of me, as I did of him.

Another of my favorite performances was a modern dance group; especially memorable, the Flame Dance. They leaped with exquisite grace, trailing yards of diaphanous flame-colored scarves that floated as if weighing nothing at all. I stayed awake for the Rochester Philharmonic Orchestra, too, but sometimes a single performer, such as the violinist Paul Kochanski, lulled me to sleep in the comfortable auditorium chair.

Isabel Helmholz, on the hospitality committee of the Concert Series, entertained many of the musicians in her home. Margie Helmholz Burchell will always be inspired, she says, remembering their houseguest, Myra Hess, playing Beethoven's "Moonlight Sonata" on their grand piano. Miss Hess was twenty-six years old when she made her debut as a British pianist with the London Philharmonic Orchestra. I remember news of her heroism in World War II. As bombs exploded over London, Myra Hess played free concerts at noon in London's National Gallery. In recognition of her example of courage to the people of London, King George VI conferred on her the honored title, Dame Myra Hess.

Another musical personality introduced to us was Madam Ernestine

On the Social Side

Schumann-Heink, a much admired contralto from Prague. After a varied musical career she became a member of the Metropolitan Opera Company in 1899. Sponsored by Isabel Helmholz, she came to Rochester in the midst of the Depression to sing a program of German lieder at the Rochester Armory. Isabel, who was slim as well as gracious, was guiding her hefty guest through a narrow passageway to the door through which the singer was to make her entrance when a distressed wail from Frau Schumann-Heink stopped her and she turned around to find the buxom lady all but stuck between the walls of the backstage scenery.

"Oh, dear!" Isabel said, "Walk sideways, Frau Heink."

The Wagnerian contralto said, "Aach! I have no sideways." That phrase is still a family joke when Helmholzes get together. Another houseguest at the Helmholzes' was the enchanting Cornelia Otis Skinner, actress and writer. Her monologues, such as "The Wives of Henry VIII," would keep any ten-year-old sleepyhead awake long after 9 o'clock.

Often, lecturers came to town with stories of adventure and distant places. A geologist who went with Admiral Byrd to the South Pole gave a lecture in Plummer Hall. Dad took Jay to hear him. A Dr. Reed told of being with a party of archaeologists exploring the Gobi Desert. Dr. Ogata, a pathologist from Japan who came to visit the Clinic, was also an amateur magician. He put on a show especially for children. He made an American flag disappear, but later, in an unexpected sweep, he brought it out of his sleeve. A Mrs. Remington spoke about Russia. Mrs. Wiley, curator of reptiles at a zoo in Chicago, captivated and appalled us with her photographs and movies of snakes. She was entertained for dinner at Dr. and Mrs. J. L. Bollman's, where my parents were charmed by the amazing lady snake handler. A Dr. Brindley, who had been adventuring in some far part of the globe, came to dinner at our house one day when we were in the midst of spring cleaning. Mother wrote, "... the sunroom furniture was piled in the dining room. I didn't mind, and he didn't. Admiral Wells blew into town, and that old peach, Stuart Pritchard."

Our youngest houseguest was Henry Big Elk, a five-year-old Osage Indian, my brother Billy's age. His mother was a patient of Dad's. Mother wrote, he was "the cutest little spud."

A most colorful lecturer was Count Von Luckner. In World War I he was a hero in his own country, Germany, but not in ours. Disguised as a Norwegian fisherman in a small boat, he sank twenty-five Allied ships. He was finally captured by the British and freed after the war. He then revamped his reputation with his exciting lecture series. Margie Burchell remembers he ended his talk with a feat for which he was famous. He tore a Minneapolis telephone book in half with one fierce jerk.

Without doubt, the most brilliant and remarkable person any of us ever met was Helen Keller, whom I met on her visit to the Mayo Clinic for a checkup. Blind, deaf and mute at the age of eighteen months, she was, in her own words, "... wild and unruly, giggling and chuckling, kicking and scratching.... uttering the choked screams of the deaf-mute." [12] With the help of her teachers and friends for life, Anne Sullivan and Molly Thompson, she learned braille and sign language and she learned to speak. She graduated from Radcliffe with honors in 1904 and traveled widely, making speeches to benefit the blind. The books she wrote were translated into more than fifty languages.

Helen Keller was sixty-one years old when she came to Rochester for gall bladder surgery. On one of those returns to Rochester, Carol Haines Anderson and two Wheaton College friends visiting her were invited to the Balfours to meet Helen Keller.

"She felt our heads to see how tall we were," Carol told me. "She called us each a different flower. Nancy Woodruff was a daisy; Barbara Rossmassler, a lily; and I a chrysanthemum."

Peg Plummer Stark also remembers meeting Helen Keller when she was home on vacation from school. As she entered the home of her Uncle Henry and Aunt Daisy Plummer she heard music. Daisy Plummer and Maud MacCarty were playing a duet on the grand piano. Two other women stood enjoying the music. At the end of the piece, Peg came into the room and Mrs. Plummer introduced her niece to Helen Keller and her interpreter, Mary Agnes "Molly" Thompson.

Peg sat beside them on the sofa. In a clear but unnatural monotone, Miss Keller asked Peg questions about her life at college and Molly Thompson tapped Peg's responses in rapid sign language into the palm of Helen Keller's hand.

I asked Peg, "How could a deaf person enjoy music?"

"Her hands were on the piano," Peg said. "She felt vibrations through the wood. She seemed very attentive."

Perhaps Miss Keller's greatest thrill in Rochester was being taken to a Minnesota-Purdue football game by Dr. C. F. Dixon in 1938. As the 52,000 fans roared and cheered and groaned, Dr. Dixon described the

On the Social Side

action on the field and Polly tapped his words into meaning in the palm of Miss Keller's hand.

"It was magnificent," Helen Keller said. "I am a Minnesota fan!"

By coincidence, as I was writing this section about Helen Keller, the mail came through my door slot with the "quote of the month" in our local Myers Park Neighborhood newsletter,

> I am only one; but still I am one. I cannot do everything, but still I can do something; I will not refuse to do that something I can do."
>
> —Helen Keller

The Mayo Clinic was a sociable place in which to work. Its many specialty sections in the early years often had group parties at the home of the section head. Olivia Haines Blackburn remembers the annual Endocrinology dinners at their house. Margie Helmholz Burchell recalled the fun of the annual Pediatrics Christmas Eve party. She helped her mother wrap gifts, silk stockings for the desk girls.

"After dinner," Margie wrote, "Uncle Sam Amberg handed out the gifts, all piled under the Christmas tree. But first, he read aloud each silly card and poem written by the giver. Sometimes he laughed so hard we missed the punch lines."

As the Clinic grew, and members of the sections became more numerous, the socializing became a matter of dinners with smaller groups. Barbara Benedict Hanlon remembers having dinner with groups of Fellows of her father's Ophthalmology Section and their wives.

Our parents, Barb reminded me, always entertained at home. "We never had a meal in a restaurant till we were away at college or on a trip with the family, headed for scenic places like Yellowstone Park or the Grand Canyon." Barbara's mother ordered groceries by phone and they were brought to the house in a horse-drawn delivery wagon. If he had room in the cart, the driver was willing to pick up children on their way home from Edison Elementary School.

Barbara returned to Rochester after wartime service with the Red Cross. She married Dr. David Hanlon, and they lived in a community of small apartments with other Fellows and their wives back from places all over the globe.

"We were a wild bunch," she said, "cosmopolitan, but poor. The war changed all of us privileged small-town pre-war innocents."

Pill Hill

Frequent mention is made in my mother's diaries of Clinic groups we invited for dinner: a venison dinner, for instance, on December 9, 1930, for twenty-three Clinic and Colonial helpers. There were lots of gamey dinners, including duck dinners for "Jim's Colonial girls," and "a duck dinner for our five lady doctors," which would have included our backdoor neighbor, Dr. Della G. Drips, whose driveway we kids always used on our way to Edison School.

In the early years, the Clinic itself hosted parties, such as a Fourth of July celebration at the Country Club. There were monthly dances for the Fellows and their wives or girlfriends. On September 9, 1930, as the country was sliding into its worst Depression, the Clinic put on a Hard Times Costume Party for the Clinic staff at the Country Club. Costumes in all degrees of shabbiness were judged by a panel of three—Marion Masson, Billy MacCarty and Leonard Rowntree. The winner was Isabel Helmholz as the Statue of Liberty. Standing tall, a flashlight aimed at the ceiling, she wore a cardboard headdress with star point spikes radiating from her brow. A burlap robe trailed over her gardening sandals.

On December 21, 1933, a Clinic party featured a play called "The World's Fair at Christmas," a hilarious take-off on the Century of Progress Exposition.

A Gay Nineties dance was staged at Mayowood, and a barn dance took place in Dr. Charlie's new barn.

During the anxious days of World War II when food rationing coupons put a limit on each household's supplies of butter, meat, sugar and eggs, the Henry Plummers had a "Dinner in a Basket" party. Each woman brought a dinner for two in a picnic basket and the men picked a basket from the assortment on the floor and went in search of the lady who brought it. Nick Kendall claimed Mother's basket and Dad chose Edna Keith's. A group of local musicians played music for dancing. Mother danced every dance. She told her diary the party was a huge success.

A Supper Club of couples, including the Pembertons, Hainses, Kendalls, Balfours, Hendersons, Plummers, Massons, Lobbs and sometimes others, began in one of the early years of my parents' marriage. They met monthly at the homes of members. It was my great pleasure, when I was old enough, to be allowed to help serve the dinner, but I had to do it right. Mother told me the system, and if I helped serve, I had to help with the dishes. I was further instructed on dinner party decorum by Mrs. Nora Giere and her uniformed helpers.

On one occasion I messed things up. Everything was ready. The mashed potatoes were hot and creamy under the beaters, waiting till the last moment to be whipped a little more and scooped into the warm serving bowl. Wanting to feel useful, I flipped the switch. Mashed potatoes flew every which way, splattering on the wall, the canisters of sugar and flour and me. Stella, the cook, grumbling in Swedish, sent me out of the kitchen.

When I was a little older, thirteen, I learned not to talk to the guests, or put the plates down recklessly, or pick them up from the wrong side or scrape them, stack them or pick one up in each hand and back into the swinging door, possibly bumping into another server with a platter of warm rolls or a pitcher of icewater. I loved being spoken to by the guests, and catching a wink now and then from one or another of my favorite mothers or fathers, like Uncle Sam Haines. He never failed to know it was I who picked up his plate or passed the peas. He leaned over to Mother one time and said in a whisper loud enough for me to hear, what a "lovely new maid" she had.

Once at the Supper Club, something happened that affected me profoundly; it is still fresh in my memory. We had changed the plates and were ready to bring in the dessert. Dr. Henry Plummer got up from the table, went to the sunroom and returned to his chair with an artifact he had spotted on a table, a heavy greenish metal incense pot in the shape of a beast, short-legged like a hippopotamus. An original artifact like that one, my brother Jay told me, came from Korea. He didn't know if ours was an original or an imitation. That was the subject of Dr. Plummer's rapt investigation.

The other serving girl and I went through the swinging door several times, bringing in the chocolate roll with whipped cream followed by demitasse cups and coffee. Everyone was listening to Dr. Plummer, who had the incense pot in his hands and was telling its history.

"Today's artists and vendors know the tourist fascination for antiquities," he said. "The Koreans make very good copies. They bury their modern imitations in the barnyard till they get a discoloration like the ancient verdigris."

On my next trip to the dining room, I was surprised to see Dr. Plummer still telling what he knew, and didn't know, about the possibly 1000-year-old relic he held in his hands. Had it once been buried in a royal tomb? So engrossed was Dr. Plummer in the object he studied, he was oblivious to the fact that his chair tilted forward on its front legs, nor did it matter to him when the chair was no longer beneath him. His forearms on the table cloth, the treasure between his palms, he knelt on the rug and talked softly of the ancient uses of the poisonous pigment, verdigris. Daisy Plummer went to him then, and he put the regal bronze creature into her hands, seemingly undisturbed that he was on his knees and everyone else was seated at the table.

Many of Dr. Plummer's devoted admirers resent the way tales of Dr. Plummer's occasional eccentric behavior were passed along as humor by people who didn't know him. It was, after all, his remarkable powers of concentration that enabled him to so deeply sink into a complex subject that he could understand and master it. For instance, he taught himself the art and craft of architecture to such an extreme that, without formal education in the field, he single-handedly charted and supervised the construction of the beautiful building that bears his name and its many advanced inner systems. When the building was up to its fourteenth floor, he was pleased to add Dr. Will's inspired afterthought, a carillon tower complete with many tons of bells.

Today, as then, Rochester's people and patients from everywhere still hear those joyful bells ring out at regular times and for special occasions. Some things never change. The young doctors of today come to the Clinic with the same zeal to learn from the Mayo staff. Other things, though, are different. "What's missing," my brother Jay says, "is the camaraderie we used to have as Fellows—how we enjoyed each other Monday nights when we gathered at the Foundation House for dinner and talks by one or more of the senior men. We knew everybody—it was fun."

Margie Burchell wrote that she and her husband, Howard, were in Rochester to celebrate the fiftieth anniversary of the Clinic's first heart catheterization. Dr. George Logan had died the week before of a massive stroke, and the Burchells attended the memorial service for him.

"Sitting in church," Margie wrote, "seeing our contemporaries come in, some bent, some markedly changed, all white-haired, I was struck with the realization that our generation had done its job, and it was up to the younger generations now. How lucky we all were, though. It seems as if ours was 'the best of times.'"

⇥{ 21 }⇤

Tracks in the Snow

> In the autumn of life one perhaps may be privileged
> to become reminiscent.
>
> Dr. W. J. Mayo, April 30, 1927[1]

AFTER Mother died of a heart attack in 1950, Dad was alone for fifteen years. Only Jay still lived in Rochester. Stan and I were married, with children to raise and jobs to keep.

Dad always worried about his youngest son Bill, who had always been attracted to dangerous sports. The house Bill bought in Los Angeles where he worked as an engineer had one bedroom, which he used as a workshop; he slept on a sofabed in the living room. On the living room floor he built a sailing kayak, following directions in a blueprint he ordered from *Popular Mechanics*. He was in his black frogman suit and a yellow life jacket in that swift little boat he had built when he died. A sudden squall overturned the kayak and he couldn't survive long in the cold Pacific Ocean.

That was in 1960. Dad was too infirm and emotionally unstrung by Bill's death to go out to California and do what had to be done. He asked Stan and me to take his place. Jay, who lived just a few blocks from Dad, was there to help him bear that grief.

"Bill saved my life once," Dad said on that first day of my last visit with him. He folded the sheet down and laced his fingers over the top button of his pajamas. "We took a drive in the Porsche to see some interesting rock formations carved by wind and water in the mesa a few million years ago. It was late in the day. Shadows were long and a glorious sunset streaked the western sky."

He told how Bill parked the car and they followed the tourist trail.

Pill Hill

Dad had walked a little too much that day, and when he got into some gravel he lost his footing and fell. "It was on a slope," he said, "and I'd have kept on sliding to the edge of the cliff, I suppose, if Bill hadn't come and caught me in his arms. We lay quite a while in those loose pebbles, just breathing."

A tear rolled down Dad's cheek to the pillow. Betty, the nurse who would be with him through lunch, whispered, "He's tired. I'd rather he didn't fall asleep yet. I'll go down and see if Mabel has his lunch ready."

Dad's eyes opened and he smiled at Betty. "No, I've got some spunk in me yet. I want to keep on talking till it gets dark."

Betty laughed. "All right, Doctor. I'll go see what Mabel's stirring up in the kitchen. You can talk your head off till I come back with your lunch." She walked down the hall to the stairs.

"I'll stay till your lunch comes up, Dad, or when Ruthie gets back with a new hair-do."

"Don't worry about me, Little Pony. I've lived a good life, had a good wife. Your mother was a corker. She loved the wild things. If she could be an animal she'd like to be a fox with a long, bushy tail, so she said. She liked poetry, and she wanted me to like it. I tried, but I never had the ear for it. She loved snow storms, breezy days and moonlight. We both did."

Without much tune he began to sing, "Every little breeze seems to whisper Louise, birds in the trees always sing of Louise...."

He took a quiet breath, and his smooth face furrowed as he struggled to contain whatever memory it was that had lured him. I stroked his forearm under the blue pajama sleeve.

Betty came up on the elevator with his lunch on a tray. She raised the head of the bed and set the lunch tray on the adjustable table in front of him. I said, "I'll go down and meet Ruthie when she comes in, Dad."

He didn't hear me. He was looking up at the ceiling when he spoke out in a strong, conversational voice. "We've certainly had a lot of snow this winter. Those tracks are fox, I think. Maybe rabbit." Betty and I glanced at each other and at the ceiling. The plaster had fine cracks here and there, the paint flecked. "And there's a deer, a young buck."

I put my hand on the sheet over my father's foot. "Are you thinking about the old days, Dad, when you used to go out hunting?"

"Yes, but the trouble is, you go out with a crowd, and they all fire, and there's not a chance of his getting away. I'd like to see that buck skip out of there fast. Come here," he said, and reached for my hand. "I'll tell you this, Dear. Every now and again, when I turn my head sharply, I see this magnificent elk looking at me. He comes to the foot of my bed."

My father's clear blue eyes were full of urgency that I should understand and believe what he said.

With a fast-beating heart I whispered, "Does he have antlers, Dad?"

"Indeed he does, a full rack. How many prongs I couldn't count. I think he wants me to follow him."

The small hairs on my arms rose as I imagined a great elk in my father's room at the foot of his hospital bed. I heard those words echo again and again—"I think he wants me to follow . . . to follow."

I heard the front door open downstairs and voices. "Ruthie just came back, Dad," I said. "I'll go down and have lunch with her. I'll see you after your nap."

I moved my suitcase into the guest room and went down to greet my stepmother. Ruthie, a former widow and patient of Dad's, was a major benefactor to the Mayo Foundation. Her gifts to the building program were given in honor of her father, Earle Perry Charlton, a founding partner of the F. W. Woolworth Company, and her former husband, Fredrick Mitchell. She also endowed a Professorship in Surgery in my father's name.

Dad married Ruth when he was eighty-four years old; she was seventy-four. In the years after Mother died Dad stayed busy with visits to and from relatives and old friends in this country and Canada and his four children and grandchildren. Two affable old farmers' widows lived on the third floor of the house. With Effie and Frieda and Mabel's good cooking he was kept well fed and the house looked after. His yardman, Noland, was a good and trusted friend.

Often Dad went to medical meetings and dinners at the Foundation House with the Clinic's Surgical Society and to the Emeritus Room in the Plummer Building to read the journals and magazines and to dictate letters to a secretary available to the emeritus staff. He and friends like Uncle John Pemberton used to cheer for Rochester baseball teams, and in winter, ice hockey competitions. At home his yellow Labrador, Trigger, sat by his chair as he read the newspaper, biographies and books of history. His favorite author was Winston Churchill. He liked to putter in the yard with his tomato plants and apple tree grafts. In the basement workshop, he fixed things.

Ruth, a short, stout little lady in pink, met me at the bottom of the stairs. She was distressed that she hadn't been able to meet my plane. Her silver-gray hair was fluffed up and back in loose waves; in front of each ear, a corkscrew curl.

Our lunch was a delicious vichyssoise, asparagus salad, homemade rolls and strawberry jam and, for dessert, an elegant chocolate mousse with whipped cream. Ruth sat in Dad's chair, and I faced the backyard with its light blanket of new snow. The button to ring for the maid used to be a lump under the rug at Mother's end of the table. Ruthie, in Dad's chair, couldn't reach the floor with her foot, and had the bell attached to a more accessible place on the table leg. During that week that bell had Mabel running back and forth for second helpings of her wonderful food as Ruth questioned me about my life and my writing. Where did I get my ideas? What was I working on now? Did I plan to write about my father? Perhaps those conversations gave her an idea; she commissioned Dr. Betty Mussey, a former assistant of Dad's, to compile what she knew of his history, and had it printed in a small volume.[2]

When finally Ruth and I got up from the table we went to see Dad. I took the stairs, and she used the little elevator she had installed when she came to live at "724." Beryl Gunderson, the afternoon/evening nurse, had arrived, taking Betty's place. Gundy, as we called her, was warm and attractive, gray-haired and petite. She had worked with my father before his retirement. Out of loyalty to her former chief, she came to help take care of him in his final years, when our old house had become a hospital with three nursing shifts and all the auxilliary services of the Mayo Clinic as close as the telephone.

"He's had a good nap," Gundy said, raising the head of the bed slightly. Ruth and I sat, one on each side of his bed. Dad's eyes stayed closed.

"Are you playing possum, Dad?" I asked, giving his hand a squeeze. With his dentures out, his thin lips curled inward over his gums. He seemed to be hardly breathing. Then he took a deep breath and stirred. His eyelids twitched and one eye slowly opened. The other seemed glued shut. "I'm still here, Dad," I said softly. "This morning you called me 'Little Pony.' I haven't been called that for so many years." I squeezed his hand.

The other eye opened, and a big grin spread across his face. "If it isn't my little chick, or have I died and gone to Heaven?"

"Oh, Jim!" Ruth exclaimed, taking hold of his other hand. "Don't say such things! Helen is here. She came to see you."

That night, as was our custom in past visits, Ruthie and I listened to the ten o'clock news on television, then went to bed. I was sound asleep when the doorbell rang. I was on the landing in my robe when Ruthie came down the hall in bare feet, her pink peignoir floating around her. "Go back to bed, Helen. It's just the night nurse, Bill. Gundy will let him in." I knew that, but I wanted to say hello to Bill.

Bill was a short, stocky former Marine, with a wife and three children. He loved my dad, and my dad loved him. Bill told me that often, in the quiet of the night, when Mrs. Masson was asleep, he and Dad had wonderful conversations about everything under the sun. They shared stories of hunting trips and dogs they had known. Bill told him the news from Vietnam and his experience in that war. Dad talked about Stan being wounded on the beach at Sicily in World War II, and the miracle that he was evacuated and brought home alive, and the new drug, penicillin, that had saved him. Dad missed masculine friendship and wanted to stay awake all night with Bill, sometimes shedding tears for happy memories. It must have given him pleasure to have that sturdy Marine named Bill at his bedside to talk to by the dim nightlight.

My six days at home went by rapidly. Once, during my visit, the doorbell late at night announced a delivery of flowers. Gladiolas in gorgeous shades of lavender and orange arrived special delivery from the greenhouse at the Charlton estate on the rocky New England coast where Ruthie had grown up. Another late-night special delivery from "Pond Meadow" was a box of a dozen jars of grape jelly made by Ruthie's delightful old butler, Louie. The jelly was made from the juice of Dad's most famous gardening success, blue-purple grapes the size of quarters. They flourished in the rich soil below the former homing pigeon loft. On that plot of ground Golden Pheasants had been raised, and white Leghorn chickens, incubated in our basement. After the chickens, the goats of my childhood romped and butted heads in that pen.

Someone was always coming or going. The doorbell announced the change of nursing shifts. The maid with the straight brown bangs let the daytime arrivals in. The two nurses discussed in private the chart of their patient's last eight hours. Once, a young Clinic doctor came to sit with

Dad. He wanted to meet and talk with the oldest living pioneer of the early days at the Mayo Clinic. He stayed on when a podiatrist came to cut Dad's toenails. An old best friend of Dad's, Art Osman, told me on the phone that he used to drop in at least once a week, but lately he couldn't get past the maid who always said no, the doctor was sleeping.

Mabel loved to take Dad's dinner tray up to him and have a few minutes to talk. On one of my visits home, she told me of a day when Dad was in a wheelchair on the screened porch, ready to go back upstairs. Gundy's arm was in a sling with a sprained wrist, and she needed help moving Dad from his chair to the smaller wheelchair that could fit in the elevator. Gundy called Mabel from the kitchen for help. Mabel, big strong Norwegian girl that she was, told me she lifted Dad with no trouble at all, as if he was no heavier than her son Fabian when he was a boy.

"I didn't want to put him down," Mabel said. "He smiled and looked at me with those blue eyes of his, and said, 'Mabel, here I am littler than you, and I never had a chance to pick you up.' God, Helen, I about cried. I leaned over and kissed him. I love your dad."

In his last years Dad had a slow-growing prostate cancer that weakened him, but rarely caused him pain. He was always alert and eager for visits from my brother Jay. He especially wanted to hear what Jay had done all day, the cases he saw, the surgery performed. Much was new in the treatment of patients since Dad retired in 1946.

One day they talked about a particular maxillectomy Jay had done. The patient, Jay said, was "a poor old charity case. He looked like a bum you might see with a tin cup on a sidewalk in New York." He came to the Clinic by himself with a long-neglected cancer of the upper jaw. Jay removed his left upper jaw including the orbit, the eye socket.

Dad was amazed. "How long did it take?" he asked. When Jay said two and a half hours, Dad could hardly believe it. "No operation should take more than an hour!" he exclaimed.

"That used to be true, but not anymore," Jay said.

Dad's success as a surgeon was partly due to the speed with which he worked. It was the tremendous advances in the safety of anesthetics that made feasible today's long, complicated operations. Jay's maxillectomy patient was dismissed from the hospital and sent home to heal with instructions on how to feed himself with only half an upper jaw. He came back a month or so later and a plate, like a denture, was made for him to close the opening. "That plate really pleased him," Jay said. "He could talk and eat a lot better."

On the last day of my visit home in 1974, I sat by Dad's bed while Gundy went down for his supper tray. My suitcase was packed. I would be driven to the airport in a few minutes. Dad turned his head on the pillow to look out the window, holding my hand. The lovely deep snow of a week ago was almost gone. He closed his eyes and then, with a struggle, opened them, as if he didn't want to fall asleep. He looked up at the white ceiling. In a few moments he spoke in a hushed, excited voice, "Look! Here she comes now, the doe. See how she lifts her slender legs high through the sedge. She has a little dry grass in her mouth."

Downstairs the grandfather clock began its fourth quarter chime. It bonged five times. Gundy came into the room with the supper tray. Mrs. Masson and the driver were ready, she said.

I kissed Dad's cheek. "I have to go now, Dad. I hate to leave, but I must; the kids will be home for Thanksgiving."

"Give them my love, Dear." He squeezed my hand.

I turned at the door. Dad was gazing at the ceiling again, his hand lifted from the sheet. I heard his soft voice as if he spoke to himself. "How fearlessly he carries his head and walks between the two spruce trees. He looks at me with a keen, forgiving eye."

I walked down the stairs, tears distorting the face of the grandfather clock and its spry moon. Would my father be here still when next I came home to Rochester? If he was not, I would know he had followed the magnificent elk, with his crown of many prongs, into the vast, serene whiteness that was falling over the forest of his dreams.

Notes

Prologue

1. "International Medical Progress," *Collect. Papers Mayo Clinic & Mayo Foundation,* 23:1020–1024, 1931, as quoted in Fredrick A. Willius, ed., *Aphorisms of Charles Horace Mayo and William James Mayo* (Rochester, MN: Mayo Foundation for Medical Education and Research, 1988), pp. 10–11.

Chapter 1

1. Helen Clapesattle, *The Doctors Mayo* (Minneapolis: The University of Minnesota Press, 1941), p. 530.
2. Mearl W. Raygor, *The Rochester Story* (1976), p. 10.
3. Ibid., p. 6.
4. Clapesattle, p. 89.
5. Ibid., p. 142.
6. Ibid., p. 252.
7. Ibid., p. 256.
8. Ibid., pp. 230–231.
9. Ibid., p. 549.
10. Ibid., pp. 408–409.
11. Ibid., p. 464.
12. Ibid., p. 436.
13. Herbert A. Bruce, MD, *Varied Operations* (Toronto: Longmans, Green and Co., 1958), p. 80.
14. Clapesattle, p. 582.

15. *Rochester Post Bulletin*, 7 July 1986, p. 5B.
16. Clapesattle, p. 530.

Chapter 2

1. "The Relative Value of the Special Senses to the Surgeon," *Ann. Surg.*, 86:1–5 (July), 1927, as quoted in Fredrick A. Willius, ed., *Aphorisms of Charles Horace Mayo and William James Mayo* (Rochester, MN: Mayo Foundation for Medical Education and Research, 1988), p. 59.

Chapter 3

1. "Perception," *Collect. Papers Mayo Clinic & Mayo Foundation*, 20: 997–1006, 1928, as quoted in Fredrick A. Willius, ed., *Aphorisms of Charles Horace Mayo and William James Mayo* (Rochester, MN: Mayo Foundation for Medical Education and Research, 1988), p. 73.
2. Helen Clapesattle, *The Doctors Mayo* (Minneapolis: The University of Minnesota Press, 1941), pp. 453–455.
3. Ibid., p. 453.
4. Ibid., p. 454.
5. Ibid., p. 455.
6. Ibid.
7. Ibid.
8. Ibid., p. 448.
9. Ibid., p. 463.
10. Ibid.
11. Ibid., p. 552.

Chapter 4

1. "The Economic Relation of the University System to the Development of a Social Democracy," *Collect. Papers Mayo Clinic & Mayo Foundation*, 25:1105–1107, 1933, as quoted in Fredrick A. Willius, ed., *Aphorisms of Charles Horace Mayo and William James Mayo* (Rochester, MN: Mayo Foundation for Medical Education and Research, 1988), pp. 64–65.

Early History of the Mayo Clinic

2. Helen Clapesattle, *The Doctors Mayo* (Minneapolis: The University of Minnesota Press, 1941), p. 533.

3. Ibid., pp. 135–136.

4. Harvey Cushing, "The Mayo Brothers and Their Clinic," reprinted from *Science*, vol. 90, no. 2332 (September 8, 1939), pp. 225–226.

5. Clapesattle, p. 556.

6. Lucy Wilder, *The Mayo Clinic* (New York: Harcourt Brace & Co., 1936), p. 73.

7. O. T. Clagett, MD, *General Surgery at Mayo Clinic: 1900–1970* (Rochester, MN: 1980), pp. 65–69.

8. O. T. Clagett, MD, *Reflections of O. T. "Jim" Clagett* (Rochester, MN: 1979), p. 167.

9. Ibid., p. 136.

10. From a Mayo Clinic pamphlet, "Exploring the Mayo Art Collection," pp. 28–29.

11. Charles William Mayo, *Mayo: The Story of My Family and My Career*, (New York: Doubleday & Co., 1968), pp. 333–334.

12. "The Debt of the University Graduate," *Collect. Papers Mayo Clinic & Mayo Foundation*, 16:1226–1230, 1924, as quoted in Fredrick A. Willius, ed., *Aphorisms of Charles Horace Mayo and William James Mayo* (Rochester, MN: Mayo Foundation for Medical Education and Research, 1988), p. 66.

13. "The Function of the University Concerns the Tomorrows, the Function of the Government, the Yesterdays and Todays," *Collect. Papers Mayo Clinic & Mayo Foundation*, 16:1223–1225, 1924, as quoted in Fredrick A. Willius, ed., *Aphorisms of Charles Horace Mayo and William James Mayo* (Rochester, MN: Mayo Foundation for Medical Education and Research, 1988), p. 66.

14. "Educational Development of Man," *Collect. Papers Mayo Clinic & Mayo Foundation*, 20:937–942, 1928, as quoted in Fredrick A. Willius, ed., *Aphorisms of Charles Horace Mayo and William James Mayo* (Rochester, MN: Mayo Foundation for Medical Education and Research, 1988), pp. 19–20.

Chapter 5

1. "In the Time of Henry Jacob Bigelow," *Journal of the American Medical Association*, 77:597–603 (August 20), 1921, as quoted in Fredrick A.

Willius, ed., *Aphorisms of Charles Horace Mayo and William James Mayo* (Rochester, MN: Mayo Foundation for Medical Education and Research, 1988), p. 51.

2. Lucy Wilder, *The Mayo Clinic* (New York: Harcourt Brace & Co., 1936), p. 80.

3. Ibid.

4. Mary Elizabeth Giffin, MD, *Her Doctor, Will Mayo* (Scottdale, PA: Herald Press, 1967), p. 121.

5. Ibid., pp. 123–125.

Chapter 6

1. "Tomorrow's Education Seen by Dr. Mayo," *Northwestern University Alumni News*, 10:17–19 (July), 1931, as quoted in Fredrick A. Willius, ed., *Aphorisms of Charles Horace Mayo and William James Mayo* (Rochester, MN: Mayo Foundation for Medical Education and Research, 1988), p. 11.

2. O. T. Clagett, MD, *Reflections of O. T. "Jim" Clagett* (Rochester, MN: 1979), p. 98.

3. Helen Clapesattle, *The Doctors Mayo* (Minneapolis: The University of Minnesota Press, 1941), p. 517.

4. Ibid., p. 97.

Chapter 7

1. "Surgery in Relation to Life Insurance," *Journal-Lancet*, 112:146–150, 1914, as quoted in Fredrick A. Willius, ed., *Aphorisms of Charles Horace Mayo and William James Mayo* (Rochester, MN: Mayo Foundation for Medical Education and Research, 1988), p. 18.

Chapter 8

1. "Education Guides the Young to Good Citizenship," *Minnesota Med.*, 19:468–470 (July), 1936, as quoted in Fredrick A. Willius, ed., *Aphorisms of Charles Horace Mayo and William James Mayo* (Rochester, MN: Mayo Foundation for Medical Education and Research, 1988), p. 57.

2. *The Charlotte Observer*, 31 May 1996, p. 2c.
3. Charles William Mayo, *Mayo: The Story of My Family and My Career*, (New York: Doubleday & Co., 1968), p. 60.
4. Ibid., p. 61.
5. "Education Guides," p. 57.

Chapter 9

1. "Problems in Medical Education," *Collect. Papers Mayo Clinic & Mayo Foundation*, 18:1093–1102, 1926, as quoted in Fredrick A. Willius, ed., *Aphorisms of Charles Horace Mayo and William James Mayo* (Rochester, MN: Mayo Foundation for Medical Education and Research, 1988), p. 21.
2. Lucy Wilder, *The Mayo Clinic* (New York: Harcourt Brace & Co., 1936), p. 73.
3. Helen Clapesattle, *The Doctors Mayo* (Minneapolis: The University of Minnesota Press, 1941), p. 149.
4. O. T. Clagett, MD, *Reflections of O. T. "Jim" Clagett* (Rochester, MN: 1979), p. 99.

Chapter 10

1. "Educational Development of Man," *Collect. Papers Mayo Clinic & Mayo Foundation*, 20:937–942, 1928, as quoted in Fredrick A. Willius, ed., *Aphorisms of Charles Horace Mayo and William James Mayo* (Rochester, MN: Mayo Foundation for Medical Education and Research, 1988), pp. 19–20.

Chapter 11

1. "Problems in Medical Education," *Collect. Papers Mayo Clinic & Mayo Foundation*, 18:1093–1102, 1926, as quoted in Fredrick A. Willius, ed., *Aphorisms of Charles Horace Mayo and William James Mayo* (Rochester, MN: Mayo Foundation for Medical Education and Research, 1988), p. 26.
2. Helen Clapesattle, *The Doctors Mayo* (Minneapolis: The University of Minnesota Press, 1941), p. 611.

3. Ibid., p. 673.
4. Ibid., p. 682.

Chapter 12

1. "The Relation of Mouth Conditions to General Health," *Journal of the American Dentistry Association*, 6:505–512 (June), 1919, as quoted in Fredrick A. Willius, ed., *Aphorisms of Charles Horace Mayo and William James Mayo* (Rochester, MN: Mayo Foundation for Medical Education and Research, 1988), p. 29.
2. Dr. Seuss, *The 500 Hats of Bartholomew Cubbins* (New York: Random House, 1938), p. 2.
3. Helen Clapesattle, *The Doctors Mayo* (Minneapolis: The University of Minnesota Press, 1941), p. 670.

Chapter 13

1. "Tomorrow's Education Seen by Dr. Mayo," *Northwestern University Alumni News*, 10:17–19 (July), 1931, as quoted in Fredrick A. Willius, ed., *Aphorisms of Charles Horace Mayo and William James Mayo* (Rochester, MN: Mayo Foundation for Medical Education and Research, 1988), p. 11.
2. Helen Clapesattle, *The Doctors Mayo* (Minneapolis: The University of Minnesota Press, 1941), p. 516.
3. Fred Hargesheimer, *The School That Fell from the Sky* (Auburn, CA: eBookstand Books, 2002).

Chapter 14

1. "Remarks Before the Association," (Abstr.) *Collect. Papers Mayo Clinic & Mayo Foundation*, 27:1212–1216, 1935, as quoted in Fredrick A. Willius, ed., *Aphorisms of Charles Horace Mayo and William James Mayo* (Rochester, MN: Mayo Foundation for Medical Education and Research, 1988), p. 62.
2. Harriet W. Hodgson, *Rochester, City of the Prairie* (Northridge, CA: Windsor Publications, 1989), p. 72.

Chapter 15

1. "War's Influence on Medicine: Presidential Address," *Journal of the American Medical Association*, 68:1673–1677 (June 9), 1917, as quoted in Fredrick A. Willius, ed., *Aphorisms of Charles Horace Mayo and William James Mayo* (Rochester, MN: Mayo Foundation for Medical Education and Research, 1988), p. 31.
2. Helen Clapesattle, *The Doctors Mayo* (Minneapolis: The University of Minnesota Press, 1941), p. 676.
3. *Beverages* (Boston, MA: Time-Life Books, 1983), p. 14.
4. Berton Roueché, *The Neutral Spirit* (Boston: Little, Brown, 1960), pp. 14–20.
5. William Congreve, *The Way of the World* (Act IV, Scene 1).
6. See Roueché, pp. 28–29.
7. Clapesattle, p. 567.
8. O. T. Clagett, *Reflections of O. T. Clagett* (Rochester, MN: 1979), p. 111.
9. Roueché, pp. 150–151.
10. *Rochester Post Bulletin*, 27 September 1937, p. 7.

Chapter 16

1. "Presidential Address," *Surg., Gynec. & Obst.*, 30:97–99, 1920, as quoted in Fredrick A. Willius, ed., *Aphorisms of Charles Horace Mayo and William James Mayo* (Rochester, MN: Mayo Foundation for Medical Education and Research, 1988), p. 60.
2. Helen Clapesattle, *The Doctors Mayo* (Minneapolis: The University of Minnesota Press, 1941), p. 562.
3. O. T. Clagett, MD, *Reflections of O. T. "Jim" Clagett* (Rochester, MN: 1979), p. 98.
4. Clapesattle, p. 571.

Chapter 17

1. Harry J. Harwick, *Forty Four Years with the Mayo Clinic: 1908–1952* (Rochester, MN: Whiting Press, 1957), p. 35.
2. Ibid., p. 35.

3. Ibid., p. 33.
4. Helen Clapesattle, *The Doctors Mayo* (Minneapolis: The University of Minnesota Press, 1941), p. 798.
5. O. T. Clagett, MD, *Reflections of O. T. "Jim" Clagett* (Rochester, MN: 1979), pp. 95–96.
6. Ibid., p. 113.
7. Ibid., p. 112.

Chapter 18

1. "The Examination, Preparation and Care of Surgical Patients," *Journal-Lancet*, 36:1–4 (Jan. 1), 1916, as quoted in Fredrick A. Willius, ed., *Aphorisms of Charles Horace Mayo and William James Mayo* (Rochester, MN: Mayo Foundation for Medical Education and Research, 1988), p. 5.
2. Helen Clapesattle, *The Doctors Mayo* (Minneapolis: The University of Minnesota Press, 1941), pp. 664–665.
3. Eben J. Carey, SC. D., MD, "Medical Science Exhibits, A Century of Progress: Chicago World's Fair, 1933 and 1934" (Pamphlet, Hall of Science, Chicago, 1931–1934), p. 120.
4. Clapesattle, p. 622.
5. *The Mayo Alumnus*, July 1973, p. 14.
6. Harriet W. Hodgson, *Rochester, City of the Prairie* (Northridge, CA: Windsor Publications, 1989), p. 35.

Chapter 19

1. "War's Influence on Medicine: Presidential Address," *Journal of the American Medical Association*, 68:1673–1677 (June 9), 1917, as quoted in Fredrick A. Willius, ed., *Aphorisms of Charles Horace Mayo and William James Mayo* (Rochester, MN: Mayo Foundation for Medical Education and Research, 1988), p. 28.
2. Lee Edwards, *Missionary for Freedom* (New York, NY: Paragon House, 1990), p. 61.
3. Rep. Walter H. Judd, *The Basic Themes for Survival* (Pamphlet, The Reserve Officers' Association of the United States, 1942).
4. Herbert A. Bruce, MD, *Varied Operations* (Toronto: Longmans, Green & Co., 1958), p. 281.

5. Fred Farris, *Times Recalled* (Whispering Pines, NC: Scots Plaid Press, 1989), p. 161.
6. Helen Clapesattle, *The Doctors Mayo* (Minneapolis: The University of Minnesota Press, 1941), p. 707.

Chapter 20

1. "Preventive Medicine," *Texas State Journal of Medicine* 24:403–405 (Oct.), 1928, as quoted in Fredrick A. Willius, ed., *Aphorisms of Charles Horace Mayo and William James Mayo* (Rochester, MN: Mayo Foundation for Medical Education and Research, 1988), p. 20.
2. Howard A. Anderson, MD, *Mayo Alumni Association, 1915–1992* (Rochester, MN: Mayo Alumni Association, 1992), p. 26.
3. Helen Clapesattle, *The Doctors Mayo* (Minneapolis: The University of Minnesota Press, 1941), p. 587.
4. Ibid., p. 578.
5. Ibid., p. 577.
6. Will Rogers, "Will Rogers Ropes 'Em for the Globe," *Rochester Post Bulletin*, 25 April 1934.
7. Charles William Mayo, *Mayo: The Story of My Family and My Career*, (New York: Doubleday & Co., 1968), p. 150.
8. Ibid., p. 151.
9. Eleanor Roosevelt, "My Day," Covington, Kentucky *Post*, 19 July 1938, p. J25.
10. Mayo, p. 135.
11. Ibid., p. 248.
12. "Helen Keller," *World Book Encyclopedia*, vol. 10, p. 209.

Chapter 21

1. "Medical Education for the General Practitioner," *Journal of the American Medical Association*, 88:1377–1379 (Apr. 30), 1927, as quoted in Fredrick A. Willius, ed., *Aphorisms of Charles Horace Mayo and William James Mayo* (Rochester, MN: Mayo Foundation for Medical Education and Research, 1988), p. 61.
2. Elizabeth Mussey, MD, *Years of Fulfillment: Dr. James C. Masson, A Short Biography*.

A Note on the Type

This book was set on the Linotype and printed letterpress by Heritage Letterpress, LLC, in Charlotte, North Carolina. The typeface is 10-point Electra, a contemporary modern face designed for the Linotype by William A. Dwiggins (1880–1956). Dwiggins created Electra in 1935, later adding the bold and an additional choice of italic.

Dwiggins designed, among many others, the four linotype faces most widely used in the United States and Great Britain during the twentieth century: Caledonia, Electra, Eldorado, and Metro.

The paper is 50-pound Glatfelter, an acid-free paper with a useful life of 300 years.